VITAMIN WEED

A 4-STEP PLAN
TO PREVENT AND REVERSE
ENDOCANNABINOID DEFICIENCY

VITAMIN WEED

A 4-STEP PLAN
TO PREVENT AND REVERSE
ENDOCANNABINOID DEFICIENCY

Michele N. Ross, PhD

GREENSTONE BOOKS
Los Angeles

Vitamin Weed: A 4-Step Plan to Prevent and Reverse Endocannabinoid Deficiency by Michele N. Ross, PhD

Published by GreenStone Books
2 Adams St,
Denver, CO 80206
www.greenstonebooks.com

Cover by Michele N. Ross

ISBN: 978-0-692-09066-4

Note: The information in this book is true and complete to the best of our knowledge. This book is intended only as an informative guide for those wishing to know more about health issues and the endocannabinoid system. In no way is this book intended to replace or conflict with the advice given to you by your own physician. The ultimate decision concerning care should be between you and your doctor and we strongly recommend you follow his or her advice. The information in this book is offered with no guarantees on the part of the author or GreenStone Books. The author and publisher disclaim all liability in connection with the use of this book.

This book is dedicated to my husband Todd, who supported me through sickness and in health.

Contents

PART ONE

What is Your Cannabis IQ?

PART TWO

Are you Endocannabinoid Deficient?

PART THREE

Cannabinoid Deficiency is the Root of

Disease

PART FOUR

The Vitamin Weed 4-Step Plan

PART ONE

What is Your Cannabis IQ?

CHAPTER 1

How an Anti-Drug Scientist Fell into Cannabis

"I'm in the business of stress management. Stress kills. Alcohol kills. Tobacco kills. Fat kills. Marijuana saves." - Neuroscientist Michele Ross, Ph.D.

Are you sick of being in pain? Are you worried about getting cancer or growing old? Are you always tired? Do you have too many prescriptions for your age? You or your loved one don't have to feel this way. This book will show you the real reason why your body is breaking down. Your doctor doesn't know anything about it because he wasn't even trained on the biggest neurotransmitter system in your body: the endocannabinoid system. I was once like you, a non-cannabis believer.

Flash back to 1998. I grew up in a strict family, and marijuana was not part of my life. In fact, I grew up in front of crack house, and my goal was to become a scientist who could end drug addiction. I thought marijuana was just something my slacker first boyfriend smoked to drive his parents mad. It was a drug that caused you to do poorly in school, made you smell bad, caused brain damage, and might even give you schizophrenia. I avoided it all costs and had my first hit off a joint in college only after drinking and being goaded by a boy I liked. I felt dizzy, confused, and scared of what I might do under the influence. I vowed never to smoke weed ever again.

STUDYING DRUG ADDICTION FOR MY DOCTORATE

Fast forward to graduate school, where I was working in a Molecular Psychiatry department studying the effects of "drugs of abuse" on the brain for the National Institute on Drug Abuse. Drugs of abuse included nicotine, found in cigarettes, THC, found in marijuana, or the scientific term cannabis, MDMA, found in ecstasy, cocaine, methamphetamine, and heroin. I still couldn't use cannabis, mostly because I worked with drugs delivered directly from NIDA like cocaine and heroin and a positive THC test would kill my career, and partly because I lived in Dallas, Texas and very few people had cannabis.

I was studying a process called neurogenesis in a brain area called the hippocampus. This brain region is important for learning and memory, and as we later found out, mood and addiction.[1,2] I was working under Dr. Amelia Eisch, and our lab wanted to know how neurogenesis, the birth of new neurons, or brain cells, contributed to mental health and drug abuse. The very first scientific paper I published was a review on how cannabinoids influence neurogenesis, and the evidence supported that activation of the endocannabinoid system likely grew cells in the adult brain, not killed them.[3] This up-ended everything I had learned about cannabis including my D.A.R.E era childhood and my college classes on neuroscience. It was like learning Santa wasn't real.

I started to learn more and more about the endocannabinoid system on my own time, since my graduate school classes in neuroscience barely touched on it. I was baffled that I was in a department of Molecular Psychiatry, and yet the endocannabinoid system, the largest neurotransmitter system that regulated every other neurotransmitter, was basically a footnote in my education. Turns out I wasn't alone, as doctors and nurses were also not taught the endocannabinoid system.

WHY I QUIT ACADEMIA AND FOUND MY OWN PATH

I kept finding instances in academia where the things that should be researched didn't get the grant money they deserved, and projects that never turned into treatments got millions of dollars. Even after landing a prestigious postdoctoral fellowship at the California Institute of Technology (Caltech) and Howard Hughes Medical Institute (HHMI), I felt empty and not convinced my daily routine of killing mice to study learning and memory was going to help anyone in the end. To add to the despair, my 100+ hour work week and other factors including the death of my little brother John to alcohol and opioid overdose contributed to my marriage failing.

When I got the call to be interviewed for a spot on the reality TV show Big Brother, I took it. If anyone had asked when I started my PhD whether I'd be the first scientist to star on a reality TV show, I would have laughed at them. After lasting 66 days and finishing fourth place on the highest rated summer TV show in 2009, I became a household name under Michele Noonan, and left my position at Caltech. This was the start of a career of unexpected twists and turns in a very public arena.

I didn't end up using cannabis again until I moved to Los Angeles, where medical marijuana had been legal since 1996. The cannabis culture was fascinating, but being a scientist, I didn't think that I could possibly use cannabis and still be a functioning executive. It wasn't enough that I knew that cannabis had medical benefits. The universe was going to show me until I couldn't ignore my true calling.

HOW I BECAME A CANNABIS USER

One morning in December of 2011, I woke up and my right hand and wrist were completely limp and in pain. This lasted for two months. A doctor informed me my right ulnar and radial nerves weren't sending messages through my arm. I needed an expensive surgery that might not work or could even cause permanent paralysis in my arm. After trying every alternative healthcare trick in the book for two months, it was a combination of cannabis & hours long massage of a "cold spot" in my arm that released the inflammation and slowly got my nerves to wake up.

I now know that I have chronic inflammation and neuropathy, and that I need daily constant consumption of cannabis, in all its forms, in order to have functioning nerves in my arms and legs. After an initial learning curve, I learned how to be a cannabis patient and not only a functioning scientist and patient advocate, but a leading one. In 2012 I met my husband Todd, who worked in the legal marijuana industry in California and Oregon as a grower, edible company founder, and mobile dispensary owner. He convinced me to jump 100% into cannabis and never look back on my old life in academia.

I published my first book, *Train Your Brain to Get Thin: Prime Your Gray Cells for Weight Loss, Wellness and Exercise*, with my co-author

Melinda Boyd in November 2012. After a stint as a Chief Scientist of a nutraceutical company formulating and marketing products in six countries, I realized cannabis – or at least CBD – should be the next superfood and marketed as a vitamin. The concept for my next book, *Vitamin Weed,* was born!

FROM CANNABIS USER TO CANNABIS ADVOCATE

In January of 2013 I founded the Endocannabinoid Deficiency Foundation with my husband to drive clinical research, education, advocacy and patient support on cannabis for specific health conditions. We changed the 501c3 nonprofit's name to IMPACT Network in 2015, and **IMPACT** Network's mission is **I**mproving **M**arijuana **P**olicy and **A**ccelerating **T**herapeutics for women worldwide. Shortly after, in July 2013, we were targeted for our advocacy, the Los Angeles Police Department (LAPD) raided our home, and false marijuana charges were filed. All charges were dropped after a lengthy court battle that ended in May 2014.

In June 2014 I was interviewed by 3-time Emmy winning journalist Amber Lyon for her new site on psychedelic science, Reset.me. She, like me, had also had experienced police interference for her advocacy of cannabis and other psychedelics. That interview was the first time I had talked about my journey from drug researcher to drug user to drug educator and brought up the concept of *Vitamin Weed.* Millions of people watched that interview, and it was clear I needed to share my story to help educate and inspire others.

Vitamin Weed went from book concept to draft in the summer of 2014 after the support from the interview and after receiving thousands of emails from patients in countries or states where medical marijuana is still illegal. These patients, desperate from suffering from chronic or terminal illnesses, begged me to send them cannabis illegally in the mail. I thought, there has to be a better way. I myself had become a medical marijuana refugee. After continuing to be harassed by the LAPD even after I had won my case, my family decided to move in October 2014 to Denver, Colorado where cannabis was legal for both medical and recreational use and police couldn't arrest me for being a patient or an advocate.

THE LONG JOURNEY BACK TO HEALTH

Winning my legal battle wasn't the only obstacle for me in God's plan. I was not using cannabis during most of 2014 due to my legal issues. Unfortunately, I had black mold and lead poisoning from my apartment in Los Angeles, confirmed by the Department of Health, and undiagnosed blood clots in my legs and lungs, a condition called deep vein thrombosis and pulmonary embolisms. The day after Christmas 2014, I suffered a heart attack due to my heart giving up from all the arteries to my lungs being blocked by clots. My lung also collapsed, and I had a 30 percent chance of living through the night in the ICU of the hospital. I lived, but had brain damage from hypoxia, or reduced oxygen to the brain over several weeks. I was on an oxygen tank and in a wheelchair, with little strength to think or do much but make it through the pain each day. In February of 2015 I was diagnosed with fibromyalgia as well as neuropathy from the damage to my nerves.

Frustrated with the lack of progress I was making in people to be normal again, I put myself in what I jokingly now call my 'cannabis coma.' I took full extract cannabis oil (FECO), also called Rick Simpson Oil (RSO), which is super concentrated in THC, the psychoactive cannabinoid that can put you to sleep if you do not have a tolerance to high doses. While I slept and healed for most of the days, my brain and nervous system started to heal. I started, little by little, to be able to move my legs and arms and start to walk a couple of minutes at a time in a walker. After months I no longer needed my oxygen tank and could walk for an hour with my walker. I finally started walking without the walker, and then with only a cane. I am so proud that I was able to walk without a cane one year after I had entered the ER for blood clots.

In December 2015, I started to launch the first IMPACT conferences on cannabis for specific conditions. I was wary of public speaking, as I could barely stand for an hour without excruciating pain, never-mind host a six-hour conference. Somehow, I made it through, and I can thank cannabis cream on my arms, legs, feet and back before and after my conferences as well as CBD tincture to wipe out the anxiety I had. I wondered what people would think of me now that I was this sick version of myself, a little slower both verbally and physically since my time on TV as a reality TV competitor swinging off of ropes and winning challenges. Over time I gained my mojo and my health back and continued to grow my nonprofit as well as start writing again. I now speak around the world on the benefits and science of cannabis.

It is with great pleasure that I introduce to you my labor of love that I once thought I would never finish due to my illnesses, but persevered through cannabis. Restoring endocannabinoid system deficiency was the key to my healthy and active life, and I will teach you all about the cannabinoids and natural chemicals in cannabis and other plants that boost your body's natural endocannabinoid system, improving your mental and physical health. *Vitamin Weed* is the key to a long, healthy, and happy life, and I can't wait to share it with you.

CHAPTER 2

Why You Need This Book

This book is arranged sequentially so that each section prepares you for the next.

Part One identifies what your knowledge level of the endocannabinoid system and cannabis is: misinformed, uninformed, novice or expert. It brings everyone up to speed by providing an in-depth review of the endocannabinoid system. Feel free to deep-dive, use this review as a reference as you continue on your cannabis journey, or continue on to Part Two.

Part Two gives you an overview of endocannabinoid deficiency: what it is, who suffers from it, what causes it, how it progresses and why modern medicine has not recognized it as a syndrome. If you find yourself relating to some of the common signs and symptoms of endocannabinoid deficiency, you should proceed to Part Three.

Part Three expands on endocannabinoid deficiency in specific diseases and how cannabis or CBD may treat those conditions. Many patients may have more than one condition that can be attributed to endocannabinoid deficiency. Find out to treat or prevent these condition in Part Four.

Part Four offers a complete lifestyle change to boost the ability of cannabinoid replacement therapy, nicknamed "Vitamin Weed," to reset your health. It explains how to use both cannabis and non-cannabis products for optimal health. Finally, it shows you how to maintain a healthy endocannabinoid system for life.

Vitamin Weed: A 4-Step Plan to Prevent and Reverse Endocannabinoid Deficiency will not tell you how to grow cannabis, make food infused with cannabis, or make topicals infused with cannabis. There are great books dedicated to these topics, and I encourage you to read *Marijuana Grower's Handbook: Your Complete Guide for Medical and Personal Marijuana Cultivation* by Ed Rosenthal, *The Cannabis Kitchen Cookbook: Feel-Good Food for Home Cooks* by Robyn Griggs Lawrence, and *The Cannabis Spa at Home* by Sandra Hinchliffe.

This book will also not tell you how to talk to your mom or your doctor about cannabis or give a basic overview of how to smoke or eat cannabis products. There are two great books that can help you with those conversations: *Waking Up to Weed* by Stephanie Byer and *Time for the Talk: Talking to your Doctor or Patient About Cannabis* by Regina Nelson, Ph.D.

You might be curious about cannabis because you heard about it on television or have a sick loved one you might want to get it for. Everyone has an endocannabinoid system, not just the seriously ill patients. Chances are you're not 100% happy with your health or the quality of your life. Optimizing your endocannabinoid system can help you live life to the maximum. Let's figure out what your cannabis IQ is so you can get the full benefits of this book.

THE VITAMIN WEED IQ QUIZ

1. **When it came to marijuana, my parents:**

    a. used marijuana and taught me how to use it responsibly.

    b. didn't talk negatively about it, but didn't use it.

    c. hate it. I'd have to hide the fact that I use it from them even as an adult.

    d. forbid me to use it and talked negatively about people who use it.

2. **The first time I smoked weed:**

    a. was in high school. I've been puffing away ever since.

    b. was in college. I still smoke every once in a while, but never buy my own weed.

    c. was in my 20s. I got sick or paranoid; it's not for me.

    d. was never. No way am I smoking something.

3. **When it comes to my cannabis habits, I'd like to:**

    a. try different ways of using it, like vaping or topicals.

    b. know the difference between strains and be more of a connoisseur.

    c. find the right strain so I can finally enjoy it.

    d. figure out how to use it discreetly without smoking it or getting high.

4. Once I decide to make a life change, I:

a. reward myself with gold stars and stick with it. Winners never quit!

b. I keep with it for 2 weeks or so, but then get so busy I gradually stop.

c. I give up after a day or 2. It's just too hard or I want instant results.

d. New Year's resolutions are a joke. Old dogs don't learn new tricks.

5. Exercise is ________:

a. a daily part of my life. Even if it's just 10 minutes.

b. something I wish I had more time for.

c. boring. I can't drag myself to the gym.

d. walking to the car counts as exercise, right?

6. When it comes to deciding what strain of cannabis to use:

a. I research what symptoms I have and THC to CBD to ratio I need.

b. I use whatever is around and don't care what it is as long as it gets me high.

c. I'm overwhelmed and end up buying nothing.

d. would like to try something with CBD but don't know where to get it.

7. When it comes to sleep, I get:

a. 7-8 hours of it daily. I feel pretty rested when I wake up.
b. 5-6 hours daily, but I make up for it by sleeping on the weekends.
c. it varies each day. I snore, have insomnia, or some other sleep problem.
d. sleep? what's that? I am a zombie.

8. I know ________ about the endocannabinoid system:

a. a lot! I know the two main type of receptors and the names of endocannabinoids.
b. not much. I know your brain makes marijuana.
c. a little. I know the difference between THC and CBD.
d. huh? enough with the big words.

9. When it comes to making food choices, I:

a. opt for healthy choices and go on a diet when I'm out of my desired weight range.
b. try not to eat fast food too often, but I am too busy to cook at home.
c. I have a lot of spoiled veggies and health food in my fridge. I have good intentions.
d. eat whatever I want. You only live once, right?

10. Everything I know about cannabis has come from:

a. researching a variety of sources that I trust as well as

my local budtender.

b. personal experience and what I read on the internet.
c. what my friends have told me or what I saw on TV.
d. what I was taught in D.A.R.E. class or read on Fox News.

ANSWER KEY

If you chose mostly As, you have a strong positive relationship with medical marijuana and understanding of the endocannabinoid system to use as a base, but you could get a boost to make *Vitamin Weed* really work in your life. Your openness towards cannabis means your brain is receptive to the tips in this book and the *Vitamin Weed 4-Step Plan*. In no time, you'll be on your way to a happier and healthier life.

If you chose mostly Bs, you have some of the basics down of healthy lifestyle and cannabis knowledge, but you have a lot of room to grow, especially on how the endocannabinoid system works. With a little work, you can strengthen your *Vitamin Weed* IQ, learn how to incorporate cannabis into your life, and retrain your body to heal itself. You won't see results overnight with the *Vitamin Weed 4-Step Plan*, but you will start seeing gradual results with big achievements by month three.

If you chose mostly Cs, you have a good grasp on healthy living and even some basics of cannabis, but you don't act on them in your life. Transforming knowledge into habits is the hardest part, but I'll help you make the smallest changes in your life to yield the maximum benefits from the *Vitamin Weed 4-Step Plan*. Your success depends on your commitment, but thankfully incorporating cannabis into your daily life isn't painful.

If you chose mostly Ds, you're pretty clueless about cannabis, the endocannabinoid system, and healthy living. Either you live in a state where medical marijuana is not legal, you don't know anyone that uses cannabis, or you've been misinformed about cannabis. Don't worry, I'll catch you up to speed! Choosing this book was the first step towards shifting your body to healthy mode. Results won't be instant with the *Vitamin Weed 4-Step Plan*, but I'll break down lifestyle changes into baby steps so you'll be more likely to make them habits and stay on the plan. The good news: you will see the biggest improvement in health out of any group with the *4-Step Plan.*

EVERYTHING YOU KNOW ABOUT MARIJUANA IS WRONG

For starters, that's not even its name. There are many slang names for cannabis: marijuana, weed, pot, ganja, and kush. Most people are familiar with the term marijuana because states that have legalized cannabis call it medical marijuana or recreational marijuana. However, marijuana is not the actual name of cannabis, and is derived from racist legal terms meant to criminalize its use, possession, and distribution. The majority of countries outside of North America use the word cannabis over marijuana and this book will also. I hope you start using the word cannabis instead or marijuana as well.

Most scientific and medical journals still use the term marijuana to describe the drug, and use terms like "illicit drug," "abused drug," "addictive drug," or "substance of abuse" to describe it. This is unfortunate because cannabis is only illicit because of laws, not because it is a harmful substance. To classify all cannabis user as addicts, or illegal drug users is just incorrect. Studies of addiction often lump cannabis users in with crystal meth, heroin, and cocaine users, and this has likely confounded results of these studies because cannabis use has a positive effect on health while other drug use is neurotoxic.

INFORMATION OVERLOAD

Cannabis is a fixture on your television and on the internet. It makes the evening news daily and recent reality docuseries include High Profits on CNN, Pot Barons of Colorado on MSNBC, and Medicine Man on TruTV. There are now 1000s of blogs on cannabis, hundreds of nonprofits, and several mainstream magazines including Cannabis Now and High Times providing information on everything from growing weed to how the endocannabinoid system works. Even rapper turned entrepreneur Snoop Dogg has his own marijuana education and lifestyle network called Merry Jane. But is it this explosion of information helpful or accurate?

After reviewing websites for simple information like what receptor does the main ingredient in cannabis, THC activate, I was appalled by the amount of misinformation online. One error I continued to find was that THC activates only CB1 receptors and CBD, the second most common cannabinoid in cannabis, only activates CB2 receptors. In reality, THC activates CB1 and CB2 receptors equally and CBD doesn't activate either CB1 or CB2 receptors. This is a very basic concept, what does cannabis do in your body, yet by careless editing in the information age, misinformation spreads virally.

Why is there so much misinformation on the internet? Many websites do not produce original information and instead show what is called an RSS feed, pulling original content from multiple websites for a constant stream of content. If one article is published with misinformation, it ends up being published on a thousand other sites, where it is cumulatively viewed by millions, and this misinformation is virally spread. Even if a correction to the original article is made, the 1000s of websites that published the article with misinformation are not corrected. Misinformation on cannabis is truly a virus without a cure.

We live in the digital age where delayed gratification is not possible. We want our information now! Writers feel the demand to publish often and publish fast. Articles are often posted to social media channels with grammar errors and scientific errors, and authors rely on reader feedback to correct. Unfortunately, an article can be shared 100,000 times or more via popular Facebook pages, and these readers will not return to read the corrected article.

Another problem is that many authors of articles on cannabis or the endocannabinoid system are self-taught. The endocannabinoid system is still not taught in medical school, so doctors are not publishing information on cannabis, and if they are, it is often rife with as many errors as articles written by people who are not health professionals. Who then is a trusted source of cannabis information? At IMPACT Network we are working to audit web pages of major cannabis magazines and nonprofits, providing a seal of approval on pages that contain accurate information on cannabis and the endocannabinoid system.

Outdated information is not an intentional source of misinformation, but many articles continue to cite studies that have since been disproven through studies using better technology or bigger patient groups. Because most articles online don't include references, it's impossible to know whether they are using facts from studies done in the last five years or whether they are quoting old information.

Lack of access to scientific journals is another reason for lack of updated and scientifically correct articles on cannabis and the endocannabinoid system. Subscriptions to journal articles for doctors and scientists is paid for by their employers but are exorbitantly high in price for patients. When access to a single five-page journal article can cost $40 dollars or a scientific book is $300, we have a problem. There are 14,189 research studies related to cannabis, 19,405 with cannabinoids, or 22,061 with the term marijuana using the government search engine PubMed. There is no way patients or cannabis educators can afford to pay for general articles to keep informed and are forced to rely on mainstream media's summaries of selected studies, which are often incorrect or skewed.

This book provides a trusted source of information on the endocannabinoid system and cannabis as well as resources to dig further on your topic of interest. If further assistance is needed you can contact the IMPACT Network for a doctor or dispensary referral or become a member to be updated with current cannabis studies, products and law changes.

BUT I'M NOT DYING: WHY CANNABIS IS STILL FOR YOU

The distinction between medical marijuana and recreational marijuana has made Americans believe there are only two uses for cannabis: get high or treat a terminal illness like cancer. In states that have legalized medical marijuana, there are huge differences in what medical conditions qualify a patient to obtain a medical card or recommendation. In California, almost any medical condition qualifies, but in most states qualifying conditions are limited to multiple sclerosis, severe chronic pain, seizures, AIDS, or cancer.

If you don't have a debilitating chronic or terminal illness, you might have a hard time convincing others or even yourself that you need cannabis. You will have an impossible time convincing people that your sick child needs it. Keep in mind medical versus recreational marijuana is a taxation scheme dreamed up by politicians. In reality, all cannabis is medicinal, because it does not cause death, has harmless side effects like increased appetite or sleepiness depending on strain used, and reduces inflammation and stress in your body.

The media has only focused on cannabis and its most abundant cannabinoids, THC and CBD. Turn on the nightly news and it is likely you'll hear a story about how CBD cured a child's epilepsy or how cannabis oil helped treat someone's cancer. In a country where cannabis is still federally illegally and medically legal in only a few states, it doesn't matter how effective cannabis is as a treatment if you cannot buy it or use it without being arrested, fired, or having your children taken away from you by Child Protective Services (CPS).

The dirty little secret of both the medical and cannabis industries is that you make your own cannabinoids in your brain and body. They're called endocannabinoids, and they are just as powerful as the cannabinoids in medical marijuana at fighting cancer, relieving pain, and all the wonderful health benefits we've attributed only to cannabis. The difference between endocannabinoids and phytocannabinoids found in cannabis? Endocannabinoids are made in your body and thus FREE and legal, and they don't make you high like THC in cannabis can.

The health benefits of endocannabinoid anandamide (AEA) have been studied and published in hundreds of scientific journals. Anandamide prevents the adhesion, proliferation, and migration of breast cancer cells, reduces proliferation of liver cancer cells, and suppress the initiation of pain, among many other benefits.[4-7]

How can you boost your levels of endocannabinoids? You can eat foods that have endocannabinoids or chemicals that boosts their production in the body. You can eliminate bad foods, substitute for toxic medications, and reduce other lifestyle factors that cause your endocannabinoid system to break down. You can manage stress to maintain your healthy endocannabinoid system. Finally, you can add phytocannabinoids, which are cannabinoids made from plants like cannabis, to your daily routine to enhance your own endocannabinoid system.

It's never too late to start using cannabinoids or boosting your body's natural endocannabinoid system. Cannabinoids can slow the onset or development of many diseases including Alzheimer's disease and cancer, while improving your quality of life. It can balance out whatever vices you have, including a bad diet, sleep deprivation, or regular alcohol use. Cannabinoids can even slow the aging process, keeping both your body and brain young. This is of great importance as our population extends life expectancy, but the final years are riddled with health problems and poor quality of life. Start taking control of your own health by using cannabis to prevent and treat disease.

CHAPTER 3

What is the Endocannabinoid System?

"[I was] surprised to a large extent that while the active compound in morphine had been isolated from opium 100 years before and cocaine had been isolated from cocoa leaves at the same time, the active component of marijuana was unknown." – Dr. Raphael Mechoulam, Godfather of Cannabinoid Medicine

The purpose of your endocannabinoid system is to maintain balance, called homeostasis. The endocannabinoid system modulates almost every physiological process of your mind and body including memory, pain, appetite, mood, and reproduction. All these processes are highly influenced by your environment, but the cannabinoid system is there to fine tune cells, put on the brakes or ramp up cell activity, and make sure no processes become pathological.

The endocannabinoid system (ECS) is the largest neurotransmitter system in your body. Cannabinoid receptors for endocannabinoids are present on almost every cell, regulating your brain, immune system, skin, and every other organ in your body. The ECS helps your body deal with physical and emotional stress. Your energy, resilience to life's obstacles, happiness, and health are all dependent on a functioning ECS.

Receptors are like locks, and neurotransmitters or hormones are the key that unlocks a chain reaction inside a cell, leading to physiological processes. The main receptors for endocannabinoids are CB1, which are found mostly in the nervous system, reproductive system, liver, connective tissues, and glands, and CB2, which are mainly found in the immune system and brain.[8] Some tissues, like the brain and eye, contain both receptors, but CB2 is found at a lower density than CB1 in these tissues.[8,9]

New receptors such as TRPV1, GPR55, GPR119 and GPR18 are being discovered that are activated by cannabinoids. In fact, there are hundreds of "orphan" receptors that have unknown functions and unknown binding partners. It is likely that many of these orphan receptors will be discovered to be new cannabinoid receptors.

Receptors for neurotransmitters such as dopamine, serotonin, glutamate, and gamma-aminobutyric acid (GABA) are typically found on the "postsynaptic" side of the synapse, which is the space between one brain cell, or neuron, signaling to another neuron. Neurotransmitters are typically released on the "presynaptic" side, cross the synapse, and bind to receptors which activates a molecular pathway that results in protein production and physiological effects.[10]

Cannabinoid receptors are the black sheep of neuroscience and operate in the opposite manner. Cannabinoid receptors are present on the presynaptic neuron, and endocannabinoids are produced in the postsynaptic neuron. The endocannabinoids travel "retrograde" back to the receptors in the presynaptic neuron where they typically inhibit release of additional neurotransmitters.

Inhibition of neurotransmitters by cannabinoid receptors does not mean the ultimate outcome of endocannabinoid signaling is no activation of a neural pathway. If cannabinoid receptors are on neurons that produce the excitatory neurotransmitter glutamate, CB1 activation will inhibit the release of glutamate and the neural pathway will not be activated. If cannabinoid receptors are on neurons that produce the inhibitory neurotransmitter GABA, CB1 activation will inhibit the release of GABA and the neural pathway will not activated via disinhibition (inhibiting an inhibitor). Most neural pathways are constantly in an inhibitory state because we do not need to be moving, eating, sleeping, etc. all the time. This means endocannabinoid disinhibition of neural circuits to activate behavior is a crucial part of our physiology.

WHAT IS A CANNABINOID?

Cannabis is the Latin term for marijuana, and comes from the Greek word for marijuana, *kánnabis*, first recorded in 440 BC by Herodotus. Cannabinoid means a component of cannabis. There are three types of cannabinoids: endocannabinoids, phytocannabinoids, and synthetic cannabinoids. Endo means "from within," and endocannabinoids are cannabinoids usually made within the body or brain of mammals. Phytocannabinoids are cannabinoids from plants such as cannabis and echinacea. Synthetic cannabinoids are either phytocannabinoids synthesized in a lab or altered to create new cannabinoid drugs for research or medicine. There are a few exceptions to these rules, as several endocannabinoids have been found in plants or fungi.[11-12]

WHO HAS AN ENDOCANNABIOID SYSTEM?

Cannabinoid receptors evolved over 600 million years ago, while cannabis evolved only 25 million years ago. All vertebrate animals, including humans, monkeys, rats, mice, birds, reptiles, fish, and even sea squirts have cannabinoid receptors as well as endocannabinoids. Thus, all vertebrates have a functioning endocannabinoid system. Certain components of the endocannabinoid system, such as specific enzymes or receptors are limited to specific vertebrate families or species.[13]

Insects, nematodes, hydra and fungi, and plants lack cannabinoid receptors.[14-16] The fact that plants and even some fungi produce cannabinoids but lack the receptors for them is highly interesting. This means phytocannabinoids are produced as either a defense mechanism to prevent animals from eating the plants, or in the case of fungi, produce to entice animals to eat them and spread their spores.

SYNTHESIS OF ENDOCANNABINOIDS

Your body makes endocannabinoids, which are the neurotransmitters your cannabinoid receptors were made for. These endocannabinoids are not stored but are synthesized on-demand.[17-18] The two most prominent endocannabinoids are anandamide (AEA) and 2-arachidonoylglycerol (2-AG), but there are new endocannabinoids such as virodhamine being discovered. Endocannabinoids are synthesized from proteins called fatty acids and act locally where they are produced.

AEA

Anandamide is normally synthesized in the brain from *N*-arachidonoyl phosphatidylethanolamine (NAPE) when phospholipase D (NAPE–PLD) is chopped in two or "cleaved."[19] α,β-hydrolase 4 (ABHD4) can also deacylate NAPE to form glycerophosphate, which is then cleaved to form AEA.[20] AEA can also be generated in a toxic environment by macrophages when phospholipase C cleaves NAPE to form phosphoanandamide, which is then dephosphorylated into AEA.[21]

2-AG

2-AG is normally synthesized in the brain from diacylglycerol (DAG), which includes the omega-6 fatty acid arachidonic acid. Diacylglycerol lipase, which comes in alpha (DAGLα) and beta (DAGLβ) forms, turns DAG into 2-AG.[22] 2-AG can also be generated by dephosporylating arachidonoyl-LPA or by a reaction involving phospholipase A1 (PLA1) and lysophopholipase C (lyso-PLC).[23-24]

RELEASE OF ENDOCANNABINOIDS

Endocannabinoids differ from other neurotransmitters because they are fat-soluble, instead of water-soluble and cannot be stored in synaptic vesicles.[25] AEA and 2-AG regulate cannabinoid signaling both temporally and spatially. AEA tonically activates cannabinoid receptors at a low level while 2-AG is a more powerful signal released when needed in specific regions.[26] A way to visualize this is AEA is like a low-watt light bulb illuminating an entire room constantly, but 2-AG is like a flashlight that provides a strong stream of light to a very small area for a short amount of time.

UPTAKE OF ENDOCANNABINOIDS

Anandamide is a type of fatty acid amide and belongs to the family of *N*-acylethanolamines (NAEs). AEA and other NAEs are transported from the synapse to inside the cell via fatty acid amide hydrolase (FAAH)-like anandamide transporter (FLAT) and fatty acid binding proteins (FABPs).[27] There are three FABP subtypes in the mammalian brain: FABP3, FABP5, FABP7.[28] FABPs help transport AEA to the FAAH enzyme where it is degraded.

The mechanism by which 2-AG is transported from the synapse inside the cell is less clear. It has been proposed that 2-AG shares the same transport system as AEA, but that is not the case, as 2-AG does not bind to FABPs.[29] An endocannabinoid membrane transporter (EMT), yet to be discovered, that transports both AEA and 2-AG is supported by recent research.[30]

BREAKDOWN OF ENDOCANNABINOIDS

FAAHs

Once transported into the cell, anandamide is quickly broken down by the enzyme FAAH and recently discovered FAAH2.[31-32] FAAH is found in the endoplasmic reticulum (ER) of cells while FAAH2 is found in lipid droplets in the cytoplasm.[33] FAAH2 prefers to break down primary fatty acid amides, such as oleamide (OEA), over NAEs such as anandamide and breaks down AEA and PEA at 40% of the rate FAAH does.[33-34] FAAH2 is produced in humans, but not mouse or rat, limiting the usefulness of rodent studies of the endocannabinoid system to elucidate human function.[35] FAAH2 is found in the heart and ovary while FAAH is not, suggesting FAAH2 may regulate endocannabinoid signaling in these regions.[35]

MAGL

2-AG has its own metabolic pathway and 85% of this endocannabinoid is broken down by the enzyme monoacylglycerol lipase (MAGL) at the cell membrane. MAGL turns 2-AG into neuroinflammatory arachidonic acid that is further degraded into neuroinflammatory prostaglandins.[36-37]

4% of 2-AG in the brain is metabolized by α/β-hydrolase 6 (ABHD6) at the cell membrane and 9% is metabolized by α/β-hydrolase 12 (ABHD12), discovered in 2007.[37-38] ABHD6 is located postsynaptically instead of presynaptically, suggesting this enzyme's role is to regulate 2-AG levels at the site of synthesis instead of presynaptically where 2-AG acts on CB1 receptors.[37] ABHD6 is found in the brain and highly expressed in the prefrontal cortex, while ABHD12 is found in the brain, prostate, fat, macrophages, and microglia.[38-39] ABHD12 may mediate inflammation and neurotoxicity during brain injury.[40]

COX-2

Anandamide and 2-AG are also broken down by cyclooxygenase-2 (COX-2), the enzyme responsible for turning arachidonic acid into inflammatory and pain causing prostaglandins.[41] Endocannabinoids are not broken down by cyclooxygenase-1 (COX-1). COX-2 breaks down AEA into prostaglandin ethanol amides (PG-EAs), also known as prostamides, and breaks down 2-AG into prostaglandin glycerol esters (PG-Gs).

There are a variety of prostamides and PG-Gs that can be formed via COX-2; each may have a variety of biological actions and therapeutic application yet to be elucidated.[42-43] Prostamides and PG-Gs do not act at CB1 or CB2 receptors and each variety may have its own set of presynaptic receptors that have not been discovered yet.[44-45] The first therapeutic application of an AEA metabolite, prostamide F2α, is in reducing eye pressure in glaucoma and has been synthesized and marketed as Lumigan (bimatoprost).[46]

Prostaglandin E2 glycerol ester (PGE2-G), produced when COX-2 breaks down 2-AG, functions in the opposite way of 2-AG in modulating neuronal activity in the hippocampus, the brain's learning and memory center.[47] In fact, PGE2-G mediates neurotoxicity in the hippocampus, producing overexcitability that can lead to neuron injury and death.[45] In times of injury or stress, COX-2's role in creating endocannabinoid metabolites will have a negative impact on learning and memory. Therapeutics targeted at inhibiting COX-2 may do more than just reduce pain and inflammation; they may suppress maladaptive learning.[47]

OTHER ENZYMES

Adding to the complex actions and pharmacology of anandamide and 2-AG is that they are also broken down by several lipoxygenases (LOXs) including 5-Lipoxygenase (5-LO,) creating a diversity of metabolites.[48] AEA and 2-AG may also be directly broken down by cytochrome P450 enzymes in the liver.[48]

ENDOCANNABINOIDS: MORE THAN JUST ANANDAMIDE

This section deep dives into anandamide and 2-AG as well as other atypical endocannabinoids.

ANANDAMIDE

Anandamide was discovered by Raphael Mechoulam in 1992 and named by "ananda," the Sanskrit word for bliss, and "amide," the chemical name for protein.[49] The chemical name for anandamide is actually *N*-arachidonoylethanolamine. AEA is the fatty acid amide of arachidonic acid and ethanolamine. The other NAEs are discussed further in this chapter below under "Atypical Cannabinoids." AEA and other NAEs are present in every mammalian cell at low levels in the range of hundreds of pmol/g in tissue but are synthesized on-demand.[50]

AEA is actually a partial agonist of the CB1 receptor and its concentration in tissues is much lower than 2-AG.[51-52] While CB1 is the receptor that mediates the high from THC, because AEA binds the CB1 receptor weaker than THC, boosting anandamide levels result in mild mood change but not euphoria. AEA also activates CB2 receptors, which may balance out any psychoactivity from the CB1 receptor.

AEA activates more than traditional cannabinoid receptors. Several orphan receptors, or receptors for which the ligand has not yet been discovered, are now being linked to cannabinoids. One of these is transient receptor potential vanilloid 1 (TRPV1) receptor, a nonselective cation channel.[53] Activation of TRPV1 receptors, also called vanilloid (VR1) receptors, on sensory nerves by anandamide mediates vasodilation, or opening of arteries.[54]

2-AG

2-AG was discovered by Raphael Mechoulam but its presence in mammals and ability to bind to cannabinoid receptors was discovered by another group in 1995.[55] Unlike AEA, which binds to both CB1 and CB2 receptors, 2-AG only binds to CB1 receptors. 2-AG is present in much higher concentration in tissue than AEA and mediates inhibition of neuronal activity in the brain via retrograde signaling.[56] In fact, 2-AG levels in the brain are three times higher than AEA.[51] 2-AG is neuroprotective and protects hippocampal neurons from inflammation by activating the CB1 receptor, which activates PPARγ to inhibit COX-2 expression.[57]

ATYPICAL ENDOCANNABINOIDS

Other *N*-acylethanolamines (NAEs) besides traditional endocannabinoids anandamide and 2-AG include *N*-palmitoylethanolamine (PEA), *N*-oleoylethanolamine (OEA), *N*-linoleoyl ethanolamine (LEA), *N*-stearoyl ethanolamine (SEA), *N*-docosahexaenoyl ethanolamine (DHEA), and homo-gamma-linoleoyl ethanolamine (HEA). This section will also review even less known endocannabinoids.

PEA

N-palmitoylethanolamine (PEA) is the fatty acid amide of palmitic acid and ethanolamine and was originally discovered in egg yolk. It is expressed widely in plant and animal tissue and has anti-inflammatory activity as well as a role in preventing neuropathic and chronic pain states. PEA tissue levels are not influenced by changes in dietary fatty acid intake, unlike other NAEs.[58] Alcohol intake does decease PEA levels in the brain.[50] PEA is metabolized by FAAH, the same enzyme that breaks down anandamide, as well as the N-acylethanolamine-hydrolyzing acid amidase (NAAA), which is highly expressed in the lung, spleen, thymus and intestine.[59]

The main target of PEA is peroxisome proliferator-activated receptor alpha (PPAR-α), a nuclear receptor that is not a cannabinoid receptor. PEA is not considered a typical endocannabinoid because it does not activate CB1 or CB2 receptors.[60] However, PEA activates orphan receptors GPR55 and GPR119, which, along with GPR18, have been identified as novel cannabinoid receptors.

PEA acts in synergy with AEA and other NAEs to provide a natural "entourage effect" similar to that seen with phytocannabinoids in cannabis.[61-62] These effects are mediated via CB1 and TRPV1.[63-64] PEA enhances the anti-proliferative effects of AEA on human cancer cells by inhibiting FAAH.[65] Long-term treatment of human breast cancer cells with PEA reduces expression of FAAH.[64]

Both PEA and SEA muscle tissue levels are elevated in patients with chronic neck and shoulder pain (CNSP) as well as chronic widespread pain (CWP).[66] PEA and SEA levels decrease during exercise in patients with chronic pain, and this is correlated with increases in pain.[66] Dietary supplementation with PEA has been shown to reduce diabetic neuropathic pain, pelvic pain, sciatic pain, and temporomandibular joint syndrome (TMJ).[67-68] An additional role of PEA is as anticonvulsant.[69-70] Finally, PEA reduces appetite after ingestion of dietary fat.[71]

OEA

N-oleoylethanolamine (OEA) is the fatty acid amide of oleic acid and ethanolamine. It is produced naturally in the small intestine, and bile acids influence its production.[72] The main target of OEA is peroxisome proliferator-activated receptor alpha (PPAR-α), similar to PEA, and together both stimulate neurosteroid synthesis and appetite.[73-74] OEA also binds to GPR119 and VR1.[75]

Boosting OEA levels is good for brain health. Increasing intake of olive oil increases brain levels of AEA as well as OEA.[76] Treatment with OEA increases formation of memories in rodents.[77] Prolonged consumption of a high fat diet may contribute to obesity by decreasing levels of NAEs including OEA in the intestine.[74]

LEA

N-linoleoyl ethanolamine (LEA) is found in brain and immune cells. Increasing intake of safflower oil, high in linoleic acid, increases LEA levels in the brain, intestine, and liver.[76] LEA weakly binds to CB1 and CB2 receptors, and both inhibits FAAAH and is broken down by FAAH. LEA from food in the intestine may increase the rewarding value of food as well as decrease consumption of it.[71]

HEA

N-homo-gamma-linoleoyl ethanolamine (HEA) is a little studied endocannabinoid found in brain and immune cells. HEA weakly binds to CB1 and CB2 receptors, and similar to LEA, is both broken down by FAAH and inhibits FAAH.

SEA

N-stearoyl ethanolamine (SEA) is the fatty acid amide of stearic acid and ethanolamine and is metabolized by FAAH, the same enzyme that breaks down anandamide. SEA reduces allergic inflammation in the skin, but other benefits have not been studied.[78]

DHEA

N-docosahexaenoyl ethanolamine (DHEA) is the fatty acid amide of docosahexaenoic acid (DHA) and ethanolamine. DHEA is present in both the brain and retina of the eye at the same concentrations as anandamide.[79-80] DHEA binds to the CB1 receptor more strongly than anandamide, and also inhibits potassium channels.[81-83] Consuming DHA increases DHEA levels and reduces inflammatory gene expression.[84-85] During brain injury and states of neuroinflammation, DHEA is produced and metabolism of DHEA creates novel anti-inflammatory chemicals.[77-86]

NALA

N-arachidonoyl-L-alanine (NALA) is a little known and studied endocannabinoid. Both NALA and DHEA inhibit growth of skin cancer cells via a mechanism that does not involve CB1 or TRPV1 receptors but involves anandamide breakdown via 5-LO.[87] This is particular interest since cancer cells often overexpress COX-2 and 5-LO, and NALA and DHEA could selectively target cancer cells while sparing healthy cells.

NADA

N-arachidonoyldopamine (NADA) activates both CB1 and TRPV1 receptors.[88-89] It is not clear yet how NADA is made near dopamine neuron terminals, but it is enriched in the brain, specifically in the hippocampus, striatum, and cerebellum.[90-91] NADA relieves pain, increases sleepiness, reduces activity, reduces body temperature, and relaxes muscles.[91-94] NADA is ant-inflammatory and also antiviral, inhibiting HIV in in vitro experiments.[95]

VIRODHAMINE

O-arachidonoyl ethanolamine, also known as virodhamine or O-AEA, is a little-known endocannabinoid created by joining arachidonic acid and ethanolamine through an ester. Virodhamine is the opposite orientation of anandamide, and is named after the Sanskrit word *virodha*, which means opposition. It is found at the same levels as anandamide in the hippocampus, the brain area that regulates memory. Virodhamine is found at 2-9 times higher levels than anandamide in regions outside the brain that express CB2 receptors.

Virodhamine inhibits CB1 receptors and activates CB2 receptors. One physiological effect of virodhamine is lowering body temperature.[96] Virodhamine also relaxes blood vessels via the endothelial cannabinoid receptors and GPR55.[97-98]

NOLADIN ETHER

2-arachidonyl glyceryl ether, also known as 2-AGE and noladin ether, is an endocannabinoid discovered by Lumír Hanus in 2001.[99] 2-AGE is found in the brain in low levels, with the highest amounts found in the hippocampus and thalamus.[100] It activates both CB1 and CB2 receptors and weakly binds to TRPV1 receptors.[101-103] 2-AGE reduces blood pressure and increases motivation to eat.[104]

CANNABINOID RECEPTORS: BEYOND CB1 AND CB2

This section deep dives into typical and atypical cannabinoid receptors.

CB1

Anandamide, 2-AG, and THC bind to cannabinoid type 1 (CB1) receptors. Other endocannabinoids, phytocannabinoids, and synthetic cannabinoids bind CB1 receptors while THCV inhibits them. The CB1 receptor was discovered in 1990. CB1 receptors signal through inhibitory G proteins, which means they usually slow down release of other neurotransmitters and reduce excitability of brain cells.[105] The number of CB1 receptors present in an organ or brain region can be impacted by age, gender, drug use, and other lifestyle factors. For example, there are lower levels of CB1 receptors in subcutaneous abdominal adipose tissue, or belly fat, in obese patients versus lean patients.[106]

CB1 receptors are found throughout the brain and body, with one exception. CB1 receptors are found in almost undetectable levels in the brainstem, the region that controls breathing, which is why it is impossible to overdose and die from using cannabis. CB1 receptors are found in the hippocampus, where they regulate learning, memory, and response to stress, in the hypothalamus where they regulate appetite, in the cerebellum and basal ganglia where they regulate movement, in the medulla where they regulate nausea and vomiting, in the cerebral cortex where they regulate higher level thinking, and in the spinal cord where they regulate sensation of pain, touch, temperature, and more. One example of CB1 receptor function outside the brain is the presence of CB1 receptors in skeletal sympathetic nerve terminals and regulate bone formation.[107]

CB2

The CB2 receptor was discovered in 1993. CB2 receptors are activated by anandamide, THC, beta-caryophyllene and other endocannabinoids, phytocannabinoids, and synthetic cannabinoids. CB2 receptors signal through inhibitory G proteins similar to CB1 receptors, but its effects on neurotransmission are a bit more variable.108 Activation of CB2 receptors, unlike CB1 receptors, does not produce the euphoria or high that that activation of CB1 receptors does, making it an interesting target for medical treatments.[109]

CB2 receptors are found in the immune system, bone, and brain. CB2 receptors are found on osteoblasts and osteoclasts, stimulating bone formation and inhibiting bone resorption.[107] One of the main roles of CB2 is to protect the skeleton against age-related bone loss.

CB2 receptors are widely expressed in the brain and mediate neuropsychiatric processes including pain, vomiting, memory, anxiety, and schizophrenic-like behaviors.110 Activation of CB2 receptors reduce anxiety, and chronic stress increases the number of CB2 receptors in the brain.[111] Short-term activation of hippocampal CB2 receptors has no effect on synaptic activity, while chronic activation for 7-10 days increases synaptic transmission.[110]

CB2 receptors modulate acute pain, chronic inflammatory pain, post-surgical pain, pain associated with nerve injury (neuropathy), and cancer pain.[112-113] Local injection of CB2 agonists inhibit inflammation and pain without the side effects of oral nonselective cannabinoids that act on both CB1 and CB2 in the brain and body.[114] CB2 receptors act in the opposite manner of CB1 receptors in terms of appetite. Inhibiting CB2 receptors boosts food intake after deprivation while stimulating C2B receptors decrease food intake.[115]

TRPV1

The transient receptor potential vanilloid type one (TRPV1) receptor, also called the vanilloid receptor (VR1) and the capsaicin receptor, was discovered in 1997. TRPV1 receptors are found in pain-sensing neurons in the body and brain, and may also regulate anxiety, learning, and memory.[116] TRPV1 receptors are important for sensing and regulating body temperature. TRPV1 receptors can be activated by temperature over 109 degrees Fahrenheit, acidic pH, capsaicin found in hot chili peppers, allyl isothiocyanate found in mustard and wasabi, anandamide, CBD, *N*-oleoyl dopamine (ODA), and *N*-arachidonoyldopamine (NADA).[117] Painkiller acetaminophen (Tylenol) breaks down into *N*-acetyl-parabenzoquinonimine (NAPQI) and para-benzoquinone (pBQ), metabolites that binds to TRPV1 receptors.[118]

Cannabinoid hyperemesis syndrome, a rare syndrome caused by using extremely high doses of cannabis for years, is marked by temperature dysregulation and involves TRPV1 receptors.[119] TRPV1 antagonists reduce pain and are a drug development target for arthritis, multiple sclerosis, and cancer; however, these drugs have an unwanted side effect of lowered body temperature or hypothermia.[120]

GPR18

N-arachidonoyl glycine receptor (NAGlγ receptor), also called the G protein-coupled receptor 18 (GPR18), was discovered in 1997. CBD, THC, anandamide, and synthetic cannabinoids including abnormal CBD activate GPR18.[121-122] Resolvin D2 (RvD2), which is a metabolite of omega-3 fatty acid docosahexaenoic acid (DHA), also activates GPR18 and is one of the mechanisms of how omega-3 fatty acids reduce inflammation.[123]

GPR18 is found in the testes, female reproductive tract, and spleen, and is found in high levels on sperm cells, where it regulates its function right before it enters the egg.[124] THC activates GPR18 more strongly than either CB1 or CB2 receptors.[125] Interestingly, cannabis use has no effect on fertility in men or women according to the newest research, but it impacts mouse sperm motility, so it is still not clear whether that is mediated by GPR18 or other receptors.[126-127]

GPR18's natural ligand, NAGlγ, is made by oxidative metabolism of anandamide or fusion of arachidonic acid and glycine.[128-129] NAGlγ acts on GPR18 to reduce pain and inflammation, increase insulin secretion, and even causes migration of microglial cells.[121,130] NAGlγ acts on GPR18 to cause migration of endometrial cells, and GPR18 antagonists may be a target for treating endometriosis.[122] Finally, activation of GPR18 via THC or NAGlγ lowers intraocular pressure and could be how cannabis relieves symptoms of glaucoma.[131]

GPR35

G protein-coupled receptor 35 (GPR35), also called CXCR8, was discovered in 1998.[132] GPR35 is activated by multiple cannabinoid compounds as wells as the chemokine CXCL17 and kynurenic acid, the metabolite of amino acid L-tryptophan.[133-135] GPR35 is found in the liver, immune system, GI tract, brain, and cardiovascular system.[135] GPR35 is involved in early onset inflammatory bowel disease (IBD), which include Crohn's disease and ulcerative colitis.[136] It is also a target to treat asthma.[137]

GPR55

G protein-coupled receptor 55 (GPR55) was discovered in 1999 and found to be widely expressed in the human brain, especially in the cerebellum.[138] GPR55 also regulates bone cell function, and is found in bone, the GI tract, adrenal glands, lung, liver, uterus, bladder, and kidney.[135,139,140] GPR55's main ligand is lysophosphatidylinositol (LPI), a lipid that controls growth and differentiation for many types of cells.[141]

GPR55 has been thoroughly researched by pharmaceutical companies. Anandamide, 2-AG, and the atypical cannabinoids PEA, OEA, and virodhamine bind to GPR55.[139] Anandamide and virodhamine are partial agonists, meaning at low concentrations they activate the GPR55 receptor and at high concentrations they inhibit it.[98] Phytocannabinoid THC also binds to GPR55, with higher efficacy than at either CB1 or CB2 receptors, and phytocannabinoid CBD inhibits GPR55.[139,142] Finally, several synthetic drugs that are antagonists at CB1 receptors including rimonabant actually activate GPR55 receptors, which may account for the undesirable side effects that lead to their removal from the market.[143]

GPR119

G protein-coupled receptor 119 (GPR119) was discovered in 2006. Anandamide, OEA and other novel synthetic and endocannabinoids bind to GPR119.[75,144,145] GPR119 is found in the GI tract, pancreas, and brain.[75] It is involved in insulin secretion, and activation of the receptor reduces food intake and body weight.[75,146-147] Therapeutically, it is a target of drugs to treat diabetes and obesity.

PHYTOCANNABINOIDS

Your body's cannabinoid receptors and endocannabinoid levels are also responsive to exogenous cannabinoids, or cannabinoids made outside the body. Exogenous cannabinoids include synthetic cannabinoids such as dronabinol, marketed as the prescription drug Marinol, and phytocannabinoids. Phytocannabinoids are cannabinoids from plants such as cannabis, also known as marijuana. Several plants, including echinacea and *Piper nigrum*, used to make black pepper, also contain cannabinoids. Chapter 16 of this book, *Vitamin Weed*, will cover the production, metabolism, and medical benefits of phytocannabinoids.

There are three species of cannabis plants: *Cannabis indica*, *Cannabis sativa*, and *Cannabis ruderalis*. A hoax story claiming a new species was discovered in Australia in 2010 was debunked. *Cannabis ruderalis* is the least studied of the three cannabis species. *C. ruderalis* was first identified in 1942 in Russia by botanist Janischewski. *C. ruderalis* is often high in CBD and can now be found growing where hemp is cultivated. It is not used recreationally.

Cannabis indica and *Cannabis sativa* are differentiated by the shape and number of leaves, height, terpene content, and other attributes. *Cannabis indica* and *Cannabis sativa* are often bred together to create hybrid strains, and in fact there has been so much breeding of species that is often difficult to find a true indica or sativa strain, even if one is labeled so by a grower or dispensary. In reality, almost all *Cannabis indica* strains have some *Cannabis sativa* and vice versa. It is no longer relevant to say indica strains cause sleepiness and sativa strains cause alertness, there is a mix of effects seen in both species now. One interesting note is that strains with high levels of THCV originated from *Cannabis indica.*[148]

Cannabis contains over 111 cannabinoids, the most predominant being THCA, CBDA and CBGA. Cannabinoids in the marijuana flower, or bud, and leaves are not psychoactive until heated. The raw cannabis plant does not contain THC or CBD. Some cannabinoids may have evolved to protect the cannabis plant form being eaten, as they may make insects sleepy or sick. All cannabinoids from cannabis (not industrial hemp), whether raw or heated form, are illegal in the United State under the Controlled Substances Act, where they are classified as Schedule 1 drugs.

SYNTHETIC CANNABINOIDS

Synthetic cannabinoids include commercial production of isolated cannabinoids and novel cannabinoid drugs made to enhance activity at receptors beyond what is produced in nature.

PRESCRIPTION DRUGS

Three cannabinoid-based prescription drugs have been approved by the Food and Drug Administration (FDA) in the United States: Marinol (dronabinol, a synthetic version of THC), Syndros, a liquid version of Marinol, Cesamet (nabilone, a novel synthetic cannabinoid similar to THC).[149] These drugs are all approved for treatment of chemotherapy-induced nausea and vomiting, and both Marinol and Syndros are approved to stimulant appetite in AIDS patients.[150]

Marinol and Cesamet are Schedule 3 drugs, while Syndros is a Schedule 2 drug because of increased risk of abusing liquid THC over pills. It's important to note that the natural source of THC, cannabis, is still Schedule 1 in the United States with no medical benefits and high potential for addiction according to the government, even though they know that is not true.

A fourth drug, Sativex, approved in multiple countries outside the United States, is a sublingual spray containing equal parts THC and CBD as well as other cannabinoids and terpenes and is used to treat spasms in multiple sclerosis (MS) patients.[151] A final drug, nabilone, is similar to THC but binds 10 times more strongly to the CB1 receptor than THC and is available in Canada.

A final drug by GW Pharmaceuticals that will likely be approved by the FDA at the end of 2018 is Epidiolex, CBD used to treat severe, orphan, early-onset treatment-resistant epilepsy syndromes such as Dravet syndrome, Lennox-Gastaut syndrome (LGS), Tuberous Sclerosis Complex (TSC) and Infantile Spasms.[152-154]

PRESCRIPTION DRUGS IN DEVELOPMENT

Many drugs that target the endocannabinoid system are being developed by private companies and are either in preclinical research stage or entering clinical trials. Some are merely cannabinoids administered in new routes, such as patches or transdermal gels. Others are modifications of CBD which elevate levels of anandamide much higher than natural CBD.

PLANT BIOREACTORS

While numerous companies are developing endocannabinoid boosting drugs that are taken orally, injected, or used transdermally as a skin patch, other companies are looking for a more natural way to boost our endocannabinoid levels. Many of our foods are fortified with vitamins; for example, our milk and bread have Vitamin D in them. In a similar way, we could fortify our foods with endocannabinoids to ensure everyone is protected from aging and disease.

Because anandamide does not occur in nature at a large enough level to be commercially extracted and put into other foods, AEA would have to be synthesized chemically in a factory. AEA is only soluble in fat, not water, so it would work best in oils or dairy foods like milk, cheese, yogurt, chocolate, or ice cream.

At the current price of $300 for 25 mg of synthetic anandamide, fortification of food with anandamide is too costly to be commercially viable. A new way to create biological chemicals like AEA is through genetically modified organisms (GMOs), saving both time and money in chemical synthesis. Yeast can be modified to produce drugs like insulin for diabetics, and groups have gotten yeast to produce cannabinoids like THC with limited success. One benefit of using GMOs to produce cannabinoids is that they do not require the use of fat soluble dairy products or oils as carriers.

In the same way, plants can be genetically modified to produce chemicals they didn't before, a concept called "plant bioreactors." Several companies are attempting to produce cannabinoids such as anandamide and THC in fruits like strawberries. Anandamide can also be extracted from these plant bioreactors and formulated into pills, and *Vitamin Weed* becomes a reality, just like Vitamin D.

There has been much negative public reaction to GMO food and several countries have begun banning GMO foods. The danger in GMO foods lies not in the fact that additional genes are added to the plants or organisms, but when the plants are genetically modified to be resistant to a new pesticide. GMO crops, including the majority of corn and soy sold in the United States, are created by Monsanto to be resistant to their pesticide Roundup. The problem is that eating these GMO foods can cause gastrointestinal distress, boost cancer risk, and cause other nasty side effects because the main ingredient in Roundup, glyphosate, is not safe for humans.[155] Even if you dutifully wash these your fruits and veggies before eating them, you're not washing off all the pesticides, and glyphosate has been found in our water and air.

Plants or yeast that make cannabinoids like anandamide or THC are not being made by Monsanto and are not being treated with Roundup pesticide. Thus, there should be no risk to humans or the environment if you eat foods or pills made from GMOs making cannabinoids.

FUTURE OF CANNABINOID THERAPEUTICS

It is important as we move forward in creating synthetic cannabinoids or modulators of the endocannabinoid system that are farther and farther away from the natural compounds produced by plants or the body that we make sure side effects, both short-term and long-term, are minimized. Modern medicine and drug development has created some incredible treatments for diseases, but it has also brought incredible mistakes that caused significant damage to human health.

LESSONS FROM RIMONABANT

Rimonabant was a first-generation inhibitor of CB1 receptors, working both in the brain and the body. It was first approved in Europe in 2006 and was taken off the market in 2008 due to psychiatric side effects in 10% of patients including suicidal thoughts that outweighed its medical benefits as a weight loss drug. It was never approved as a drug in the United States.

A second generation of CB1 inhibitors have been developed, this time working only on peripheral cannabinoid receptors and not crossing the blood-brain barrier. These second-generation drugs, like AM6545, do not have the same psychiatric side effects rimonabant does but reduce elevated metabolic parameters including cholesterol and insulin.[156] Rimonabant also induced nausea and vomiting, while AM6545 has minimal nausea side effects. AM6545 only decreased weight in mice that are obese due to a high-fat diet, and not normal mice.[156] This is important because it shows CB1 inhibitors will not be abused by normal weight or underweight patients looking to drop 10 pounds in a week.

MAGL

Chronic blockade of MAGL, the enzyme that degrades 2-AG, is limited as a potential therapeutic for endocannabinoid deficiency because it antagonizes the endocannabinoid system. Chronic treatment with MAGL inhibitors cause physical dependence to drugs, reduces endocannabinoid-mediated synaptic plasticity important for learning, and CB1 receptor desensitization.[157] Acute inhibition of

MAGL raises levels of 2-AG and causes a side effect of hypomotility,which is reduced movement, commonly referred to as "couch-lock."[158]

Interestingly joint inhibition of MAGL and FAAH are being investigated as a treatment for opiate dependence, which includes physical or mental dependence on prescription painkillers as well as heroin.[159] MAGL inhibition is associated with alleviation of most opiate withdrawal symptoms, but has effects similar to using THC, while treatment with FAAH inhibitors is less effective at alleviating opiate withdrawal.[159]

FAAH

The future for chronic blockade of FAAH, the enzyme that degrades anandamide, as a therapeutic is much brighter. Chronic treatment with FAAH inhibitors causes anandamide to accumulate and activate more cannabinoid receptors, which leads to antidepressant, anti-anxiety and pain-relieving effects within 1-4 weeks of treatment.[160] Blocking FAAH also facilitates extinction of aversive memories.[161] Interestingly FAAH inhibitors are effective at relieving pain and inflammation as THC.[162]

It is important to note that inhibition of FAAH increases levels of all NAEs, including the atypical endocannabinoids PEA and OEA, and thus behavioral effects of FAAH inhibitors may be partly due to increase in these proteins, and activation of PPAR receptors, in addition to anandamide.[77,163]

FLAT

Blockade of FLAT, the transporter that brings anandamide into the cell to be broken down, may be useful to boost anandamide, control pain, and reduce drug dependency. FLAT is not associated with the psychotropic and THC-like effects of AEA.[164] Future research is needed to determine if FLAT inhibitors are a therapeutic target with more tolerable side effects than FAAH inhibitors.

FABPs

Inhibition of FABPs is associated with reduction in inflammatory, visceral, and neuropathic pain while elevating anandamide levels in the brain.[28] Anandamide uptake into the cell is not dependent on the activity of the enzyme that breaks it down (FAAH), suggesting FABP inhibitors may be more efficient boosters of AEA levels that FAAH inhibitors.[165] Boosting AEA through inhibition of transport does not result in a high or increase drug-taking behaviors like THC does.[164] This makes FABP inhibitors a preferred target for reducing pain and inflammation.

PART TWO

Are You Endocannabinoid Deficient?

CHAPTER 4

What is Endocannabinoid Deficiency?

"There's evidence now to show that diet can positively influence the endocannabinoid system and its balance." - Dr. Ethan Russo

What if your government lied to you about your health? What if there was a cheap blood test covered by health insurance that could diagnose the real root of your health problems? What if there was a cheap vitamin you could buy at your pharmacy to replace your expensive prescription medications with their toxic side effects.

VITAMIN D

This little miracle vitamin is Vitamin D. For decades the United States government reported that Americans were receiving enough Vitamin D through their diet or made in their body through sun exposure. The reality was that the Western Junk Food Diet was devoid of any vitamins or minerals, obesity was increasing, and Americans were hiding in their homes and offices, away from the sun, and slathering on UV-blocking sunscreen when they were outside.

Vitamin D deficiency isn't just rampant and severe in the United States, it is a global pandemic, even in seemingly healthy adults.[166] Up to 50% of humans are deficient in Vitamin D, with a higher incidence rate in chronically ill patients. Vitamin D deficiency has been linked with multiple sclerosis, migraine, depression, weight gain, cancer, Crohn's disease and ulcerative colitis.[167-169]

Vitamin D deficiency may start at birth, making a lasting impact on health. Vitamin D deficiency in pregnant mothers is even correlated to neurodevelopmental disorders like schizophrenia and autism in their children.[170,171] Finally, there was a 15x increase in Vitamin D deficiency in children between 2008 and 2014.[172]

There was an 83x increase in Vitamin D testing billed to Medicare from 2000 to 2010, making it Medicare's fifth most commonly ordered test. Yet there's still no consensus from the Institute of Medicine on what the safe levels of Vitamin D supplementation in pill form is for achieving optimal blood levels. A group of scientists have even formed a Vitamin D council to create awareness of Vitamin D deficiency. One thing is for certain, the Recommend Daily Allowance (RDA) of 600 IU a day of Vitamin is clearly insufficient.

WHAT ELSE IS OUR GOVERNMENT HIDING?

It's up to patients to take their health in their own hands and throw out the misinformation the government feeds the public. What other simple changes could patients make to boost their health instead of popping pharmaceuticals like Tic Tacs? Since we were lied to about Vitamin D deficiency, isn't it possible we are also being lied to about other forms of deficiency, like endocannabinoid deficiency?

NUTRITIONAL DEFICIENCY

Vitamins and minerals found in our diet are key to some of our most basic bodily functions, including keeping organs like your heart and kidneys working. Running low on certain essential nutrients can cause mild symptoms like fatigue, trouble sleeping, muscle cramps, or joint pain. Severe deficiency in some basic vitamins and minerals for an extended period of time can mimic severe diseases and even result in seizures or long-term damage to organs.

ESSENTIAL VITAMINS AND EFFECTS OF SEVERE DEFICIENCY

Vitamin A (Retinol)	hyperkeratosis, night blindness, keratomalacia
Vitamin B1 (Thiamine)	Wernicke-Korsakoff syndrome, Beriberi
Vitamin B2 (Riboflavin)	corneal vascularization, cheilosis, angular stomatitis
Vitamin B3 (Niacin)	dermatitis, GI problems, nerve dysfunction, glossitis
Vitamin B5 (Pantothenic Acid)	fatigue, depression, insomnia, vomiting, burning feet
Vitamin B6 (Pyridoxine)	anemia, seizures, neuropathy, dermatitis
Vitamin B7 (Biotin)	anemia, anorexia, hair loss, depression, rashes
Vitamin B9 (Folic Acid or Folate)	anemia, confusion, neural tube birth defects

Vitamin B12 (Cobalamin)	anemia, confusion, ataxia, paresthesia
Vitamin C (Ascorbic Acid)	scurvy
Vitamin D (Cholecalciferol)	bone issues (rickets, osteomalacia), muscle weakness
Vitamin E (Alpha-tocopherol)	neurological issues, red blood cell hemolysis
Vitamin K (Phylloquinone)	excessive bleeding, osteopenia

ESSENTIAL MINERALS AND EFFECTS OF SEVERE DEFICIENCY

Calcium	osteoporosis, fatigue, muscle cramps, numbness, arrhythmia
Copper	anemia, neuropathy, myelopathy
Iodine	goiter, IQ reduction, breast sensitivity
Iron	anemia
Magnesium	fatigue, nausea, vomiting, numbness, muscle cramps, seizures
Manganese	slow healing
Potassium	muscle cramps, abdominal pain, constipation, arrhythmia

Selenium	hypothyroidism
Sodium	nausea, poor balance, headaches, confusion, seizures
Zinc	loss of smell, taste or appetite, slow healing and growth

NEUROTRANSMITTER DEFICIENCY

Our brain and peripheral nervous system control all our physiological processes, and a chemical imbalance in the brain wreaks havoc on the body. Brain cells, called neurons, use neurotransmitters to chemically talk to each other between synapses, the gap between neurons.

Many diseases are known to be caused by a deficiency in a type of neurotransmitter or its signaling. Parkinson's disease is caused by deficiency in dopamine, the neurotransmitter responsible for movement and motivation. Depression is suggested to be a deficiency in serotonin and is treated with antidepressants that raise serotonin levels. Alzheimer's disease is caused by deficiency in acetylcholine, a neurotransmitter that modulates memory, decision making and wakefulness. It makes sense then that there are diseases caused by deficiency in endocannabinoids, the natural marijuana-like neurotransmitters produced by our brain and body.

ENDOCANNABINOID DEFICIENCY

Dr. Ethan Russo coined the term Clinical Endocannabinoid Deficiency (CECD) to describe a pathological deficit in endocannabinoid system function causing other disease states.[173] Most of the disease states related to CECD are marked by chronic pain, dysfunctional immune systems, fatigue, and mood imbalances. This is not surprising as the endocannabinoid system regulates most of these physiological processes.

Interestingly, the cluster of diseases related to acquired CECD are related to stress. Many stress-related disorders have no known cause. With no molecular mechanism previously attributed to these disorders, there were no effective pharmaceutical treatments for patients who suffer from them, and doctors did not take these disorders seriously. Finally, patients can breathe a sigh of relief. Their symptoms are not in their head. It makes sense that a deficiency in the largest neurotransmitter system that regulates all the other neurotransmitter systems would cause such a myriad of symptoms that would be hard to treat with pharmaceuticals only targeting one neurotransmitter at a time.

The link between CECD and disease is stronger for some disorders than others. Treatment with endocannabinoids, made in your brain, or phytocannabinoids, like THC found in marijuana, is associated with a decrease in migraine severity as well as serotonin pathways associated with migraines.[174-175] Fibromyalgia is another disease where symptoms become worse with stress. Clinical research has shown cannabis is a better treatment for fibromyalgia than any other pharmaceutical on the market. Irritable Bowel Syndrome (IBS), a disorder marked by cycles of gastrointestinal pain, diarrhea, constipation, food sensitivity, and mood alteration, is also both stress-related and linked to the endocannabinoid system.

Part Three of this book discusses major diseases associated with CECD and specific advice on how to treat them.

CAUSES OF ENDOCANNABINOID DEFICIENCY

OVERVIEW

There are several ways in which your body can have a deficiency in endocannabinoid signaling. First, there might not be enough endocannabinoids synthesized. This would mean you have low levels of endocannabinoids anandamide (AEA) or 2-arachidonylglycerol (2-AG), but normal levels of cannabinoid receptors. Second, there might not be enough cannabinoid receptors, possibly because the genes that encode cannabinoid receptor type 1 (CB1) or cannabinoid receptor type 2 (CB2) are blocked, or methylated. Third, there may be too much of the enzymes that break down endocannabinoids. This means your body is making enough AEA and 2-AG, but too much fatty acid amide hydrolase (FAAH) or monoacylglycerol lipase (MAGL). Finally, there may be enough endocannabinoids and cannabinoid receptors, but there is not enough signaling happening downstream of the receptor.

There is a broad range of subjective and physiological responses to cannabis use, and this is due to many factors including medication use, diet, lifestyle, medical conditions, and genetics. A personalized medicine approach to treating endocannabinoid deficiency must be employed due to the complex nature of restoring balance to the endocannabinoid system which regulates all other neurotransmitter systems.

IT STARTS IN CHILDHOOD

There are two types of endocannabinoid deficiency: congenital and acquired. Congenital CECD means your endocannabinoid system has been abnormally functioning since birth. This type of CECD is harder to treat because not having enough endocannabinoids during brain development and childhood causes your brain to mature in a dysfunctional manner. Even if endocannabinoid levels are later restored, some health problems will not be repaired. Acquired CECD occurs later in life and is easier to treat because your brain and immune system has matured normally. All that is lacking is proper endocannabinoid levels in adulthood, which can be restored with time.

Congenital endocannabinoid deficiency can stem from endocannabinoid deficiency in the mother during pregnancy and/or during breastfeeding. Endocannabinoids are essential for development of the brain and immune system and 2-AG is even found in breastmilk.[176-178] Cannabinoid receptors are found on immature neurons, or brain cells, meaning they require cannabinoid signaling to travel to the right location in the brain and mature. Children that are not breastfed or are not breastfed long enough for proper immune system and brain development may also develop congenital CECD.

A mother deficient in endocannabinoids may end up with a fetus that has reduced endocannabinoid signaling. One way epilepsy may develop in the neonatal brain is from increased excitability of neurons, which can occur when cannabinoid receptors are expressed at a lower rate than normal.[179] One could argue epilepsy is the most extreme case of endocannabinoid deficiency; because it starts while the brain is still developing, the effects are more severe than endocannabinoid deficiency that occurs later in life. Future research is warranted on whether cannabinoid treatment of mothers with a fetus at genetic risk for developing epilepsy or other brain conditions prevents development or decreases severity of the diseases.

Endocannabinoid deficiency in the fetus may also develop if the mother has a poor diet deficient in fatty acids that are the building blocks of endocannabinoids. Low omega-3 fatty acid consumption in mothers was correlated with low IQ in their children.[180] Supplementation with fatty acids that build endocannabinoids as described later in this book can be a strategy for pregnant women that want to boost their endocannabinoid system without cannabis use.

Infection in newborns like the flu may be linked to endocannabinoid deficiency later in life. Increasing inflammation in newborn rat pups increased FAAH and anandamide levels as well as decreased CB1 receptors when they grew up to be adolescents.[181] The same rats were less social than normal, and this behavioral issue was normalized by treatment with a FAAH inhibitor that boosted anandamide levels.[181]

Researchers do not know what normal levels of endocannabinoids are in the brain and blood of children. Children, with a rapidly developing brain, are likely more sensitive to the effects of endocannabinoid deficiency than adults. CECD during childhood may be linked to cognitive problems like ADHD, depression, or cognitive problems in future research.

IT'S IN YOUR DNA

You might be able to blame your parents for your endocannabinoid deficiency. Polymorphisms, or mutations, in genes that encode cannabinoid receptors, the enzymes that make endocannabinoids, or the enzymes that break down cannabinoids can result in either too much endocannabinoid signaling or too little endocannabinoid signaling.

The genes in your DNA are the recipes to make proteins that make up your cells, like receptors and enzymes. There are multiple types of mutations in your DNA that change the recipe and end up with a botched final product; the table below "Types of Mutations," defines them. Missense mutations are often called "single nucleotide polymorphisms" or SNPs and are biomarkers for many diseases. SNPs occur on average once every 300 nucleotides, and there are about 10 million SNPs in the human genome. Repeat expansion mutations often come in pairs of three, called trinucleotide repeats or triple repeats.

TYPES OF GENETIC MUTATIONS

Missense	Results in a change in one amino acid in the resulting protein
Nonsense	Results in incomplete production of a protein
Insertion	Adds extra DNA, which may increase or decrease protein function
Deletion	Removes extra DNA, which may change protein function

Duplication	DNA is repeated one or more times, changing protein function
Repeat Expansion	DNA sequences are repeated multiple times

Mutations in endocannabinoid system genes that contribute to disease or impact how lifestyle choice effect our health is discussed in detail throughout this book.

ENDOCANNABINOID SYSTEM GENES

FAAH	CNR1
FAAH2	CNR2
MGLL	ABHD6
DAGLA	ABHD12

GENDER

Women may be more likely to have endocannabinoid deficiency as they are more likely to suffer from chronic illnesses related to CECD including depression and fibromyalgia. Constantly cycling reproductive hormones as well as pregnancy offer unique influences on the endocannabinoid system that are not present in men.

MENSTRUAL CYCLE

Anandamide reaches peak blood levels during the menstrual cycle at ovulation, the same time estrogen and gonadotrophin levels peak.[182] During menstruation, anandamide levels are low, and may contribute to the mood changes, pain, and cramps associated with menstruation. Women that are on hormonal birth control do not ovulate, and likely have lower levels of endocannabinoids as their normal baseline.

PREGNANCY

Endocannabinoid deficiency may result in ovulation not occurring and inability to get pregnant. High blood levels of anandamide at ovulation and low levels at embryo implantation are associated with successful pregnancy.[183] High anandamide levels may prevent pregnancy, and thus a drop in AEA levels could signal timing for optimal in vitro embryo transfer.[184] CBD applied intravaginally and/or taken orally may be able to boost effectiveness of birth control methods in the future.

Low levels of FAAH in lymphocytes of healthy women at 7-8 weeks of pregnancy correlated with spontaneous abortion within 10 days.[185] Levels of cannabinoid receptors and the anandamide transporter had no correlation with spontaneous abortion. Anandamide levels in the uterus are constant during the first 5 days of pregnancy and drop off after day 6.[186] Blood levels of anandamide in the second and third trimester are significantly lower than the first trimester of pregnancy.

Blood levels of anandamide increase one and half times during labor from 1.2 to 1.82 nm, and the greater the rise in anandamide blood levels the shorter the duration of labor.[187] This suggests anandamide is involved in the physiological process of labor. A woman who is endocannabinoid deficient due to poor diet or stress may have lengthy labor. Anecdotally, eating cannabis edibles speeds up labor, potentially validating this hypothesis.

GENDER EFFECTS OF CANNABINOIDS

Women are more sensitive to the effects of cannabinoids than men, likely because they have a higher percentage of body fat and cannabinoids are fat soluble. There are no gender differences in the way cannabinoids influence the following processes: stress response, impulsivity, learning, memory and hypothermia.[188] Women may have fewer cannabinoid receptors in brain regions than men, but studies suggest the signaling pathways downstream of activated receptors are more active.[189] This suggests women have more efficient cannabinoid receptors. Overall the influence of gender on endocannabinoid deficiency and endocannabinoid system function are complex.

AGE

Old age can create an endocannabinoid deficiency in someone who was not deficient before or worsen an existing endocannabinoid deficiency. Aging reduces the expression of both CB1 and CB2 receptors in rodents, although the study needs to be confirmed in humans.[190] Aging also causes low levels of 2-AG in the cerebral cortex due to changes in levels of the enzymes that synthesize and metabolize 2-AG.[191] It is suggested that the main effects of aging are mediated by changes in CB1 signaling, especially on GABA neurons, and not by CB2 signaling.[192]

It is suggested that reduced signaling of the endocannabinoid system in the brain is responsible for neurodegeneration, something that will be explored more in Chapter 7: Aging and the Endocannabinoid System.

DIET

Endocannabinoids are synthesized from fatty acids, so it is possible that if you don't get enough fat in your diet you could be deficient in endocannabinoids. Simply eating foods with endocannabinoids will not cure endocannabinoid deficiency, because the endocannabinoids will be degraded by the intestine and liver before they could make their way to the brain, although they can be active in the gut.[193] One way to solve this problem is to administer endocannabinoids in ways that bypass the liver and intestine, such as a rectal suppository or transdermal patch, or to consume precursors to endocannabinoids in the diet.

Supplementing the diet with endocannabinoid precursors can boost endocannabinoid levels in the brain, similar to how people boost levels of serotonin by taking its precursor 5-HTP. Supplementing baby pigs with formula that contained precursors to endocannabinoids, specifically arachidonic acid (AA) and docosahexaenoic acid (DHA), boosted levels of AA, DHA and other NAEs in the brain.[84] Mice fed linoleic acid, a precursor to arachidonic acid, had increased levels of endocannabinoids anandamide and 2-AG in the liver, gained weight.[194]

Arachidonic acid is an omega-6 fatty acid, which has often been demonized in the media because it can be converted to inflammatory prostaglandins instead of anandamide and 2-AG. Omega-3 fatty acids are considered anti-inflammatory, and nutritionists suggest keeping your ration of omega-6 to omega-3 ratio close to 1. Unfortunately, people who consume Western diets usually eat a fatty acid ratio of 16:1, meaning they eat 16 times more omega-6 fatty acids than is healthy.

There is some confusion that supplementation with arachidonic acid will cause further harm to your health because it adds to the omega-6 to omega-3 ratio instead of lowering it. Clinical research has shown that arachidonic acid supplementation, in combination with high omega-3 fatty acid intake, is safe and has no impact on cardiovascular or immune system health.[195]

Currently the majority of Americans consume their arachidonic acid from the linoleic acid precursor, which comes from fast or junk foods containing corn, soy and vegetable oils. Reducing unhealthy sources of linoleic acid and replacing them with healthier sources of arachidonic acid as well as eating or supplementing with omega-3 fatty acids is a good strategy to improve endocannabinoid levels in your brain.

BODY WEIGHT

Sometimes too high levels of endocannabinoids in the bloodstream is as bad as too little endocannabinoids. In fact, high levels of endocannabinoids can indicate compensation for decreased cannabinoid receptors or some other issue with endocannabinoid system function.

Appetite, fat burning, and weight gain are regulated by the endocannabinoid system. Anandamide and 2-AG are produced by fat cells, where they stimulate fat burning via CB1 receptors and are controlled by leptin and insulin.[196] Patients with a common mutation in the FAAH gene who produce more anandamide also had higher levels of DHEA and OEA, which are fat-burning hormones.[197]

The relationship between endocannabinoid levels in the brain, blood, and saliva and body weight is complex. Obesity is associated with higher than normal endocannabinoid levels of both anandamide and 2-AG.[198] Blood levels of 2-AG but not AEA are correlated with body mass index (BMI), belly fat, waist size, and fasting insulin levels in obese men.[199] Cerebrospinal fluid (CSF) levels of 2-AG but not AEA are negatively correlated with CSF leptin levels, but not BMI.[200]

Endocannabinoids AEA and 2-AG as well as atypical cannabinoids palmitoylethanolamine (PEA) and oleoylethanolamine (OEA) were measurable in saliva and their level correlate with obesity.[201] Blood levels of AEA and 2-AG were elevated in obese women and were not changed after 5% body weight loss, suggesting these changes are a cause rather than a consequence of obesity.[202] Higher endocannabinoid levels were associated with reduced FAAH expression in fat tissue. CB1 and FAAH expression were reduced in obese postmenopausal women.[202]

Endocannabinoid levels are also elevated in overweight patients with type 2 diabetes.[203] Insulin decreases blood endocannabinoid levels but is less effective in patients that are insulin-resistant.[203] 2-AG levels are reduced in obese (OB) patients with type 2 diabetes (OBT2D) but not in OB patients compared to normal weight patients.[196] OEA and PEA levels in subcutaneous adipose tissue (SAT) of OBT2D patients were elevated compared to normal patients.[196]

Finally, patients that reduce obesity through bariatric surgery have a reduction in blood levels of anandamide compared to levels preoperatively.[204] This is not a reflection of endocannabinoid deficiency, but in fact normalization of the endocannabinoid system.

EXERCISE

Your activity level can determine your endocannabinoid levels. Healthy amounts of exercise boost endocannabinoid levels and brain function, while skipping out on exercise or performing marathons regularly may decrease endocannabinoid levels.

Exercise is an acute stressor that raises both levels of the stress hormone cortisol and endocannabinoid levels. Ninety minutes of intense exercise in fit men boosted anandamide levels during exercise and 15 minutes afterwards.[205] In fact, a rise in endocannabinoid levels, combined with an increase in endorphins and dopamine levels, is responsible for the phenomenon known as "runner's high." Patients who regularly exercise have higher levels of the enzyme FAAH that breaks down anandamide compared to inactive patients, and this helps maintain endocannabinoid balance.[206]

Exercise boosts CB1 receptors in an area of your brain known as the periaqueductal gray matter (PAG), where it reduces perception of pain.[207] Finally, exercise also increases the number of CB1 receptors in an area of your brain known as the hippocampus, which is responsible for a boost in spatial memory.[208]

UV EXPOSURE

Melanin is the pigment that both protects your skin cells from damage from UV-radiation as well creates pigmentation or "tan." The endocannabinoid system is fully functional in melanocytes, the cells that create melanin. Exposure to UVB light, whether from the sun or indoor tanning beds, can stimulate production of anandamide and 2-AG.[209-210] It's possible that people who do not have enough UVB light exposure may actually boost their risk of skin cancer because endocannabinoids aren't being produced in those cells, and anti-cancer signaling is not happening.

How do you know if you aren't getting enough light for your health? Vitamin D is produced in the skin when exposed to light. Sadly, the majority of Americans are Vitamin D deficient, especially in the winter. We don't spend time outside, we avoid indoor tanning due to misinformation about the harms of UV light, we use sunscreen that blocks the wavelength of light needed for Vitamin D production, and we sit next to windows that block UVB rays. To find out if you are deficient in Vitamin D, you can order a blood test that measures Vitamin D levels through your doctor or online through companies like Life Extension.

SLEEP

Some patients have medical conditions that interfere with sleep, such as obstructive sleep apnea, muscle spasms, or chronic pain, while others just skimp on getting their 7-8 hours of sleep nightly. Patients with obstructive sleep apnea have increased anandamide levels in their blood, and this correlates with the oxygen deprivation they are experience while sleeping.[211] In healthy patients that are sleep deprived, the endocannabinoid system attempts to compensate by increasing endocannabinoid levels include 2-AG. This is pathological, as it also increases hunger and weight gain.[212] You might be familiar with this phenomenon if you've ever pulled an "all-nighter" and went through bags of junk food.

On the flip side, a healthy endocannabinoid system promotes deep, refreshing sleep we all desperately need in our busy lives. Patients with a common mutation in the FAAH gene that increases the amount of anandamide in the body have improved sleep quality compared to those without the gene.[213] Endocannabinoids promote both non-REM and REM sleep and restore sleep in a model of insomnia.[214] It appears blocking CB1 receptor activity boosts wakefulness while activating the CB1 receptor promotes sleep.[215] Prevent endocannabinoid deficiency to improve sleep quality, avoid insomnia, and wake up refreshed.

CIRCADIAN RHYTHM

Circadian rhythms are physiological processes or behaviors that follow a 24-hour cycle and are set by light and dark in the organism's environment as well as changing seasons. Organisms have an internal body clock that regulates when they sleep and eat or produce certain hormones. The endocannabinoid system contributes to a wide range of important physiological processes including sleep/wake cycles, feeding, temperature regulation, motivation, gastrointestinal function, and endocrine function so it is not surprising levels of endocannabinoids change throughout the day.[216-220]

The question that remains is whether endocannabinoids are regulated by the internal body clock, or endocannabinoids regulate the internal body clock. Levels of endocannabinoids anandamide and 2-AG and atypical endocannabinoids fluctuate with circadian rhythm, as do CB1 receptor number in certain brain regions, and expression of enzymes that synthesize and break down endocannabinoids.[221-224] It is unclear whether endocannabinoid deficiency dysregulates circadian rhythm.

Interestingly, some medical conditions that are linked to abnormal circadian rhythms and sleep patterns are also linked to issues with endocannabinoid system function. These include mental health disorders depression, bipolar depression, and schizophrenia, as well as Alzheimer's disease and insomnia.[225] Cannabinoid treatment does not alter normal circadian rhythms, but does prevent shift to artificial circadian rhythms, such as those that might be present in psychiatric disease.[226] Cannabinoids act on CB1 receptors that are highly expressed in the suprachiasmatic nucleus (SCN), the brain region that acts as the body's clock and controls circadian rhythms.[226]

SMOKING CIGARETTES

Smoking cigarettes causes an inflammatory environment for your brain, lungs and whole body. Nicotine is but one of thousands of chemical components of cigarette smoke that damage your lungs and deplete your levels of glutathione. Nicotine even prevents chemotherapy from killing cancer cells.[227]

It is unclear whether smokers have lower levels of anandamide or 2-AG to begin with. Endocannabinoid deficiency combined with cigarette smoking may be what triggers lung cancer. Boosting anandamide prevents lung cancer tumors from growing, as CB1 receptors are expressed on lung cancer cells.[228]

ALCOHOL USE

Alcohol use causes endocannabinoid deficiency. Every time you drink, alcohol blocks release of anandamide in your brain.[229-230] Alcohol does not change the amount of anandamide produced or its breakdown, it merely just prevents it from getting to the synapse where it could bind to CB1 receptors.[230]

Alcohol use decreases anandamide and 2-AG levels in multiple areas of the rodent brain.[230] Alcohol also decreases CB1 receptor number and function in the amygdala, a brain associated with fear and anxiety.[231-232] The brains of humans with alcoholism were imaged using positron emission tomography (PET), and researchers found CB1 receptor number was decreased in multiple brain regions similar to what was seen in rodents.[233]

COCAINE ABUSE

Cocaine use can cause long-term changes in endocannabinoid system function. 2-AG production in the brain is reduced in rodents after a single exposure to cocaine and remains reduced with regular cocaine use.[234] Anandamide production increases after regular cocaine use, but this is likely a compensation for other brain changes.[234]

STRESS

The role of stress in reducing endocannabinoid system function is complex, depending on whether we are looking at blood levels or brain levels of endocannabinoids as well as short-term versus long-term stress.

ACUTE STRESS

Activation of cannabinoid receptors in an area of the brain known as the periaqueductal gray (PAG) reduce the "fight or flight" response that is expressed as panic, anxiety, and gastrointestinal distress in humans.[235] When you are exposed to the same stressor repeatedly, your body adapts to the stressor and reduces its response to it. This process, called habituation, requires the endocannabinoid system.

The body ramps up 2-AG but not anandamide in response to acute stress. One study found blood levels of 2-AG were increased in both depressed and healthy patients immediately after the Trier Social Stress Test (TSST) and recovered to normal levels 30 minutes later.[236] Anandamide blood levels did not change immediately after or 30 minutes after the TSTT test.

Exposure to acute (short-term) stress increases the activity of FAAH, decreasing the amount of anandamide at the CB1 receptors in the basolateral amygdala (BLA), the brain area responsible for emotional responses and important for development of anxiety and PTSD.[161] This results in increased anxiety, but without repeated stress the BLA returns to normal and anxiety goes away.

Patients with a mutation in the FAAH gene that results in less FAAH activity and increased anandamide show a reduced response to stress in the BLA.[237] Thus, boosting anandamide levels can be a healthy way to deal with daily stressors. If you are already endocannabinoid deficient, you may not be as resilient in the face of stress, and long-term anxiety or depression issues may result.

CHRONIC STRESS

The most common and potent factor in endocannabinoid deficiency is chronic stress. Chronic stress results in endocannabinoid deficiency and dysfunction. The endocannabinoid system maintains the hypothalamic-pituitary-adrenal (HPA) axis, which is responsible for our physiological and behavioral express of stress responses. In fact, the endocannabinoid system is known as a "gatekeeper" to the body's stress response, preventing burnout of the norepinephrine system and HPA axis.

Chronic stress increases corticosterone levels and disrupts endocannabinoid signaling in the amygdala, resulting in anxiety.[238] Chronic stress prompts release of corticotropin-releasing hormone (CRH), which activates CRH receptor type 1 (CRHR1), increasing expression of FAAH, resulting in decreased anandamide levels in the amygdala.[239-240]

Epigenetic modifications of genes, such as acetylation or methylation, can cause long-term changes in expression of genes and in effect, permanently silence or turn them on. Chronic stress can induce epigenetic modifications of multiple genes, including the CB1 receptor (CNR1) gene.[241] This results in long-term endocannabinoid system dysfunction and is in seen in stress disorders such as PTSD in the form of increased CB1 receptor expression despite depressed anandamide levels.[242-243]

CHRONIC STRESS DURING CHILDHOOD

Patients with a mutation in the FAAH gene have reduced FAAH and increased anandamide levels. These patients, when exposed to repeated stress or trauma during childhood, are more likely to develop anxiety or depression as an adult than patients without the mutation that were exposed to childhood stress.[244] The researchers suggest having high levels of anandamide combined with childhood stress causes lifelong abnormal stress response due to lower levels of CB1 receptors during brain development.[244]

MEDICAL CONDITIONS

Numerous medical conditions have been linked to endocannabinoid deficiency in both human and rodent studies. Part Three of this book explores these medical conditions in detail.

MEDICAL CONDITIONS LINKED TO ENDOCANNABINOID DEFICIENCY

fibromyalgia	post-traumatic stress disorder (PTSD)
endometriosis	migraine headache
cancer	irritable bowel syndrome (IBS)
anxiety	schizophrenia

MEDICATIONS

We are an overmedicated country. 70% of Americans take at least one prescription drug, and 20% of Americans take more than 5 prescription medications.[245] It is likely that these drugs impact our endocannabinoid system some way.

HORMONAL BIRTH CONTROL

One of the most widespread prescription drugs used by women is hormonal birth control. Over 14 million American women take hormonal birth control each month to prevent unwanted pregnancy or for other reasons like preventing heavy periods.[246] In fact, over 80% of American women who have had sex have used "the Pill" at some point in their life according to the Guttmacher Institute. While some forms contain estrogen, many contain synthetic progesterone, also known as progestin. Progesterone lowers anandamide levels, possibly by increasing fatty acid amide hydrolase (FAAH) expression.[186] The side effects many women associate with birth control pills, such as depressed mood, anxiety, headaches, increased sensitivity to pain, nausea, or the worst, decreased sex drive (libido), may actually be due to endocannabinoid deficiency.

YOUR BIRTH CONTROL PILL CONTAINS PROGESTERONE IF IT CONTAINS ONE OF THESE EIGHT FORMS OF PROGESTIN

Desogestrel	Cyclessa, Mircette
Drospirenone	Beyaz, Yasmin, Yaz
Ethynodiol Diacetate	Continuin, Demulen, Femulen, Luteonorm, Metrodiol, Ovulen
Levonorgestrel	Lybrel, Seasonale, Seasonique, Trivora
Norethindrone	Loestrin, Norinyl, Ortho-Novum
Norethindrone Acetate	Junel
Norgestrel	Ovral
Norgestimate	Ortho Tri-Cyclen Lo

Progesterone-only birth controls pills (POPs) are also called the "mini-pill" because they lack estrogen. They contain less progestin than combination birth control pills.

Depo-Provera is an injection containing only progestin and no estrogen. The vaginal ring NuvaRing and the subdermal (under the skin) implant Nexplanon both contain the progestin Etonogestrel, which is the active metabolite of the inactive progestin Desogestrel. The contraceptive "Patch" called Ortho Evra contains the progestin Norelgestromin.

If you are currently taking or have a long history of using hormonal birth control, you can find out what your options are in Chapter 13 on eliminating things that harm your endocannabinoid system.

CHEMOTHERAPY

Each year 650,000 cancer patients receive chemotherapy in the United States according to the Center for Disease Control (CDC). Chemotherapy is associated with late effects, aka side effects that can appear years after treatment has ended. These include early menopause, osteoporosis, infertility, heart problems, and increased risk of other cancers. Treatment with chemotherapy such as vincristine, oxaliplatin, paclitaxel, or bortezomib for cancer often causes lasting neuropathy (CIPN), or nerve pain, which may be mediated by deficits in endocannabinoid signaling.

Levels of anandamide and 2-AG are upregulated in the spinal cord after administration of chemotherapy, suggesting the body is attempting to restore a deficit in endocannabinoid signaling.[247] Boosting endocannabinoid levels by inhibiting FAAH or MAGL reduces neuropathy quick and effectively, matching or exceeding efficacy of traditional drugs used to treat neuropathy such as morphine, gabapentin, and amitriptyline.[247]

CHAPTER 5

Signs and Symptoms of Endocannabinoid Deficiency

"A number of very common diseases seem to fit a pattern that would be consistent with an endocannabinoid deficiency, specially these are migraine, irritable bowel syndrome, and fibromyalgia. They have some things in common."
– Dr. Ethan Russo

Now that you know what endocannabinoid deficiency is, it's time to find to find out how severe yours is so that you know how rigorously you need to follow the *Vitamin Weed 4-Step Plan*. Let's start off with this quiz that identifies pre-existing conditions you have that could influence your severity of endocannabinoid deficiency.

THE ENDOCANNABINOID DEFICIENCY QUIZ

Instructions: Enter the appropriate response number to each statement in the columns below. Use the values in the rating scale below:

0 = Never or None

1 = Rarely or Mild

2 = Sometimes or Moderate

3 = Always or Severe

PRE-EXISTING CONDITIONS

_____ I have depression.

_____ I have anxiety.

_____ I have schizophrenia.

_____ I have post-traumatic stress disorder (PTSD).

_____ I am not overweight or obese.

_____ I have traumatic brain injury (TBI).

_____ I suffer from migraines.

_____ I have a history of alcohol or drug abuse (not counting cannabis).

_____ I use birth control pills or other form of hormonal contraception.

_____ I have Irritable Bowel Disease (IBD), which can be Crohn's disease or Ulcerative Colitis.

_____ I have fibromyalgia.

_____ I have multiple sclerosis (MS).

_____ I have Chronic Fatigue Syndrome (CFS).

_____ I have epilepsy.

_____ I have autism.

_____ I have cancer.

_____ I have arthritis.

_____ I have anorexia.

_____ I have Celiac disease.

_____ I am menopausal or post-menopausal.

_____ I am over the age of 60.

_____ **TOTAL**

This quiz helps you understand what pre-existing factors might be contributing to or be a result of your endocannabinoid deficiency. This total here is not as important as understanding the total number of conditions that might be improved by boosting your endocannabinoid system.

For a more in-depth look at what the causes and symptoms of

endocannabinoid deficiency, including pre-existing conditions and lifestyle choices, my website www.drmicheleross.com hosts a full Endocannabinoid Deficiency Questionnaire. While not meant to be a stand-alone diagnostic tool, this questionnaire can be helpful in identifying the presence and degree of endocannabinoid deficiency and monitor the status over time so you can see how the *Vitamin Weed 4-Step Plan* is working for you.

SYMPTOMS OF ENDOCANNABINOID DEFICIENCY

Now that you know what might be influencing your endocannabinoid system, you also need to acknowledge that your level of endocannabinoid deficiency could change day to day depending on your stress levels, phase of your menstrual cycle, diet, and more. Endocannabinoid deficiency, just like iron or vitamin deficiency, isn't always a chronic, incurable state. Let's explore what the symptoms of endocannabinoid deficiency are so you can treat them with the *Vitamin Weed 4-Step Plan.*

INFLAMMATION

Cannabinoids are anti-inflammatory, so when the body is in a state of chronic inflammation, it is likely that endocannabinoid levels are low. Inflammation in the brain plays a role in many diseases, including amyotrophic lateral sclerosis (ALS), Parkinson's disease, Alzheimer's disease, multiple sclerosis, schizophrenia, AIDS, dementia, and autism. When your body is inflamed, prostaglandins are released that cause pain. If you have chronic pain, whether it be in your back, pelvis, or joints, and you don't know what the cause is or just haven't received a diagnosis yet, you might be deficient in endocannabinoids.

PAIN

Chronic pain is the easiest sign of endocannabinoid deficiency while acute pain can reflect an acute deficiency. You feel better after you take a Tylenol or NSAID because these OTC painkillers activate the endocannabinoid system. Chronic cluster, migraine and tension headaches, lower back pain, abdominal pain, pelvic pain, joint pain, and temporomandibular joint syndrome (TMJ) are all signs your body is inflamed and endocannabinoid deficient. A low pain threshold, seen in disorders like fibromyalgia, is also a sign of endocannabinoid deficiency.

NAUSEA AND VOMITING

Appetite, nausea, and vomiting are all regulated by the endocannabinoid system. Patients with lower endocannabinoid levels in their blood and high levels of stress in response to motion were more likely to have motion sickness, resulting in nausea and vomiting.[235] Feeling ill with nausea, vomiting, diarrhea, or abdominal pain after eating could also be a sign you have a GI disorder like Irritable Bowel Syndrome or Irritable Bowel Disease and are endocannabinoid deficient.

FOOD PATTERNS

What or how you eat can influence the function of your endocannabinoid system, as outlined in the previous chapter on causes of endocannabinoid deficiency. If you have no appetite, it takes you forever to finish a meal, or you suffer from anorexia, you might be deficient in endocannabinoids. In fact, the best treatment for anorexia is cannabis and Marinol, which is prescription THC, was

FDA-approved to increase appetite in HIV/AIDS patients.

If you feel better after going on a gluten-free, dairy-free or vegetarian diet but you don't stick with it, you might have a food sensitivity. If you have one of more food allergies or sensitivities, especially one that developed later in life, you might have a leaky gut and endocannabinoid deficiency. If you are constantly craving sugar and sweets, you could have ECD from a systemic candida fungal infection, and Chapter 14 on Priming Your Endocannabinoid System will tell you how to fight it.

SLEEP PATTERNS

A regular schedule of 7-8 hours of sleep each night is key to a healthy endocannabinoid system. Signs you are not sleeping well, besides a diagnosed sleep disorder, include jaw pain from grinding your teeth at night, having trouble falling asleep, and having trouble staying asleep or getting up multiple times to go to the bathroom. Chapter 15 on Stress Management deep dives into your quality of sleep and what you can do to improve it.

ENERGY PATTERNS

Your energy levels during the day and how you cope with them are signs and causes of endocannabinoid deficiency. Alertness, sleeping, waking and motivation are mediated by acetylcholine, serotonin, and dopamine, neurotransmitters all regulated by the endocannabinoid system. If you always feel tired no matter how much you sleep, can't wake up in the morning, are always running fifteen minutes late, or don't have the energy to clean the house or do other chores, you might have a sluggish endocannabinoid system. Downing two or more cups of coffee or other caffeine-containing drinks like soda or energy drinks, especially after noon, is a sign you can't stay awake, you are experiencing physiological stress and burnout, and your endocannabinoids are depleted.

Your activity levels are also reflective of your health If you don't have the energy or time to exercise regularly, but you feel better, although a little bit sore, when you do exercise, you could be endocannabinoid deficient. That good feeling from working out hard, or "runner's high," is partially due to anandamide. If walking more than five minutes is exhausting, and you haven't been diagnosed with obesity or a medical condition that would make you winded, like fibromyalgia, the culprit might be endocannabinoid deficiency.

BRAIN PATTERNS

Cannabinoid receptors are highly concentrated in your brain, especially in regions that modulate learning, memory, and attention. If you have trouble focusing, remembering names, places, or events, constantly lose things, or have a short attention span, you could be deficient in endocannabinoids. If you are impulsive, have been diagnosed with attention deficit disorder (ADD) or attention deficit hyperactivity disorder (ADHD), or use legal or illegal stimulants such as Adderall or methamphetamine (also known as speed), your brain chemistry is likely imbalanced, and you could benefit from cannabinoid treatment.

MOOD PATTERNS

Cannabinoid receptors in brain regions like your hippocampus, amygdala, thalamus, and prefrontal cortex regulate release of neurotransmitter important for mood like serotonin and GABA. If you suffer from anxiety or depression, constantly feel stressed out or overwhelmed, are often irritable or angry, feel lonely or bored often, or have mood swings, you could be endocannabinoid deficient. An addiction to drugs, alcohol, gambling, sex or even cigarettes can reveal a brain imbalance endocannabinoid deficiency.

MENSTRUAL CYCLE PATTERNS

Being a woman means you have constantly changing levels of hormones, whether it's due to your menstrual cycle, pregnancy, or menopause. Because anandamide levels are linked to estrogen, you can be endocannabinoid deficient during different phases of your life or even in different weeks due to your moon cycle. If you have premenstrual syndrome (PMS) each month for week before your period, have painful periods, excessive bleeding, or endometriosis, you could be endocannabinoid deficient. Being on hormonal birth control can also throw your endocannabinoid system balance off. Missing your period because you are perimenopausal, menopausal, or postmenopausal is also a possible sign of endocannabinoid deficiency. Finally, missing your period because of stress or undereating is a definite sign you are endocannabinoid deficient.

IMMUNE PATTERNS

A healthy endocannabinoid system will help the body fight infection, but an underactive one could either cause a lack of an immune response or a hyperactive or autoimmune response. Getting colds or flus regularly could be a sign your immune system is suppressed. Swollen or aching lymph nodes could be a sign that your body is actively fighting an infection.

Most fibromyalgia patients and patients with other types of autoimmune disorders are infected with multiple types of viruses, such as herpes or Epstein-Barr virus (EBV).[248] If you have oral herpes simplex virus (HSV-1), also known as cold sores, which 50-80% of Americans have, or genital herpes (HSV-2), your immune system is constantly trying to fight the illness and is never successful. This chronic state of immune hypervigilance can cause endocannabinoid deficiency.

TEMPERATURE REGULATION

Feeling cold all the time, fluctuating between too hot and cold, and not being able to feel whether the temperature of the air or a surface is hot or cold could all be signs your body cannot regulate temperature properly. Atypical cannabinoid receptor TRPV1 regulates both response to temperature as well as perception of body temperature. Endocannabinoid deficiency caused by wrong number of TRPV1 receptors or anandamide deficiency could cause temperature dysregulation, often seen in menopause, fibromyalgia, and cannabis hyperemesis syndrome.

SKIN CONDITIONS

Cannabinoid receptors are present in the skin, where they regulate touch, temperature, inflammation, healing, itch, oil production, and more. When there is endocannabinoid deficiency, conditions like rashes, hives, acne, dry skin, athlete's foot, and chronic itch can occur. Restoring endocannabinoid balance through topical application of cannabis can provide immediate relief and combining it with internal ingestion of cannabinoids and lifestyle changes can provide long-term relief.

TESTS FOR ENDOCANNABINOID DEFICIENCY

There are several ways to measure endocannabinoid levels: blood (serum), cerebrospinal fluid (CSF), and tissue. These three modes of testing do not always correlate with each other, as endocannabinoids can be released locally in a tissue or organ like the uterus, but not impact body levels as measured by blood.

Discrepancies between research studies correlating endocannabinoid levels to diseases may come about due to differences in how the endocannabinoid levels are taken, when they are taken, how big the population of patients is they are measuring, and what medications the patients have used. Endocannabinoid levels in blood versus CSF versus brain or liver tissue are very different and not all levels are altered in each disease. For example, in schizophrenia, studies have found increases in CSF levels of AEA but not blood levels.[249]

Studies of endocannabinoid levels in tissue, taken from human that have died (post-mortem) or rodents, often contradict each other. Researchers have now identified the way brain tissue is collected after death and the way protein are extracted can influence whether endocannabinoids are broken down before they can be measured.[250] This means that endocannabinoid levels in recent studies are more accurate than older ones.

BLOOD TESTING

Endocannabinoid levels in blood are influenced by circadian rhythm, a fact not discovered until recently.[251] Older studies may not have controlled for time of blood collection, and thus may have found no change in blood levels when there was actually a change or vice versa. Further confounding comparisons between studies is that many psychiatric conditions, like schizophrenia, have alterations in circadian rhythm. Endocannabinoid levels are also influenced by menstrual cycle and hormonal birth control in women, meaning studies of endocannabinoid levels in humans will not produce meaningful data until researchers control for these factors.

Blood testing for endocannabinoid levels could diagnose endocannabinoid deficiency quickly and cheaply, while providing a reason for health insurance to cover cannabinoid treatment. Currently there are no commercial tests for blood levels of endocannabinoids. IMPACT Network is working with blood testing labs to make commercialization of these tests a priority, because they exist in the context of laboratories.

IMPACT Network compares blood testing for anandamide to testing for vitamin D. The government tells Americans they are getting enough vitamin D, but blood testing has shown almost 90% of the population is deficient, especially in winter when they are exposed to less sun. Because the government has ignored the importance of the endocannabinoid system, there are no recommended blood levels of anandamide. IMPACT Network hopes to establish those blood levels and give sick patients access to a blood test to establish their endocannabinoid deficiency.

DNA TESTING

Mutations in endocannabinoid genes can also lead to endocannabinoid deficiency. Several companies now sell genetic testing for millions of genes, and separate companies will analyze those SNPs for relevance to health conditions and medication sensitivities. I use 23andMe's $199 genetic testing which requires a quick and painless saliva sample. You can purchase it at www.23andme.com.

A wide range of companies will try to interpret the raw gene data 23andMe provides you with, but most lack updated information on and relevance of SNPs in endocannabinoid system genes and disease. While 23andme tests for FAAH, FAAH2, CNR1, CNR2, MGLL, DAGLA, ABHD6, and ABHD12, information on these genes is absent or inaccurate from most of the DNA interpretation services like LiveWello or Promethease.

My company Infused Health has partnered with Endocanna Health to provide low cost automated as well as personalized interpretations of your genetic data and how it corresponds to cannabinoid response and treatment options. DNA testing is just one piece of the puzzle in finding your optimum cannabinoid balance for life.

DON'T IGNORE ENDOCANNABINOID DEFICIENCY

Endocannabinoid deficiency and a lack of homeostasis in the body is a breeding ground for inflammation, disease, and aging. Pathological processes in the body, left unchecked, will eventually kill you. Your death may be caused by cancer, cardiovascular disease, autoimmune disorders, or depression, all diseases mediated by the endocannabinoid system.

Adrenal fatigue will develop as your body struggles to deal with chronic high or low levels of cortisol, your stress hormone. Patients with adrenal fatigue also don't make enough DHEA, a hormone that other hormones such as estrogen and testosterone are made from. This can cause infertility, early menopause, skipped periods, lack of sex drive, and other issues related to hormone imbalance.

People with endocannabinoid deficiency are more likely to become ill in response to a stressor, more likely to experience more severe symptoms, and more likely to recover slower than people with functioning endocannabinoid systems. Endocannabinoid deficiency impacts more than your response to pain or illness. This impacts your emotional health and your resilience to bounce back and adapt to life's challenges. Some people just can't recover when they've lost their job or a love one. They fall into a depression, lose touch with friends, or become unemployed or underemployed.

CHAPTER 6

Why Your Doctor Doesn't Know About Endocannabinoid Deficiency

"It is an unfortunate reality of 2016 that many doctors still lack the basic knowledge about cannabis, cannabinoids, and the endocannabinoid system that would enable them to have an informed discussion with their patients, and that the knowledge gap gives rise to stigmatization, alienation, and a fracture of the doctor–patient relationship."[256] - Dr. Mark Ware, Executive Director of the Consortium for the Investigation of Cannabinoids.

In order for doctors to care about a disease, there must be a pharmaceutical treatment for it. Doctors prescribe stimulants like Adderall for ADHD, which is considered a deficiency in dopamine function. Doctors prescribe anti-depressants like Prozac for depression, which is considered a deficiency in serotonin function. So why don't doctors prescribe cannabis for endocannabinoid deficiency?

FEDERAL LAW

Doctors cannot prescribe cannabinoid therapies for endocannabinoid deficiency in the United States because cannabis is still a Schedule 1 drug with no medical benefit according to Federal law. This is unfortunate because there have been tens of thousands of studies showing there is medical benefit to cannabis products and, as of 2017, 75 million Americans now have state legal access to marijuana in some form, whether medical or recreational. Science and federal law clearly are contradicting each other.

Many doctors are afraid of losing their medical license for recommending cannabis in state where medical marijuana is legal. Some doctors simply are uneducated about the endocannabinoid system, as only 12% of American medical school teach anything about the endocannabinoid system, despite it being the biggest neurotransmitter system in the human body. Or maybe they are misinformed about the safety of cannabis, believing it to be more addictive than the highly addictive prescription painkillers they dole out to patients. Other doctors simply refuse to believe the medical benefits, possibly because they or their teenaged children partake in cannabis to get high.

The one loophole is that synthetic THC, called dronabinol and marketed as Marinol, is Schedule 3 in the United States so doctors can prescribe it without fear of prosecution. Because Marinol does not have other cannabinoids like CBD to balance out the psychoactive effects, patients prefer smoking cannabis to taking the pill. A recent study found patients disliked inconsistent onset and duration of Marinol, side effects and lack of full-benefits attributed to using whole plant cannabis in methods such as smoking. Marinol is much more expensive than cannabis. Bottom line: patients want whole plant cannabis, not synthetic versions that are less effective and less safe.

NO WAY TO PROFIT

Perhaps the biggest reason doctors don't prescribe cannabis is because pharmaceutical companies don't profit from it, and they in turn don't. Doctors are marketed to daily by pharmaceutical representatives and paid generously to present on the efficacy of a drug to the medical community. These opportunities are non-existent for the cannabis industry because of its illegality on the federal level.

When a patient comes in showing signs of depression, the doctor's first mode of action isn't to suggest exercise, healthy diet, and OTC serotonin precursor 5-HTP. The doctor will immediately recommend a prescription antidepressant, and if that doesn't work, continue down the line of available pharmaceuticals. In the same way, it is not surprising that even if doctors are educated on the endocannabinoid system and the role it plays in diseases, they will not suggest cannabinoid treatment and always recommend a pharmaceutical drug.

Big Pharma is much bigger than the Cannabis or Nutraceutical industries. Chemotherapy and other cancer treatments were a $110.6 billion dollar global industry in 2013 according to BCC Research. Chemotherapy alone is a $24.3 billion dollar market, having doubled in five years as our population is both growing and aging. Because doctors aren't incentivized to cut costs for health insurance providers, recommending cannabis, an inexpensive yet less proven way of treating cancer, is too risky for most doctors.

MISEDUCATION

Most doctors have learned all the myths of cannabis: that it's highly addictive, that it's the gateway drug to harder drugs like heroin and methamphetamine, that it causes brain damage, that marijuana smoking causes lung cancer, and that marijuana use during pregnancy results in fetal marijuana syndrome. Many trusted sources of information for doctors, such as the National Institute on Health (NIH) and National Institute on Drug Abuse (NIDA), have persisted to present outdated or even propaganda information on marijuana.

It's often hard to unlearn wrong facts than to learn new things. In fact, being presented with facts that disagree so strongly with what you have learned is a recipe for cognitive dissonance: rejecting the new facts entirely and doubling on your old beliefs. This is why doctors, when presented with research headlines or stories from patients that cannabis is beneficial, often reject what should be indisputable evidence.

TRASHCAN DIAGNOSIS

Even if CECD is recognized by the healthcare industry as a legitimate syndrome, it likely to be disregarded by traditional doctors as a "wastebasket diagnosis." Also known as a "trashcan diagnosis" is a diagnosis given when the doctor can't figure out was disorder the patient really has, if any. Wastebasket diagnoses include fibromyalgia, candida (yeast) overgrowth, leaky gut, chronic fatigue syndrome, endometriosis, and gastroesophageal reflux. Wastebasket diseases do not get funding for research and aren't taken seriously by doctors.

Patients that suffer from chronic pain, gastrointestinal symptoms, fatigue, and headaches are often give a trashcan diagnosis like fibromyalgia when their doctor is simply sick of testing for what is wrong with the patient or thinks the patient's symptoms are "in their head." Lazy doctors may just diagnose CECD and prescribe cannabis when the patient is in fact really sick and needs intensive medical treatment for a rare disorder.

YOUR DOCTOR MIGHT SUPPORT IT

On a positive note, some doctors are now embracing medical marijuana. These including pediatricians that found cannabinoid products control epileptic seizures better than any pharmaceutical and oncologists dealing with cancer patients. Alternative healthcare providers like acupuncturists, chiropractors, and massage therapists are also more likely to accept and even recommend cannabinoid therapy for their patients.

According to a 2013 study published in the New England Journal of Medicine, 76% of doctors approve the use of marijuana for metastatic breast cancer, and 82% of oncologists believe marijuana provides medical benefits according to a 2014 survey by WebMD.[252]

A 2016 survey of medical students at the University of Colorado found they were more likely to believe marijuana was an appropriate treatment for a qualifying condition if they grew up in Colorado, which has a history of accepting medical cannabis use, or they had used cannabis themselves.[253] Slightly more medical students in this survey than a 2013 survey of doctors in Colorado would recommend marijuana to a patient themselves, which means the younger generation is slightly less conservative than its elders.[254]

YOUR DOCTOR MIGHT EVEN RECOMMEND IT

The problem is that your doctor's hands are tied by government red tape. Doctors cannot prescribe medical marijuana to their patients because it is still considered a "Schedule 1" drug with no medical benefit and high potential for abuse, despite thousands of published studies to the contrary. To give you a feel of how out of place THC, CBD, and medical marijuana as flower or the plant are on this Schedule 1 list, here are the other Schedule 1 drugs: heroin, bath salts, khat (cathinone), methaqualone (Quaaludes), mescaline (peyote), LSD (lysergic acid diethylamide), GHB (gamma-hydroxybutyric acid), ecstasy (MDMA), and psilocybin (magic mushrooms).

Doctors cannot prescribe medical marijuana in state where it is legal, but they can "recommend" it, which leads to a medical card authorizing a patient to purchase cannabis from an authorized dispensary or caretaker, or to grow their own cannabis. Many doctors are prohibited from recommending cannabis to their patients due to the very real possibility of losing their job, federal funding for research, or their malpractice insurance.

The qualifying conditions for a medical marijuana recommendation vary greatly by each state, and doctors may support the use of cannabis for a medical condition but be legally barred from recommending it for that patient. For example, autism is a qualifying condition in only one state, Illinois, yet case studies and preclinical research suggest the endocannabinoid system is greatly involved in the pathology of this brain disease. The sad part is that pharmaceutical drugs are often prescribed "off-label" for many conditions for which they were not clinical studied when the drug was first FDA-approved. Medical cannabis is not allowed the same "off-label" recommendation, even though it is a safer treatment that most pharmaceuticals.

Interestingly, the 2013 survey of Colorado doctors found only 31% had ever recommended medical marijuana to a patient, and out of those, only 1% had recommended medical marijuana to more than 50 patients.[254] This suggests while doctors are become more open to medical marijuana, few are suggesting this regularly as a first-line therapy.

REASONS WHY YOUR DOCTOR IS AFRAID TO RECOMMEND IT

INCONSISTENT PRODUCT QUALITY

Lack of quality products and dosing information was a barrier for recommending medical marijuana according to 46% of oncologists surveyed.[255] The biggest variable in patient response is the cannabis product. I'll walk you through how the same product from the same dispensary can yield a different result depending on what day you buy it.

A cannabis joint can vary in the strain used, which means the THC, CBD, and other cannabinoid levels will vary depending on what someone rolled up. There can even be toxins like mold or pesticide residue, which accounts for many of the negative effects people can feel from cannabis, including nausea, headache, or anxiety. Even when the same strain is used every time a patient smokes a joint, the same strain can vary in THC level from harvest to harvest due to little changes like weather, plant stress, or a change in grower.

To make things even more confusing, some cannabis strains are mislabeled, meaning that someone could be selling Sour Diesel when it's really Girl Scout Cookies! The consumer certainly can't see or smell the difference between the strains, so they are dependent on the grower or dispensary to do their due diligence on verifying strains. Unfortunately, there are few tools that can cheaply identify the cannabinoid and terpene profile and match it to a standard strain to combat "counterfeit" strains trying to be sold for a higher price or simply mislabeled strains. Because there is no federal government oversight on what is sold to cannabis customers, like there is for alcohol and tobacco (Alcohol and Tobacco Tax and Trade Bureau), there are no consumer protections. Your best protection is to work with a grower or dispensary you or your patient trusts, and never purchase black market products.

NO DOSING PROTOCOLS

Doctors are afraid to recommend medical marijuana as a treatment because unlike pharmaceuticals, there are no clear dosage guidelines. Instead, there are many questions: How many mg of THC and/or CBD is a patient supposed to eat if they have a migraine? What about brain cancer? Will it interact with their other medications? What's the difference between oil containing CBD isolate and hemp oil containing CBD and other terpenes?

With many unanswered questions, and the looming fear of medical malpractice lawsuits, suspension of their medical licenses by state medical boards, or at the very worst, raids by the Drug Enforcement Administration (DEA), doctors are right to be hesitant to provide treatment protocols for marijuana. However, numerous alternative medicine treatments exist including diets, supplements, acupuncture, transcranial magnetic stimulation, and doctors often are permissive or even suggest patients try these treatments. Cannabis should be considered another tool in the toolbox when traditional treatments aren't working.

Trial and error is still the approach used in many fields of medicine, including psychiatry. A psychiatrist will put a patient on an antidepressant, wait one month to see if it works, adjust the dose if it doesn't and wait another month, then switch to antidepressant #2, #3, #4 and so on. There's hope: cannabinoid medicine leaders have developed new cloud-based software programs to collect cannabis treatment data and analyze with artificial intelligence (AI) to come up with treatment protocols in future years.

TALK TO YOUR DOCTOR ABOUT CANNABIS

Don't be scared to start the conversation about cannabis with your doctor. It's not illegal to ask your doctor about any treatment, and they can't report you even if you are in state or country where marijuana is not yet legal.

Ask your doctor if they heard about it for your medical condition. In the best-case scenario, the doctor has, can recommend cannabis for you, and even has some guidance on treatment options. In the worst-case scenario, your doctor knows nothing or won't discuss it with you. If you have the one bad apple doctor who is judgmental or rude to you over discussing your current or possible cannabis use, it's time to find another doctor that respects you. So, be brave, what's the worst that could happen?

Doctors won't change their mind about cannabis if patients aren't honest about using cannabis for their medical conditions or don't prod their doctors to read up more so they can discuss treatment options with them. Keep in mind right now 61% of patients get their information about medical benefits of cannabis from a budtender at a dispensary, but 31% prefer a medical professional.[257] Cannabis use will only become mainstream medicine if this is a conversation happening at the doctor's office.

It is the patients that will close the gap in cannabinoid medicine knowledge. You're taking the first step, by educating yourself through reading this book. Remember to pass this book along, even to your doctor, it could save someone's life.

PART THREE

Cannabinoid Deficiency is the Root of Disease

CHAPTER 7

Aging and the Endocannabinoid System

"I've been trying to find a drug that will reduce brain inflammation and restore cognitive function in rats for over 25 years; cannabinoids are the first and only class of drugs that have ever been effective. I think that the perception about this drug is changing and in the future people will be less fearful." - Neuroscientist Gary Wenk, Ph.D.

Cannabinoid medicine offers benefit for patients without any chronic pain or illness. All patients have one thing in common: they are aging. Cannabinoid medicine offers the ability to slow the aging process and possibly prevent the degenerative diseases that make our final years lack the quality of our younger years. I'll outline one huge aspect of aging for women, menopause, under Chapter 11: Women's Health and the Endocannabinoid System.

This chapter will outline the involvement of endocannabinoid deficiency and the mechanism of cannabis treatment for the following disorders that occur in the final years of life: Alzheimer's disease and Parkinson's disease.

ALZHEIMER'S DISEASE

Alzheimer's disease impacts 5.1 million Americans, 66% of which are women. By 2050 there will 13.8 million Americans living with the disease as we continue to live longer and longer. 1 in 3 seniors dies with Alzheimer's disease or a similar form of dementia. Risks factors for developing Alzheimer's disease include old age, a family history, having the ApoE4 gene, having a history of traumatic brain injury, heavy smoking of cigarettes, and maintaining an unhealthy diet.

Alzheimer's disease, the most common form of dementia, is characterized by progressive loss of memory and cognitive function. There are seven stages of disease progression, from no impairment to moderate decline to very severe decline. Alzheimer's disease is a deficiency in acetylcholine, a neurotransmitter that modulates memory, decision making and wakefulness. It is also characterized by brain plaques which are clumps of beta-amyloid, a protein found in cell membranes of brain cells. Beta-amyloid plaques cause brain inflammation and block signaling between neurons. Finally, neurofibrillary tangles form when tau protein collapses and cannot transport nutrients throughout the neuron, causing cell death.

Symptoms of Alzheimer's disease include:

- memory loss
- difficulty planning or solving problems
- vision problems
- forgetting events, conversations and appointments
- believing things that are not true

- misplacing items, often in inappropriate locations
- inability to multitask
- getting lost in familiar places like the supermarket
- forgetting the names of family, friends, foods and other familiar things
- asking the same questions over and over again
- mood swings or depression
- irritability and aggression

Common treatments of Alzheimer's disease include cholinesterase inhibitors that increase acetylcholine including Aricept (donepezil), Exelon (rivastigmine), and Razadyne (galantamine), and the NMDA antagonist Nameda (memantine). Other drugs such as sleep medications Ambien (zolpidem) and Lunesta (eszopiclone) or anti-anxiety medications Klonopin (clonazepam) and Ativan (lorazepam) are used to treat behavior issues associated with Alzheimer's disease, but have serious risks to the patient.

ROLE OF THE ENDOCANNABINOID SYSTEM IN ALZHEIMER'S DISEASE

Endocannabinoid dysfunction or deficiency likely plays a role in development and progression of Alzheimer's disease. One study at UCLA that started in 2013 is looking at the interaction between cannabis use and the APOE4 gene on structure of the hippocampus and cognitive function in patients over 55 to see if cannabis users have a lower or greater risk of developing Alzheimer's disease, especially if they carry the gene that increase risk of it.[258] So far, no studies have shown mutations in endocannabinoid genes lead to

Alzheimer's; however it is not clear that studies were looking for such a correlation.

Cannabinoid receptors are at high levels in the healthy brain in the hippocampus, the brain region important for learning and memory and decrease with age. One very small study found while brains of Alzheimer's patients had even less CB1 receptors than healthy brains of the same age, the regions of lower CB1 receptors did not correlate with location of amyloid-beta plaques or tangles.[259] CB2 receptor level is actually increased in the brains of Alzheimer's patients, most likely to combat the neuroinflammation occuring.[260-261] There is evidence that CB1 and CB2 receptors are nitrosylated and have defective downstream signaling, resulting in endocannabinoid deficiency.[260]

Activation of CB2 receptors in the brain can reduce activation of migroglia that promote inflammation and excitotoxicity, and promote adult neurogenesis, or the birth of new brain cells.[262-263] CB2 receptor deficiency in a rodent model increases amyloid-beta and plaque formation, indicating the role of CB2 in protecting the brain against the development of Alzheimer's disease.[264] CBD reduces inflammation and gliosis in a mouse model of Alzheimer's disease, as well as promotes neurogenesis and neuron survival by increase anandamide in the brain.[265-267]

The endocannabinoid system can protect against Alzheimer's disease outside the traditional cannabinoid receptors. Inhibiting breakdown of endocannabinoid 2-AG by using a MAGL inhibitor causes a reduction in beta-amyloid in a mouse model of Alzheimer's disease.[268] This reduction in beta-amyloid is not caused by actions of 2-AG at either the CB1 or CB2 receptor, but rather, 2-AG acts through PPARγ receptors to inhibit BACE1, the enzyme that breaks amyloid precursor protein (APP) into beta-amyloid.[269] Increasing 2-AG also reduces neuroinflammation and neurodegeneration and improves spatial memory.[270-271]

CLINICAL RESEARCH ON CANNABIS AND ALZHEIMER'S DISEASE

The U.S. government holds a patent #6630507 awarded in 2003 on "Cannabinoids as Antioxidants and Neuroprotectants." In the abstract of the patent, it states that "The cannabinoids are found to have particular application as neuroprotectants, for example in limiting neurological damage following ischemic insults, such as stroke and trauma, or in the treatment of neurodegenerative diseases, such as Alzheimer's disease, Parkinson's disease and HIV dementia." The fact that cannabis is a Schedule 1 drug listed by the government as having no medical benefits is at completed odds with this patent that clearly shows cannabinoids can reduce neurodegeneration in Alzheimer's disease.

Several clinical trials have completed or are in progress on the role of cannabinoids in treating behavioral aspects of Alzheimer's disease. One study that is currently recruiting at John Hopkins University is investigating synthetic THC (Marinol) as a treatment for agitation in Alzheimer's disease.[272] This follows up on the small pilot study that found Marinol increased appetite and reduced severity of disruptive behavior in Alzheimer's patients.[273] One case study found Marinol stopped treatment-resistant dementia-associated sexual disinhibition that was disruptive in a nursing home.[274] Another study at Sunnybrook Health Sciences center is recruiting patients for a study on nabilone, a THC analogue, in reducing agitation, sleep issues, and other symptoms of dementia.[275]

APPLICATION OF CANNABINOID MEDICINE TO ALZHEIMER'S DISEASE

Vaporizing CBD strains or taking CBD oil or pills can relieve anxiety and agitation associated with Alzheimer's disease. For patients who do not respond to CBD-only products THC can be added to improve efficacy. THC and CBD combination therapy often works best, due to the fact that CBD reduces psychoactivity of THC and extends the amount of time cannabinoids are in the body.[265]

When patients over the age of 65 were treated with anti-inflammatory NSAIDs for 2 years, they were less likely to develop Alzheimer's disease 8 years later.[276] Taking anti-inflammatory cannabinoids CBDA and CBD should also have the same neuroprotective effect, although clinical trials have yet to test this.

RISKS OF TREATING A PATIENT WITH ALZHEIMER'S DISEASE WITH CANNABINOID MEDICINE

Some antipsychotics, anti-anxiety drugs, and anti-depressants are broken down by the p450 liver enzyme CYP3A4, which is inhibited by CBD. Taking both CBD and these specific drugs may increase or (in rare cases) decrease the amount of drug that is absorbed, leading to unwanted side effects like sedation or agitation.

CBD or THC use may induce short-term memory deficits in some patients. This can be offset by consuming caffeine, taking the cognitive supplement citicoline, or using peppermint oil or alpha-pinene. Finally, for those patients who will not avoid THC products, advise them to keep the THC dosage low, not mix it with alcohol or other drugs, and not consume it in a new place or with new people.[277]

PARKINSON'S DISEASE

Parkinson's disease impacts 1.5 million Americans and 23,000 die each year. 96% of patients are over the age of 50 and men are more likely to develop Parkinson's disease than women. Risk factors for developing Parkinson's disease include genetics, exposure to toxins like paraquat pesticide, illnesses and old age. Caffeine, green tea, and aerobic exercise may prevent the development of Parkinson's disease. Parkinson's disease is a deficiency in dopamine, a neurotransmitter that modulates pleasure, motivation, smell, balance, and movement.

Parkinson's disease is characterized by loss of smell, tremor, speech changes, writing changes, problems with balance, rigidity, slow movement (bradykinesia) and freezing. Additional issues experienced by patients include sleep disorders, problems swallowing, depression and other mood changes, cognitive difficulties, bladder issues, constipation, fatigue, blood pressure changes, pain, and changes in libido or sexual performance. Brain changes include the presence of alpha-synuclein enriched Lewy bodies that clump and can't be broken down by cells.

Common treatments of Parkinson's disease include drugs that raise dopamine levels, such as carbidopa-levodopa, which converts into dopamine once it crosses the blood-brain barrier and dopamine agonists such as Mirapex (pramipexole), Requip (ropinrole), Neupro (rotigotine), and Apokyn (apomorphine). Monoamine oxidase B (MAO-B) inhibitors prevent the breakdown of dopamine and include Eldepryl or Zelapar (selegiline) and Azilect (rasagiline). Catechol-O-methyltransferase (COMT) inhibitors also block breakdown of dopamine and include Comtan (entacapone) and Tasmar (tolcapone).

Amantadine is a drug given to relieve symptoms of early-stage Parkinson's disease as well as to control side effects of Parkinson's drugs such as carbidopa-levodopa. Finally, surgical methods including deep brain stimulation (DBS) and stem cell transplantation also help Parkinson's patients, as so massage, acupuncture, meditation, yoga, dance, music and art therapy.

ROLE OF THE ENDOCANNABINOID SYSTEM IN PARKINSON'S DISEASE

Endocannabinoid levels and CB receptors decrease with age and menopause.[190] Less cannabinoid signaling may mean less neuroprotection for dopamine cells, less ability to break down Lewy bodies, and other issues. No mutations in genes that regulate the endocannabinoid system have been identified in Parkinson's disease; however it likely that researchers have not pursued that as a possible mechanism of Parkinson's disease yet. CB1 receptors are not found on dopamine neurons in the striatum or substantia nigra that control movement; however CB1 receptors are present on other types of neurons such as GABA neurons that control dopamine neurons in these regions.[278-279]

CLINICAL RESEARCH ON CANNABIS AND PARKINSON'S DISEASE

Both CBD and cannabis containing THC have been found to relieve symptoms of Parkinson's disease. While only 4.3% of Parkinson's patients used cannabis in one survey study, that found to be among the most effective complementary and alternative medicine (CAM) treatments used.[280] Another survey of Parkinson's patients using cannabis found 46% found some benefit; 45% had improvement of bradykinesia, 31% had improvement of resting tremor, and 14% had improvement in levodopa-induced dyskinesia.[281] One clinical study found smoking cannabis with THC in it improved motor symptoms, tremor, bradykinesia, sleep, and pain in patients with Parkinson's disease.[282] In a rodent model of Parkinson's disease, the cannabinoid THCV reduced motor impairment and neurodegeneration.[283]

A pilot study being conducted at University of Colorado School of Medicine by Dr. Maureen Leehey found Epidiolex (CBD from GW Pharmaceuticals) significantly improved total Movement Disorder Society (MDS) and Motor MDS scores in Parkinson's patients, but not rest tremor.[284] One clinical study found 300 mg of CBD a day improved quality of life but not motor symptoms in Parkinson's patient, possibly due to it being in the lowest range necessary to see improvements in Parkinson's patients.[285] Another study found CBD treatment decreased symptoms of rapid eye movement (REM) sleep behavior disorder in Parkinson's patients.[286] Finally, psychosis in Parkinson's disease is also treated by 150 mg of CBD a day for 4 weeks.[287]

More research needs to be done on different dosages, ratios, and routes of administration of THC and CBD in Parkinson's patients.[288] Currently Michael J. Fox Foundation for Parkinson's Research funds research on marijuana and Parkinson's in Israel and full supports the use of the compound in patients.

APPLICATION OF CANNABINOID MEDICINE TO PARKINSON'S DISEASE

Taking CBD in pill or tincture form can be explored as a complementary treatment, whether to relieve anxiety, decrease REM sleep behavior disorder symptoms, or psychosis. Anecdotal evidence exists for Parkinson's disease patients smoking or vaporizing cannabis and being able to move normally without tremor within minutes. Despite not knowing the best strains or dosages to use, it is likely that vaporizing cannabis, in particular cannabis strains with CBD in it, will not harm a Parkinson's disease patient. Cannabis should be vaporized instead of smoked because toxins from burning cannabis, like ammonia, could cause further harm to dying dopamine cells.

RISKS OF TREATING A PATIENT WITH PARKINSON'S DISEASE WITH CANNABINOID MEDICINE

Drugs used to treat Parkinson's disease do not interact with CBD because they are not broken down by the same p450 liver enzymes that CBD inhibits. CBD or cannabis use may induce short-term memory deficits in some patients. This can be offset by also consuming caffeine, taking the cognitive supplement citicoline, or using peppermint oil or alpha-pinene.

CHAPTER 8

Cancer and the Endocannabinoid System

"The results we are obtaining are telling us that cannabinoids may be useful for the treatment of breast cancer. We started to do experiments in animal models of glioblastoma, brain tumors, and we observed that the cannabinoids were very potent in reducing tumor growth."

- Cancer scientist Dr. Christina Sanchez

Each of us has mutated cells and the seeds of cancer growing within us. It's up to us to take cancer prevention into our own hands and create an environment where cancer cannot survivor or thrive. A healthy endocannabinoid system prevents cancer growth and migration and promotes cell death. This chapter will outline the involvement of endocannabinoid deficiency and the mechanism of cannabis treatment for the following aspects of cancer care: cancer prevention, cancer treatment, treatment of side effects of chemotherapy or radiation therapy, and cancer survivorship.

CANCER PREVENTION

41% of men and 38% of women will develop cancer as some point during their lifetime in the United States. More people are surviving cancer than ever before and survivors have long-term health problems that are often not addressed. Cancer prevention is more important now than ever to prevent years of pain and suffering. Thankfully, cancer prevention can be easily managed through digital healthcare, lifestyle modification and cannabinoid medicine.

ENDOCANNABINOIDS AND DNA REPAIR

A common misconception is that our body ages and develops cancer as we get older because our DNA gets more mutations. In reality we age because our body's ability to repair DNA mutations gets limited with age. Healthy people have the same rate of DNA mutations in their 20s as they do in their 80s, our DNA mechanic just doesn't come by as often, and the mutations start to snowball. DNA can be damaged in a multitude of ways including exposure to UV radiation from the sun, radiation from medical imaging including x-rays, pollution, viruses and chemicals including cigarette smoke and hydrogen peroxide.

The reality is that most of us look healthy but are a mess inside. The American lifestyle of junk food, no sleep, and little exercise means most people's bodies are in a chronic state of inflammation. Chronic inflammation causes cells with DNA mutations to divide before they are repaired, creating a copy of the DNA mutated cell. With twice the number of DNA mutations to repair, the body's DNA repair machinery cannot keep up, and mutated cells exponentially grow, resulting in tumors. By the time cancer is large enough to be detected or cause symptoms, it has been growing inside of us for ten years or more. The American lifestyle turns our bodies into cancer incubators, and we are unable to turn on our own cellular defense system to destroy it.

Exposure to UV light from indoor tanning beds or the sun is a carcinogen responsible for 90% of non-melanoma skin cancers, which accounts for 15,000 deaths a year in the United States alone.[289] Interestingly chemical sunscreen and wearing hats in the sun have done little to reduce these type of skin cancers and there are 3.5 million new case a year in the U.S. If avoiding UV radiation is impossible for most Americans, we must focus on bolstering DNA repair instead of avoiding DNA mutations.

COX-2 is produced in cancer cells and by in skin cells exposed to UV radiation. Pre-treatment with COX-2 inhibitors prevents UV-radiation induced skin tumors. Prophylactic treatment with raw cannabis juice or CBDA extracts may be a real way for people with high cancer risk or sun exposure to protect themselves against carcinogens they can't avoid.[289]

ENDOCANNABINOIDS AND CANCER GENE EXPRESSION

Endocannabinoids have health benefits independent of typical cannabinoid receptors CB1 and CB2 or atypical receptors like TRPV1. Anandamide increases gene expression of nuclear factor erythroid 2–related factor 2 (Nrf2), a protein that binds DNA and regulates expression of other antioxidant proteins. Boosting anandamide may be especially important in fighting the effects of aging, as Nrf2 expression decreases with age and likely contributes to neurodegeneration, cardiovascular disease, and cancer in the elderly.

Drugs that that stimulate the Nrf2 pathway are being investigated to treat diseases caused by oxidative stress and characterized by injury and inflammation. These diseases include autism, Alzheimer's disease, Parkinson's disease, diabetes, multiple sclerosis, cancer, and many more. In fact, Biogen received FDA approval in 2013 for Tecfidera, a Nrf2 activator formulated as dimethyl fumarate, to treat multiple sclerosis.

Boosting levels of anandamide through diet or other lifestyle changes is more efficient than taking any individual antioxidant supplement. Nrf2 is the "master regulator" of the antioxidant response, regulating expression of hundreds of genes, including antioxidant enzymes as well as clusters of genes that control a broad range of functions including immune response, cognitive function, addiction, tumorigenesis, and tissue remodeling. Dysregulation of Nrf2-related genes provide the link between oxidative stress and inflammation and over 200 human diseases.[290]

Nrf2 activating strategies include drugs, foods, dietary supplements and exercise. Nrf2 activators can be used to prevent disease, prevent disease recurrence, or slow disease progression.[291] Like any treatment, Nrf2 activation must be done in moderation. Excessively high consumption of Nrf2 activators could promote the survival and growth of cancer cells. However, consumption of foods or supplementation with low doses of Nrf2 activator will be in the range that promotes health without stimulating tumorigenesis.

One thing Nrf2 activators are not ideal for is treatment of cancer, as it may actually interfere with traditional chemotherapy and radiotherapy treatments that aim to kill, not strengthen tumor cells.[291] In fact, Nrf2 is overexpressed in many type of cancer cells, promoting their survival. It is unclear whether Nrf2 activation combined with cannabis treatment alone for cancer would be beneficial.

ROLE OF THE ENDOCANNABINOID SYSTEM IN CANCER PREVENTION

Endocannabinoid deficiency could contribute to cancer. Anandamide inhibits breast cancer proliferation, and low levels of anandamide in a patient may provide an environment for breast cancer to thrive. In fact, blood levels of anandamide were reduced in patients with a variety of cancers, while 2-AG and OEA levels were increased correlating with the number of metastases and disease stage.[292] Daily CBD use to boost anandamide levels could theoretically reduce breast cancer risk, but this would need to be tested using longitudinal studies.

CBD has anti-inflammatory actions and antioxidant actions which can prevent cancer cells from thriving and multiplying. CBD also increases anandamide levels and binding to TRPV1 receptor mediates apoptosis of cervical cancer cells.[293] CBD also upregulates 680 genes that are anti-cancer and down regulates 524 genes that are pro-cancer, including Id-1.[294]

CBD is also an antagonist at the GPR55 receptor which may mediate anti-cancer effects. Activation of GPR55 was recently found to promote growth of colon cancer, and it is assumed a GPR55 antagonist would slow colon cancer growth.[295] Activation of CB1 receptors, whether through THC or anandamide, reduced inflammation in colon which may also protect against colon cancer.[296]

CBDA, which is what the plant makes before it is decarboxylated into CBD, is a selective COX-2 inhibitor and NSAID. COX-2 inhibition is a mechanism by which drugs like Celebrex are being investigated for cancer prevention and treatment. It is possible that CBDA may also prevent and treat cancer through COX-2 inhibition. Very little research has been performed on this topic. An early study found CBDA inhibits migration of human breast cancer cells, but through inhibition of cAMP-dependent protein kinase A, not COX-2 inhibition.[297]

THC may also prevent development of cancer. A study found rodents treated with THC for two years were less likely to develop uterine, breast, pancreas and pituitary gland cancer.[298] CBN, THC and delta-8-THC all inhabited the growth of lung cancer cells in another study.[299] Finally, THCA, or THC before it is decarboxylated, may also be protective against cancer growth.[300]

CLINICAL RESEARCH ON CANNABIS AND CANCER PREVENTION

Longitudinal clinical research studies on cannabinoids for cancer prevention have not performed due to the Schedule 1 nature of cannabis and limited funding for medical benefits of cannabis. My nonprofit IMPACT Network and other organizations are attempting to launch registries that will track CBD and cannabis use and look at cancer incidence or recurrence over the long term. Does daily or weekly CBD or cannabis use result in less risk of cancer? Does daily CBD use prevent cancer in a pair of twins with the same DNA and lifestyle where one uses CBD and one doesn't? What dosage of CBD or CBDA is required to lower cancer risk? These are all questions that need to be answered and will over the next decade or two. Until then, it is not likely that CBD or cannabis use increases cancer risk, so consider cannabis a tool in your toolbox for wellness and perhaps even cancer risk management.

APPLICATION OF CANNABINOID MEDICINE TO CANCER PREVENTION

Juicing raw cannabis with THCA and/or CBDA in it may decrease inflammation as well as promote apoptosis of cancerous cells without psychoactivity or other side effects. While THC is the most potent cannabinoid for killing cancer cells, it may not be the optimal cannabinoid for daily cancer prevention due to its psychoactivity and other side effects. CBD may be the best weapon in cancer prevention. CBD not only promotes an environment where cancer cannot thrive, but it turns off and on genes key to cancer and has broad actions. Taking 5-10 mg of CBD once or twice a day could be a way to manage your cancer risk. If you know you have genes for cancer or a strong family history of cancer, you may want to take higher dosage of CBD.

RISKS OF USING CANNABINOID MEDICINE TO ATTEMPT TO PREVENT CANCER

It is important to note that cannabis users, especially those that only smoke marijuana, do get diagnosed with cancer just like stress-free, clean-eating yoga teachers do. Sometime our family genes are stacked against us, or we are exposed to some environmental toxin or virus we are not aware of. The doses of THC required to treat cancer are usually much higher than those used to prevent cancer or prevent its recurrence.

Because long-term effects of CBD, CBDA, THCA, or other cannabinoids have not been studied, it is not backed by science whether taking daily cannabinoids will decrease, increase or have no effect on developing cancer in general or specific cancers. Therefore, taking cannabinoids to prevent cancer is a follow-at-your-own-risk protocol.

As outlined in other chapters, CBD is a potent inhibitor of p450 liver enzymes CYP3A4 and CYP2C9. If you are taking a medication that says do not take with grapefruit, and you take CBD in tincture, pill, capsule, or edible form, you could end up with too much of your medication in your bloodstream and have unwanted side effects. This could happen with common drugs including warfarin, taken by millions to prevent blood clots, and antidepressants like Zoloft. Ways to mediate that risk include lowering your dose of medication under your doctor's guidance or lowering your dose of CBD to a dose that causes minimal inhibition of p450 enzymes.

CANCER TREATMENT

Cancer is characterized by abnormal cells that growth uncontrollably and spread to other tissues, where they kill surrounding healthy tissue. Cancer is the second-leading cause of death in the United States, and almost 50% of Americans will receive a cancer diagnosis at some point in their life. Cancer can be caused by genetic mutations, such as BRCA genes in breast cancer, but also usually has a second "hit" such as virus, stress, smoking, or exposure to environmental toxins.

Signs of cancer include fatigue, lumps, weight loss or gain, unexplained bleeding or bruising, persistent cough, trouble breathing, skin changes or sores, changes in bladder and bowel habits, difficulty swallowing, hoarseness, persistent muscle and joint pain, persist fevers and night sweats, and persistent discomfort after eating.

Common cancer treatments vary for the type of cancer and the stage. Treatments include chemotherapy, radiation, surgery, prescription creams, immunotherapy, hormone therapy, medication, and even stem-cell transplant.

Drugs used to treat cancer that are broken down by the CYPA34 p450 liver enzyme and can interact with CBD include:

- Cytoxan (cyclophosphamide) - leukemia and lymphoma
- Xalkori (crizotinib) - lung cancer
- Sprycel (dasatinib) - leukemia
- Tarceva (erlotinib) - pancreatic cancer, and lung cancer
- Zortress, Afinitor (everolimus) - kidney, pancreas, brain, and breast cancer
- Gleevec (imatinib) - leukemia and other cancers
- Tykerb (lapatinib) - breast cancer and other cancers
- Tasigna (nilotinib) - leukemia
- Votrient (pazopanib) - kidney cancer and soft tissue sarcoma

- Nexavar (sorafenib) - liver, kidney, and thyroid cancer
- Sutent (sunitinb) - kidney cancer, GI tract tumors, and pancreas tumors
- Caprelsa (vandetanib) - thyroid cancer
- Zelboraf (vemurafenib) - melanoma (skin cancer)

According to a 2013 study published in the New England Journal of Medicine, 76% of doctors approve the use of marijuana for metastatic breast cancer, and 82% of oncologists believe marijuana provides medical benefits according to a 2014 survey by WebMD.[252] Most doctors still recommend it only for palliative care, not for shrinking tumor size or preventing metastasis. Cancer patients are more likely to use cannabis in a state where it has been legalized for medical and/or recreational use.[301]

ROLE OF THE ENDOCANNABINOID SYSTEM IN CANCER TREATMENT

Cannabinoids including THC can kill cancer cells through a broad range of mechanisms that make them superior treatments to chemotherapy or radiation in some cases. Cannabinoids can stop tumor growth and cancer cell migration, or metastasis. Cannabinoids can induce a type of cell death called apoptosis only in cancer cells without killing surrounding healthy cells, while chemotherapy causes necrosis and inflammation, killing healthy cells.[302] Cannabinoids can also prevent angiogenesis, or the growth of new blood vessels that would provide nutrients to a tumor. Finally, cannabinoids can work synergistically with some chemotherapies.

CBD has more actions than at typical cannabinoid receptors CB1 and

CB2. CBD interacts with PPAR receptors to reduce angiogenesis and metastasis of cancer cells.[303] CBD has anti-inflammatory actions and antioxidant actions which can help healthy cells survive cancer treatments. CBD also upregulates 680 genes that are anti-cancer and down regulates 524 genes that are pro-cancer, including Id-1.[294] CBD can also stimulate brain cell growth, while chemotherapy and radiation treatment kill newborn hippocampal cells and further exacerbate cognitive issues in cancer and cancer survivorship.

Synthetic cannabinoids are also being used to target cancer in preclinical research. Breast cancer cells express CB2 receptors, and when they are removed, the breast cancer cells die, indicating they are important for their survival.[304] O-Quinone is a synthetic CB2 receptor agonist that is effective against triple-negative breast cancer.[305] JWH-015 is another synthetic CB2 receptor agonist that reduces breast cancer growth and metastasis.[304]

CLINICAL RESEARCH ON CANNABIS AND CANCER TREATMENT

More than 23,000 patients will be diagnosed with a brain or spinal cord cancer in 2016.[306] Gliomas are brain tumors than express mostly glial tissue and are the most common type of brain tumor. Gliomas have a poor prognosis with a 5% five-year survival rate. GW Pharmaceuticals is developing a proprietary CBD:THC combination product to treat glioblastoma in combination with standard treatment temozolomide, which successfully completed a Phase 1 study and finished Phase 2 trials.[307] 83% of glioblastoma patients using the CBD:THC drug survived one year compared to 53% of patients on placebo.

Several clinical trials have completed or are in progress looking at palliative use of cannabis in cancer. One study that is not yet recruiting is looking at a strain of low THC/high CBD cannabis for pain and inflammation in lung cancer patients undergoing radiation therapy.[308] Another study found Sativex, a 1:1 CBD to THC spray, reduced pain in cancer patients whose opioids did not fully control their severe pain.[309]

Dexanabinol, also known as HU-211, is a new synthetic cannabinoid that doesn't activate CB1 or CB2 receptors, but rather is an antagonist at NDMA receptors.[310] Dexanabinol is being investigated in combination with chemotherapy in patients with advanced tumors to see if tumor size decreases.[311] It also was studied for brain cancer[312] Interestingly, patients using natural cannabis products report greater relief of cancer or cancer-treatment symptoms than those treated with synthetic cannabinoids.[313]

CLINICAL RESEARCH ON CANNABIS AND TREATMENT OF SIDE EFFECTS OF CANCER TREATMENT

Chemotherapy and radiation can cause short-term side effects such as nausea and vomiting, and long-term effects such as chemotherapy-induced neuropathy or nerve pain and cognitive issues. A brand new study looked at 2970 cancer patients treated with medical cannabis between 2015 and 2017 in Israel, with over 50% of the patients being stage 4. 25% of patients died during the study, 18% stopped using cannabis, and out of the remaining 60%, 96% found cannabis improved their symptoms including sleep, pain, nausea, and lack of appetite.[314]

A review of 28 randomized controlled studies with 1,772 participants found general benefits of cannabinoids for chemotherapy-induced nausea and vomiting. Out of these 28 studies, 14 used nabilone, 9 used Marinol (THC), 4 used levonatradol, a synthetic analogue of THC developed by Pfizer that 30 times more potent than THC but never FDA approved, and 1 study used Sativex (nabiximols), a 1:1 ratio of CBD to THC.[315] Raw cannabinoids THCA and CBDA are actually more potent inhibitors of nausea and vomiting than THC or CBD. THCA is actually a stronger stimulant of appetite than THC.

Several clinical trials have completed or are in progress looking at cannabis and side effects of chemotherapy. One study that has completed looked at whether cannabis use during chemotherapy exacerbates chemotherapy-related cognitive impairment (CRCI).[316] Another study looked as nabilone for the treatment of pain in patients with chemotherapy-induced neuropathy.[317]

APPLICATION OF CANNABINOID MEDICINE TO CANCER TREATMENT

Treatment of cancer with cannabis is personalized medicine and should not be pursued without the guidance of a true professional. Your doctor may not know how to use cannabis besides telling you smoking it may increase your appetite or help with pain. You will need to consult a certified cannabis coach, cannabis nurse, or other vetted expert.

When people hear cannabis for cancer treatment, they are often told about "Rick Simpson Oil (RSO)" or "Phoenix Tears," named after Rick Simpson, who put his metastatic skin cancer into remission in 2003 with his oil. RSO is actually full extract cannabis oil (FECO), a highly concentrated form of THC taken daily for a total of 60g in 60 ml of oil over a total of 3 months. While many patients claim complete remission of their cancer or significant tumor size reduction, others have found their tumor grew in size or died during treatment. Because RSO has not been studied in clinical trials or studies, and is not commercially made in a standard manner, it is not clear whether this protocol is appropriate for all or any types of cancer. A patient that uses this method is do-at-your-own-risk, and this is not the only way to treat cancer.

Some patients may require more CBD and less THC due to estrogen-positive breast cancer, which may actually increase in size or metastasize with high doses of THC. Some patients may not be responsive to any cannabis treatment at all, perhaps because their subtype of cancer doesn't express typical cannabinoid receptors. Sometimes cancer patients with the same cancer, same stage, require completely different dosages or cannabinoid ratios. There is no one size-fits-all with cannabis for cancer.

Finally, rectal suppositories with THC and/or CBD are a great way to absorb very high amounts of THC needed to kill cancer without getting high. Rectal suppositories are also the preferred way to locally treat colon or prostate cancer. Vaginal suppositories may be helpful for treating uterine, cervical, endometrial, or bladder cancer in women. Little research on efficacy and safety of vaginal or rectal suppositories in cancer patients has been done, but anecdotal evidence of efficacy is overwhelming.

Future research needs to explore whether topical application of cannabis creams can reduce tumor size in breast, skin, and other cancers close to the skin surface. Injection of cannabinoids into tumors or CBD given intravenously (IV) to replace chemotherapy may be other ways cancer is treated in the future.

RISKS OF TREATING CANCER WITH CANNABINOID MEDICINE

Cannabinoid treatment protocols for specific types of cancer are still being developed, and it is truly personalized medicine. Because cannabis is not FDA-approved to treat cancer, you have to make the decision that cannabis treatment is appropriate for you in addition to your current treatments or as a stand-alone treatment.

As outlined in other chapters, CBD is a potent inhibitor of p450 liver enzymes CYP3A4 and CYP2C9. If you are taking a medication that says do not take with grapefruit, and you take CBD in tincture, pill, capsule, or edible form, you could end up with too much of your medication in your bloodstream and have unwanted side effects. This could happen with common drugs including warfarin, taken by millions to prevent blood clots, and antidepressants like Zoloft. The chemotherapy drugs that interact with CBD were listed in the first part of this section. Chemotherapy and CBD drug interactions are real and can be dangerous. Ways to mediate that risk include lowering your dose of medication under your doctor's guidance or lowering your dose of CBD to a dose that causes minimal inhibition of p450 enzymes.

One concern parents have is whether cannabis is safer for pediatric cancer. The answer is yes. In fact, a survey of 654 pediatric oncologists in legal medical marijuana states found 92% were willing to help pediatric cancer patients access medical marijuana.[255] The issue isn't that your child's oncologist won't support it, but that they don't know what product or dosage to recommend to you, and 43%

don't even know that cannabis is illegal at the Federal level.[255]

Pediatrician Dr. Bonnie Goldstein reported treating a 16 year old with stage 4 osteosarcoma (bone cancer) with 500 mg CBD and 500 mg THC daily, and scans showed no evidence of cancer after 3 months and in complete remission one year later. A case report details another physician successfully treating a child withe terminal acute leukemia with cannabis oil.[318] Children tolerate high doses of THC much better than adults, partly because their endocannabinoid system has not matured yet and the downstream pathways that are turned on when cannabinoid receptors are activated are not as strong as in adults. There are anecdotal reports of children not only tolerating hundreds of milligrams of THC, a dose that would put most adults to sleep for many hours or even days, but functioning on it.

CANCER SURVIVORSHIP

There are over 15.5 million Americans living with a history of cancer. Cancer survivorship focuses on the health and quality of life of a cancer patient after treatment through the end of life. Cancer is a chronic illness, and cancer survivorship is more than just physical health; it's psychological health, social health, and financial health, as cancer causes major changes to a person's lifestyle. Patients undergoing cancer treatment often have a ton of support that goes away once cancer is "beaten." Finally, cancer patients often grieve and have to cope with the fact that they have an incurable disease.

Cancer survivors have to manage their risk of cancer recurrence as well as deal with side effects or lasting damage from their cancer treatments. For example, most people don't realize cancer survivors struggle with fatigue, chronic pain, skin issues, sleep issues, cognitive issues similar to chemo fog, sexual dysfunction, and organ problems. Cancer survivors become socially withdrawn and are less likely to pursue healthy habits like proper diet, exercise, and quitting smoking or drinking. Cancer survivorship programs are often not supported by health insurance, or patients don't know they exist when they are free or reduced in price. Few cancer survivors are supported in their post-treatment phase.

ROLE OF THE ENDOCANNABINOID SYSTEM IN CANCER SURVIVORSHIP

Low levels of endocannabinoid levels will likely create an environment where cancer can again thrive and multiply. No cancer treatment kills 100% of cancer cells in your body, and new mutations could always occur in cells creating new tumors. Certain cancers have a higher rate of recurrence than others, and it's up to you to manage your risk through smart lifestyle choices as well as incorporating cannabinoid medicine. Little research has been done on endocannabinoid levels in cancer survivors or whether mutations in endocannabinoid genes reduce or increase cancer recurrence or mortality, but the future is exciting.

CLINICAL RESEARCH ON CANNABIS AND CANCER SURVIVORSHIP

We currently do not have data for whether cannabis, CBD or other cannabinoid use prevents recurrence of cancer or prevents mortality. IMPACT Network and other groups hope to perform these studies in the future.

APPLICATION OF CANNABINOID MEDICINE TO CANCER SURVIVORSHIP

Few traditional treatments are targeted for cancer survivors. Cannabinoid medicine can successfully treat many of the issues cancer survivors face. CBD can be used with or without caffeine to improve focus and attention and beat symptoms of chemotherapy-related cognitive impairment (CRCI) that persist years after treatment, impacting 14-85% of patients. CBD and other cannabis products can be used to treat anxiety, depression, sleep and fatigue issues that are often seen in cancer survivors. Cannabis cream topicals for skin pain or rashes, and cannabis lubes, topicals, or suppositories can be used to reduce vaginal dryness and pain during sex. Finally, cannabis as an alternative to HRT for menopause since breast cancer & ovarian cancer survivors are banned from using HRT.

RISKS OF TREATING A CANCER SURVIVOR WITH CANNABINOID MEDICINE

Because long-term effects of CBD, CBDA, THCA, or other cannabinoids have not been studied, it is not backed by science whether taking daily cannabinoids will decrease, increase or have no effect on cancer recurrence in general or specific cancers. Therefore, taking cannabinoids to prevent cancer recurrence is a follow-at-your-own-risk protocol.

As outlined in other chapters, CBD is a potent inhibitor of p450 liver enzymes CYP3A4 and CYP2C9. If you are taking a medication that says do not take with grapefruit, and you take CBD in tincture, pill, capsule, or edible form, you could end up with too much of your medication in your bloodstream and have unwanted side effects. This could happen with common drugs including warfarin, taken by millions to prevent blood clots, antidepressants like Zoloft, and opioids like fentanyl and oxycodone. Ways to mediate that risk include lowering your dose of medication under your doctor's guidance, or lowering your dose of CBD to a dose that causes minimal inhibition of p450 enzymes.

CHAPTER 9

Mental Health and the Endocannabinoid System

"I think we're desperately seeking new treatments for PTSD," she said. "Our hypothesis is that we believe cannabis will reduce the severity of the PTSD symptoms. But we don't know that ... it needs to be tested." - Dr. Sue Sisley, researcher on the first clinical trial on marijuana in U.S.

Mental illness touches every family. 1 in 5 American adults experience mental illness sometime in the year, with 1 in 25 adults experiencing severe mental illness that reduces their ability to work, go to school, and/or take care of his or her family. Sadly, many patients never receive a diagnosis or proper treatment for their mental illness due to lack of health insurance, being underinsured, or stigma about being labeled. Those that do get treatment may take years to find a medication that works for them or they make suffer unbearable side effects like sexual dysfunction. Finally, many patients are treatment-resistant, and never find something that works for them.

Thankfully cannabinoid medicine as emerged as a new treatment for mental conditions, one that may be especially effective for those with treatment-resistant forms. Cannabinoid medicine as a treatment for mental health makes sense because several brain regions that control emotional regulation, including the basolateral amygdala, prefrontal cortex, and hippocampus, all contain high levels of endocannabinoid receptors. A balance of endocannabinoid signaling is necessary for proper mental health, as upregulation of the endocannabinoid system can result in inappropriate fear responses, and downregulation of the endocannabinoid system can result in not enough emotional response as well as increased response to rewarding stimuli such as drugs.[319]

This chapter will outline the involvement of endocannabinoid deficiency and the mechanism of cannabis treatment for the following mental health disorders: anxiety, depression, bipolar depression, post-traumatic stress disorder (PTSD), and schizophrenia.

ANXIETY

Anxiety disorders are characterized by frequent, excessive, and intense worries and fears about normal situations. There are several types of anxiety disorders: general anxiety disorder, panic disorder, separation anxiety disorder, social anxiety disorder, and phobias.

Symptoms of anxiety include:

- feeling nervous, tense or restless
- feeling a sense of panic, danger or doom
- increase heart rate
- hyperventilating or rapid breathing
- excessive worrying
- trouble concentrating

- feeling tired or weak
- sweating
- shaking or trembling
- having trouble falling or staying asleep
- gastrointestinal problems such as upset stomach or vomiting
- avoiding people, places, or things that cause anxiety

Common treatments of anxiety are similar to depression and PTSD, including therapy and medication. Therapies include: cognitive-behavioral therapy (CBT), exposure therapy, interpersonal therapy (IPT), acceptance and commitment therapy (ACT) and eye movement desensitization and reprocessing (EMDR). Antidepressants are used to treat anxiety and include the following classes: selective serotonin reuptake inhibitors (SSRIs), selective norepinephrine inhibitors (SNRIs) and tricyclic antidepressants. Anti-anxiety medications are also known as benzodiazepines and include: Valium (diazepam), Klonopin (clonazepam), Ativan (lorazepam) and Xanax (alprazolam). Alternative therapies are also used to treat anxiety, including: transcranial magnetic stimulation (TMS), yoga, acupuncture, and meditation.

ROLE OF THE ENDOCANNABINOID SYSTEM IN ANXIETY

The endocannabinoid system regulates anxiety that is healthy and unhealthy. Activation of cannabinoid receptors in an area of the brain known as the periaqueductal gray (PAG) reduce the "fight or flight" response that is expressed as panic, anxiety, and gastrointestinal distress in humans.[235] When you are exposed to the same stressor repeatedly, your body adapts to the stressor and reduces its response to it. This process, called habituation, requires the endocannabinoid system.

The endocannabinoid system is like armor against the physical and emotional stressors of life. For patients that have endocannabinoid deficiency due to genetic causes or lifestyle choices, or for those who have impaired endocannabinoid system signaling due to months of chronic stress, their acute stress response goes into overdrive, making them incapable of handling the tiniest stressors.

There may be a link between mutations in genes that control the endocannabinoid system and anxiety. A SNP in the FAAH2 gene located on X chromosome causes anxiety.[320] It is likely that future research will show SNPs in genes that endocannabinoid system will mediate both endocannabinoid deficiency and responsiveness to cannabis treatment for anxiety.

CLINICAL RESEARCH ON CANNABIS AND ANXIETY

Cannabidiol, abbreviated CBD, is useful for both acute stress in healthy patients as well as patients with anxiety disorders. 300 mg of CBD reduced anxiety after but not before a simulated public speaking (abbreviated SPS) test in healthy volunteers.[321] Patients with Social Anxiety Disorder (SAD) who had never been treated with any medication had reduced anxiety and cognitive impairment during an SPS test when they took 600 mg of CBD 1 hour before.[322] Patients with SAD who took 400 mg of CBD had reduced anxiety as well as brain activity in areas that regulate mood and cognition as measured by SPECT.[323]

A clinical trial on sublingual CBD tincture taken three times daily for a month for anxiety will be launched at Harvard University in 2018. The dose of CBD in this study will be 28 mg/day.[324]

APPLICATION OF CANNABINOID MEDICINE TO ANXIETY

Anecdotal evidence exists for vaporizing or smoking high-CBD cannabis strains or taking sublingual CBD to reduce acute stress episodes. For scheduled episodes of high anxiety, such as a public speaking engagement, patients with anxiety may benefit from an oral dose of CBD in the range of 300-600 mg 1 hour before the stressful event. Daily low dose CBD therapy of 25 mg may be helpful to manage anxiety and prevent acute episodes.

RISKS OF TREATING A PATIENT WITH ANXIETY WITH CANNABINOID MEDICINE

There are several risks of treating a patient with cannabis or CBD products if they have anxiety. First, if a patient is on any prescription medications that are contradicted with grapefruit, they should also avoid products with CBD in it or adjust their dosage under the care of their doctor. CBD can inhibit liver p450 enzymes in the same fashion as grapefruit does, increasing or (in rare cases) decreasing the amount of drug that is absorbed. Taking CBD or cannabis containing CBD with Zoloft may cause an overdose or side effects such as nausea, mood swings, agitation, itchy skin and dizziness, particularly in patients such starting Zoloft. CBD may also interact with Prozac, BuSpar, Valium, and Halcion.

Second, CBD may induce short-term memory deficits in some patients. Recent animal research suggests this may be offset by taking caffeine as well.[325] Finally, products with THC may worsen anxiety, especially in social or stressful situations. A single oral dose of 10 mg in healthy patients produced anxiety and dysphoria, whereas 600 mg of CBD produced no measurable effect compared to placebo.[326] Products containing high CBD and low THC should be recommended. Finally, for those patients who will not avoid THC products, advise them to keep the THC dosage low, to not mix it with alcohol or other drugs, and to not consume it in a new place or with new people.[277]

DEPRESSION

Depression, also known as major depressive disorder, is a mood disorder that causes long-term feelings of sadness and withdrawal from daily activities. Depression is relatively common in the United States, with 17% of Americans having the condition at some point in their life. 7% of American adults had a least one major depressive episode in 2015 according to the National Survey on Drug Use and Health. A staggering 350 million people worldwide have depression.

Symptoms of depression include:

- Feeling sad, empty, hopeless or teary without cause
- Feeling irritable, frustrated, or angry without cause
- Feeling anxious, agitated, or restless
- Feeling guilty or worthless
- Trouble focusing, remembering, or making decisions
- Slow movement or thinking
- Lack of energy and tiredness

- Losing interest in everyday activities
- Change in appetite
- Change in sleep patterns or sleep quality
- Substance abuse
- Unexplained physical health issues like headaches or joint pain
- Suicidal thoughts, suicide attempts or suicide

Common treatments of depression include antidepressants and therapies, including psychotherapy, electroconvulsive therapy (ECT), and transcranial magnetic stimulation (TMS). Antidepressants are categorized into the following classes:

- Selective serotonin reuptake Inhibitors (SSRIs) including Prozac, Paxil, Zoloft, Celexa and Lexapro.
- Serotonin-norepinephrine reuptake inhibitors (SNRIs) including Cymbalta and Effexor.
- Norepinephrine-dopamine reuptake inhibitors (NDRIs) including Wellbutrin.
- Tricyclic antidepressants including amitriptyline and Vivactil.
- Atypical antidepressants and monoamine oxidase inhibitors (MAOIs) such as Parnate.

ROLE OF ENDOCANNABINOID SYSTEM IN DEPRESSION

Traditional treatments for depression have focused on modulating neurotransmitters like serotonin, dopamine, or norepinephrine. One class of neurotransmitters, endocannabinoids, are a novel therapeutic target. Endocannabinoids like anandamide and 2-AG regulate the pre-synaptic release of all other neurotransmitters. This means treating a patient with a treatment that stimulates cannabinoid receptors or boosts endogenous endocannabinoids may regulate serotonin or other neurotransmitter involved in the etiology of depression.

Marijuana use and depression are often comorbid. The endocannabinoid system helps us forget. Signs that your body is deficient in endocannabinoid signaling are negative thinking, inability to focus, nightmares, depression, and even PTSD. Since depression is often linked with focus on negative thoughts, it makes sense that cannabis can be used to help patients forget negative thought patterns.

In addition, depression and pain are often comorbid, with a co-occurrence of up to 80%.[327] As cannabis is an effective treatment for pain, many patients with pain who use cannabis may also see reduction in their symptoms of depression.

Marijuana use during depression has often been classified as substance abuse or cannabis use disorder (CUD) in the literature. Several clinical trials have looked at antidepressant treatment to treat comorbid depression and cannabis use disorder, however results have shown no effect on either disorder.[328-330] Instead of looking at cannabis use in a patient with depression as substance abuse, we should look at this as a form of self-medication. In fact, if a patient had a deficiency in the level of their natural endocannabinoids, it would follow that cannabis might relieve many of their depression symptoms.

Women may be more prone to endocannabinoid deficiency than men, especially because their endocannabinoid levels are linked with their menstrual cycle and estrogen levels. Women are also more likely to suffer from depression than men, and this may be due to endocannabinoid deficiency, both due to menstrual cycle stages as well as menopause. In fact, women with major depression have lower blood levels of anandamide and 2-AG.[236]

There may be a link between mutations in genes that control the endocannabinoid system and depression. A single nucleotide polymorphism, or SNP, in the CNR1 gene, which codes for the CB1 receptor, is associated with depression.[331] This suggests a role for the cannabinoid receptor type 1 in mood disorder. In addition, the same SNP is associated with antidepressant treatment resistance, especially in women with depression and comorbid anxiety and better response to citalopram in males with depression.[332]

A SNP in the CNR2 gene, which codes for the CB2 receptor, is associated with higher depression scores on the Hamilton Depression Rating Score (HDRS).[332] A different SNP in the CNR2 gene is associated with depression as well as alcoholism in Japanese men.[333]

A common SNP in the FAAH gene is associated with major depression in Caucasians.[331] FAAH is an enzyme that breaks down anandamide, and a SNP in the FAAH gene may boost levels of anandamide in the brain. In this case, too much anandamide may be as detrimental as not enough anandamide.

CLINICAL RESEARCH ON CANNABIS AND DEPRESSION

There have been no clinical trials of cannabis or CBD products in prevention or treatment of depression. A 2016 study found three months of medical marijuana treatment reduced self-reported symptoms of depression, reduced sleep disturbance, and improved quality of life.[334]

APPLICATION OF CANNABINOID MEDICINE TO DEPRESSION

Benefits of using cannabis over antidepressants and other medications include less side effects, and no risk of overdose or death. In some instances, antidepressant use can increase the risk of suicide, and that has not been reported with cannabis use.

Sativa strains can be helpful for depression during the day, as they can increase energy, creativity, and communication. Indica strains may be helpful at night, as it can help slow racing negative thoughts and help patients go to and stay asleep. Finally, using strains that have some CBD in them may be helpful to balance amotivational effects of THC as well as lower abuse potential.[335-336]

Finally, there's more to cannabis medicine than just cannabinoids when it comes down to treatment of depression and anxiety. Terpenes are chemicals that contribute to the smell of cannabis, but also have their own medicinal actions. For example, beta-caryophyllene (BCP) is a terpene found in many essential oils as well as cannabis. BCP acts as an atypical cannabinoid, activating CB2 receptors. In rodents, BCP's activation of CB2 receptors reduces anxiety and depression.[337] Strains rich in this terpene may be helpful to patients with depression.

RISKS OF TREATING A PATIENT WITH DEPRESSION WITH CANNABINOID MEDICINE

There are several risks of treating a patient with cannabis or CBD products if they have depression. First off, if a patient is on any prescription medications that are contradicted with grapefruit, they should also avoid products with CBD in it or adjust their dosage under the care of their doctor. CBD can inhibit liver p450 enzymes in the same fashion as grapefruit does, increasing or (in rare cases) decreasing the amount of drug that is absorbed. Taking CBD or cannabis containing CBD with Zoloft may cause an overdose or side effects such as nausea, mood swings, agitation, itchy skin and dizziness, particularly in patients such starting Zoloft. CBD may also interact with Prozac, BuSpar, Valium, and Halcion.

Second, if a patient is currently using Effexor XR (also known as venlafaxine), combining Effexor XR with cannabis can reduce the effectiveness of the antidepressant as well as increase the risk of cannabis use disorder due to increasing severity of marijuana withdrawal.[329-330] If a patient is currently on Effexor XR and would like to try CBD or cannabis products, it is recommended that he or she switches to a different antidepressant first to reduce addiction risk.

POST-TRAUMATIC STRESS DISORDER

Post-traumatic stress disorder (PTSD) is a mood disorder that develops in response to a traumatic event. The severity or type of traumatic event does not ensure that the exposed patient will get PTSD. Patients with PTSD are at increased risk of suicide, and more than 22 veterans a day take their own lives.

Male veterans are the demographic most commonly diagnosed with PTSD due to VA doctors being more educated on symptoms than other medical professionals. However, rape victims, police, ER nurses, 9/11 survivors, and many other demographics are also at high risk for PTSD due to chronic or acute stress. In fact, women are more likely to experience PTSD at some point in their lifetime, with incidence for women at 9.7% and men at 3.6%.

Symptoms of PTSD may occur within three months of a traumatic event but can also appear years after the event. Symptoms can vary in frequency and intensity over time and may go away permanently. PTSD symptoms can be grouped into four types: intrusive memories, avoidance, negative changes in mood and thinking, and changes in arousal symptoms.

Intrusive memories include:

- Flashbacks of the traumatic event
- Recurring and disturbing memories of the traumatic event
- Disturbing dreams about the traumatic event
- Panic induced by reminder of the traumatic event

Avoidance symptoms include:

- Avoiding talking or thinking about the traumatic event
- Avoiding people, places or activities that remind you of the traumatic event

Symptoms of negative changes in mood and thinking include:

- Feeling emotionally numb or unable to experience positive emotions
- Lack of interest in activities once enjoyed
- Feeling negative about self or other people
- Memory loss or problems including details of traumatic event
- Difficulty maintain close relationships
- Feeling hopeless about the future

Changes in arousal symptoms include:

- Irritable or aggressive behavior
- Angry outbursts
- Substance abuse
- Self-destructive behavior such as gambling or reckless driving
- Trouble sleeping
- Trouble concentrating
- Startling easy or easily scared
- On guard for danger or emergency situations
- Feelings of guilt and shame

Psychotherapy, including cognitive or talk therapy, exposure therapy, and eye movement desensitization and reprocessing are used to treat PTSD. The antidepressants Zoloft and Paxil are FDA-approved for treatment of PTSD, but many other antidepressants are used off-label for PTSD with various levels of efficacy. Anti-anxiety medications, sleep medications including Minipress, Ambien (zolpidem) and OTC drugs are also used for PTSD.

ROLE OF ENDOCANNABINOID SYSTEM IN PTSD

Marijuana use and PTSD are often comorbid. The endocannabinoid system helps us forget. Since PTSD is characterized by inability to forget traumatic experiences, that cannabis is used by patients to treat PTSD.

Marijuana use during PTSD has often been classified as substance abuse or cannabis use disorder (CUD) in the literature. Instead of looking at cannabis use in a patient with PTSD as substance abuse, we should look at this as a form of self-medication. In fact, if a patient had a deficiency in the level of their natural endocannabinoids, it would follow that cannabis might relieve many of their PTSD symptoms.

There are documented cases of endocannabinoid deficiency in PTSD. After the 9/11 attack on the World Trade Center, many New Yorkers developed PTSD, and this was associated with reduced blood levels of the endocannabinoid 2-AG years later.[338] Low levels of the endocannabinoid anandamide in these patients was also associated with high retention of traumatic memories associated with the attack.[338]

In addition, 2013 study found reduced levels of anandamide in patients with PTSD, particularly in women.[339] These patients had increased number of CB1 receptors, as measured using PET scan to compensate for their anandamide deficiency.[339] A follow up study found increased number of CB1 receptors in the amygdala, the brain center for emotional processing, is associated with increased attention to threat or perceived threat.[243]

Genetics play a huge role in response to therapy and medications for PTSD. For example, a SNP in the gene for BDNF, which encodes brain derived neurotrophic factor, results in low levels of BDNF and poor response to exposure therapy.[340] A common SNP in the CNR1 gene, which encodes the CB1 receptor, is associated with increased severity of fear in PTSD patients.[341]

CLINICAL RESEARCH ON CANNABIS AND PTSD

Cannabis is effective to treat sleep disturbances which both exacerbate PTSD symptoms and are main symptom themselves. Nabilone, a synthetic version of THC, has been validated for use with PTSD in several clinical studies. A max dosage of 3 mg of THC for seven weeks reduced frequency and intensity of nightmares in military personnel with PTSD in a small pilot study.[342] An average final dose of 4 mg of THC for an average length of 11 weeks decreased PTSD-associated insomnia, nightmares, PTSD symptoms, and chronic pain in prisoners.[343] Finally, in a pilot study of 10 patients with PTSD on stable medication, adding 5 mg of THC twice a day reduced frequency of nightmares and improved both sleep quality as well as frequency of nightmares.[344]

Clinical trials on the safety and efficacy of cannabis strains with varying potencies of THC and CBD are underway in both Canada and the United States. The American study has been spearheaded by advocate for veterans Dr. Sue Sisley.

Finally, cannabis treatment of pediatric patients with PTSD may be safe. A case report was published in 2016 on a ten-year-old girl with

PTSD who showed reduced anxiety and sleep improvement after treatment with 25 mg of CBD before bedtime as well as sublingual CBD spray administration when anxious.[345]

APPLICATION OF CANNABINOID MEDICINE TO PTSD

To improve sleep quality and reduce insomnia and nightmare, THC should be eaten in edible, tincture, or pill form before bedtime. Start with a low dose of 1 mg if possible, and increase dosage slowly over time until desired effects are seen. In patients that wake up and still feel the effects of THC in the morning, try starting treatment after dinner to combat the delay in onset of action. A max dosage of 5 mg of THC taken orally should be observed as to not trigger psychosis.

There is significant anecdotal evidence that smoking medical marijuana can improve mood and focus, and reduce substance abuse and negative thinking in patients with PTSD. Strains of cannabis that are sativa as opposed to indica can promote these outcomes as well as reduce substance abuse risk. In addition, strains containing some amount of CBD in addition to THC may be helpful in reducing anxiety without inducing psychosis.

RISKS OF TREATING A PATIENT WITH PTSD WITH CANNABINOID MEDICINE

There are several risks of treating a patient with cannabis or CBD products if they have PTSD. First, if a patient is on any prescription medications that are contradicted with grapefruit, they should also avoid products with CBD in it or adjust their dosage under the care of their doctor. CBD can inhibit liver p450 enzymes in the same fashion as grapefruit does, increasing or (in rare cases) decreasing the amount of drug that is absorbed. Taking CBD or cannabis containing CBD with Zoloft may cause an overdose or side effects such as nausea, mood swings, agitation, itchy skin and dizziness, particularly in patients such starting Zoloft. CBD may also interact with Prozac, BuSpar, Valium, Halcion, and methadone.

If a patient is taking medications that may interact with CBD, an alternative is available. Nabilone, aka synthetic THC, has been available as a prescription in Canada since 1981 and has a very low abuse potential and minimal interaction with p450 enzymes.[346] Marinol is the equivalent in the United States, as well as cannabis products that contain THC.

Finally, cannabinoid hyperemesis syndrome has been reported in heavy users of cannabis, including veterans with PTSD. Cannabinoid hyperemesis is characterized by cyclical nausea, vomiting, and abdominal pain that is relieved by multiple hot baths or showers. The syndrome is distinct from cannabis withdrawal, and in fact using cannabis results in additional nausea and vomiting. The syndrome is rare, and average duration of cannabis use before onset of symptoms is 16 years.[347] For patients that display this syndrome, cannabis is not advised.

CHAPTER 10

Pain and the Endocannabinoid System

"Examples of the patients' responses were as follows: 'I wish I had received this treatment when I was first diagnosed with fibromyalgia,' 'I returned to be the same person as before,' 'I regained my health," and 'This is a miraculous treatment.' "
– Dr. George Habib, author of Medical Cannabis for the Treatment of Fibromyalgia

Twenty-five million Americans experience chronic pain, which is defined as pain every day for three or more months. Over 40 million American adults have pain that requires some treatment but may not fit the definition of chronic pain due to a shorter duration than 3 months or episodic nature of pain. Chronic pain costs America over $600 billion annually in healthcare costs as well as lost productivity in the workforce. Solutions like cannabis must be introduced to improve quality of life for patients and reduce burden on our healthcare system.

The United States is in the midst of rapidly growing opioid epidemic where more than 115 Americans are dying each day from an opioid overdose.[348] New York City reported the opioid epidemic cost the city over $500 million dollars. Sadly, 94% of patients in treatment for opioid addiction said they chose to use heroin because they could not afford or obtain prescription opioids.[349] The addiction, deaths, and impact to families and communities is devastating. Cannabis provides an alternative to opioid treatment for pain as well as a treatment for opioid abuse itself.

There are many conditions involving acute or chronic pain that cannabis can effectively treat, however, inclusion of all of them would require a series, not a single book. This chapter will outline the involvement of endocannabinoid deficiency and the mechanism of cannabis treatment for the following conditions involving chronic pain: migraine headache, back pain, and fibromyalgia.

MIGRAINE HEADACHE

36 million Americans, approximately 12% of the country, suffer from migraine. Migraine is a medical condition with enormous personal and socioeconomic costs, impacting one in four American households.[350] Specifically, these costs reached $17 billion in the United States in 2005 and resulted in work loss for almost all sufferers.[351-352] Sadly, in 2012 the National Institute of Health (NIH) funded only $8 million for migraine-related research. This is a fraction of 1% of the total NIH research budget, despite over 30% of women suffering from migraine. Migraine headache is characterized by a throbbing headache that typically affects one side of the head and is often accompanied by nausea and disturbed vision. Migraines can last hours or days and can range from minor to so disabling a patient needs to go to the hospital to terminate it. Migraines can begin anytime in life and can be triggered by stress, alcohol, food and food additives, loud noises, bright lights, sleep changes and hormonal changes like menstruation,

pregnancy, or menopause.

Migraines have four stages: prodrome, aura, headache and post-drome. Not all patients experience all stages. Some patients are aware of when a migraine is about to happen, a phenomenon called aura. Auras happen before or with headache, and can include tingling on one side of face, arm or leg, blind spots or flashes of lights.

Symptoms of migraine headache include:

Prodrome (one to two days before migraine):

- increased yawning
- increased thirst and urination
- neck stiffness
- food cravings
- rapid mood changes
- constipation

Aura (before or during migraine):

- seeing flashes of light, shapes or bright spots
- vision loss
- difficulty speaking
- hearing music or noises
- uncontrollable twitching
- pins and needles feeling in arms or legs
- weakness or numbness in face or one side of the body

Headache (during migraine):

- throbbing or pulsing pain on one or both sides of head
- nausea and vomiting
- blurred vision
- lightheadedness or fainting
- sensitivity to light, sounds, smell or touch

Post-drome (24 hours after migraine):

- sensitivity to light and sound
- fatigue
- euphoria
- moodiness
- dizziness
- confusion

Common treatments of migraine headache include triptans, which increase serotonin. Triptans include: Axert (almotriptan), Relpax (eletriptan), Frova (frovatriptan), Amerge (naratriptan), Maxalt (rizatriptan), Imitrex or Alsuma (sumatriptan), and Zomig (zolmitriptan). Midrin (acetaminophen isometheptene-dichloralphenazone), Cafergot (erogtamine tartrate), Migranal Nasal Spray (dihydroergotamine) are also used to treat migraines. OTC medications used include Excedrin Migraine (aspirin, acetaminophen and caffeine), Motrin Migraine and Advil Migraine (ibuprofen). Finally, nausea and vomiting associated with migraine are treated with drugs prescribed in addition to the treatments above: Compro (prochlorperazine), Reglan (metoclopramide), Thorazine (chlorpromazine), Inapsine (droperidol).

Drugs to prevent migraine include Botox, anti-seizure medications including Neurontin (gabapentin), Topamax (topiramate), Depakote (valproic acid), antidepressants including amitriptyline and Aventyl (nortriptyline), and drug used to treat high blood pressure including calcium channel blocker verapamil and beta-blockers propranolol, metropolol, and timodol. Alternative therapies are also used to treat migraine and include: transcranial magnetic stimulation (TMS), biofeedback, yoga, acupuncture, and meditation. Finally, a new FDA-approved device called Cefaly is a headband TENS unit worn once a day for 20 minutes to prevent migraine.

ROLE OF THE ENDOCANNABINOID SYSTEM IN MIGRAINE HEADACHE

It has been proposed that migraine HA may be rooted in endocannabinoid deficiency, and that this concept explain why the condition is responsive to cannabis treatment.[353] Patients with chronic migraine HA have reduced levels of fatty acid amide hydrolase (FAAH), the enzyme that breaks down the endocannabinoid anandamide (AEA), suggesting an adaptive behavior of the endocannabinoid system.[354] Finally, migraine HA is often comorbid with conditions also linked to endocannabinoid deficiency, including irritable bowel syndrome, fibromyalgia, and psoriasis.[353]

Although identification and validation of biomarkers has facilitated diagnostic tests for many medical conditions, there is no diagnostic for migraine.[355] No study has measured plasma levels of endocannabinoid AEA in patients with migraine HA. Determining levels of plasma endocannabinoids in healthy patients and demonstrating a deficiency in endocannabinoids in patients with migraine HA would provide health insurance companies with a reason to coverage cannabinoid treatment for migraine HA.

Serotonin plays a key role in migraine HA, as serotonin agonists selective for the 5-HT_{1B} and 5-HT_{1D} receptors, called triptans, are effective for migraine HA.[356] Buspirone, a partial 5-HT1A agonist, is also effective for reducing headache frequency but not intensity and more often used to treat anxiety.[357-358] 5-HT_{1A} hypersensitivity may explain increase incidence of migraine attacks during periods of anxiety as well as explain migraine subtypes.[359-361]

Evidence suggests THC, the psychoactive component of cannabis, but not CBD, regulates serotonin release from blood platelets, modulating migraine.[175] It has not been reported whether novel cannabinoids in marijuana such as cannabichromene (CBC) or tetrahydrocannabivarin (THCV) regulate serotonin release from platelets. Cannabis strains with THC are also effective in reducing nausea, which is present in up to 50% of patients with episodic migraine.[362]

A number of preclinical studies suggest cannabinoids may be useful in the treatment of migraine. Both CB1 and CB2 receptors are involved in migraine. Mutations in the cannabinoid receptor 1 gene (CNR1) are associated with migraine in humans.[363] Endocannabinoids acting at the CB1 receptor in the periaqueductal gray (PAG) regulate trigeminovascular pathways that contribute to the severe throbbing nature of pain in migraine.[364] Rodents given anandamide had reduced pain in an animal model of migraine.[365]

Finally, activation of CB2 receptors reduces pain in an animal model of migraine.[366]

CLINICAL RESEARCH ON CANNABIS AND MIGRAINE HEADACHE

Pilot data suggests cannabis or cannabinoids in cannabis are effective for migraine.[367] A case study of five patients who used dronabinol, which is synthetic THC, with or without additional marijuana products, showed a reduction in migraine frequency.[368] A survey of over 1400 medical marijuana patients in California found 18% were using medical marijuana to treat migraine.[257] A recent study found Colorado patients using medical cannabis in edible or smokable form had a significant reduction in frequency of migraine.[369]

APPLICATION OF CANNABINOID MEDICINE TO MIGRAINE HEADACHE

Cannabis can be used in many ways to prevent and treat headache. Vaping cannabis can provide almost instantaneous relief of headache for an hour or two without the health risks of smoking. However, it does not provide all-day relief, nor is this method good for preventing headaches. In order to prevent headaches, steady-state levels of cannabinoids need to be achieved through CBD and/or THC transdermal patches, tinctures or pills containing a 1:1 to ratio of CBD to THC, or frequent application of transdermal pens to the wrist,

THC or CBD applied topically to the back of neck (BON) can be absorbed through the skin and into unmylineated neurons that are close to the surface, where they reduce pain and other migraine symptoms. This topical regional neuro-affective (TRNA) approach was created by Dr. Ronald Aung-Din, the creator of Migraderm, which an oral migraine medication turned into a topical cream at a compounding pharmacy applied BON. CBD is now applied to the BON via his new product Cannidex, but any cannabis or CBD topical should be somewhat effect for reducing muscle tension locally as well as transdermally impacting nerves that signal pain.

Anecdotal evidence suggests patient using cannabis strains such as "Durban Poison" or "Durban Haze" containing the rare cannabinoid THCV experience reduced migraine. THCV appears to be well-tolerated and not psychoactive at a 10 mg oral dose in humans.[370-372] The mechanism of how THCV works is still unclear. THCV is suggested to be a neutral antagonist at the CB1 receptor, which means it binds to the receptor but does not activate it.[373] THCV can activate CB2 receptors in vitro and decrease signs of inflammation and pain in mice via CB1 and/or CB2 receptor activation.[374] THCV can also enhance serotonin receptor 5-HT_{1A} activation, may also impart antipsychotic effects.[375] As migraine is often comorbid with mental illness, another explanation for relief from migraine seen by using cannabis enriched in THCV may be due to these antipsychotic effects. THCV also shows potential to reduce nausea, which is often a symptom of chronic migraine.[376-377]

RISKS OF TREATING A PATIENT WITH MIGRAINE HEADACHE WITH CANNABINOID MEDICINE

CBD can inhibit liver p450 enzymes in the same fashion as grapefruit does, increasing or (in rare cases) decreasing the amount of drug that is absorbed. Taking CBD or cannabis containing CBD with Zoloft (sertraline) may cause an overdose or side effects such as nausea, mood swings, agitation, itchy skin and dizziness, particularly in patients such starting Zoloft. CBD may also interact with Prozac, BuSpar, Valium, and Halcion.

BACK PAIN

Back pain is classified as acute if it lasts less than six weeks and chronic pain if it lasts three months or more. Causes of back pain include injuries such as falls, car accidents, or strains from heavy lifting, arthritis, fibromyalgia, endometriosis, osteoporosis, scoliosis, and bulging or ruptured disks in your spine. Over 80% of Americans will experience an episode of severe lower back pain in their lifetime.

Unfortunately, back pain is a $100 billion dollar a year industry in the United States, fueled by unnecessary or dangerous surgeries, injections, opioid painkillers, and alternative therapies such as chiropractic adjustments. Many times, the treatments do not help, and in the case of surgeries and opioids, can actually increase pain. In 2017, the American College of Physicians issued new recommendations that limit prescribing OxyContin and Vicodin for back pain because of their high potential for abuse and overdose.

Symptoms of back pain include:

- shooting, stabbing, or burning pain in the upper, middle, or lower back or any combination of regions
- pain that spreads down one or more legs (sciatica)
- back spasms
- inability to bend over or twist back

Common treatments of back pain include medications, physical therapy, and surgery. Medications used include OTC pain relievers, such as aspirin, ibuprofen (Advil and Motrin), naproxen (Aleve), and acetaminophen (Tylenol), prescription anti-inflammatories including meloxicam, celecoxib (Celebrex), piroxicam (Feldene), diclofenac (Voltaren), etodolac (Lodine), and indomethacin (Indocin), prescription muscle relaxants including cyclobenzaprine (Flexeril), carisopodol (Soma) and baclofen, and antidepressants including amitriptyline.

Prescription opiates like oxycodone and morphine (MS-Contin) are now used as a last resort for severe acute pain and discouraged against use for chronic back pain. Injections of corticosterone, topical OTC or prescription pain relieving or numbing creams, ice packs, heating pads, chiropractic treatments, physical therapy, yoga, massage, and acupuncture are also used to treat chronic back pain. Surgery, such as to relieve back pain from herniated disks, is used as a last resort.

ROLE OF THE ENDOCANNABINOID SYSTEM IN BACK PAIN

Pain is processed in brain regions such as the periaqueductal gray (PAG), thalamus, medulla, and amygdala, as well as the spinal dorsal horn. Activation of CB1 receptors can suppress processing of pain in any of these regions, while blocking these receptors can cause hypersensitivity to pain. CB1 and CB2 receptor activation can also reduce inflammation and overexcitability that leads to muscle spasms through alpha-3 glycine receptors.[378]

Treating back pain and other forms of severe chronic pain with cannabis is preferable to opioids besides the obvious reasons of less risk of overdose and addiction.[379] The lowest dose of opioids, taken for three weeks, causes inflammation and other changes in the brain and spinal cord that are almost identical to clinical depression.[380] In fact, long-term use of opioids often leads to depression and more pain in patients, not less pain. Cannabis has the ability to treat the source of the pain, while improving depression, not causing it.

There may be a link between mutations in genes that control the endocannabinoid system and perception of pain. SNPs in FAAH are associated with decreased pain sensitivity when exposed to cold and decreased need for post-operative oxycodone pain relief in women with breast cancer.[381] However, no studies have specifically looked at perception of back pain and mutations in endocannabinoid system genes.

CLINICAL RESEARCH ON CANNABIS AND BACK PAIN

Patients are now using cannabis as a substitute for prescription drugs, mainly opioid painkillers.[382-383] A study from the Journal of the American Medical Association (JAMA) found cannabis use for chronic pain, including back pain, is supported by high-quality evidence.[384]

Another study surveyed marijuana patients, 66% of whom had a history of chronic pain. Patients reported 75% symptom relief from using cannabis for their condition.[385] GW Pharmaceuticals has performed the most clinical research on cannabis, with several double-blind placebo-controlled studies on CBD, THC or 1:1 CBD to THC ratio products for different forms of pain used to approve drugs like Sativex. GW Pharmaceutical's studies have found that Sativex, the 1:1 CBD to THC product was effective for several types of chronic pain.[386]

APPLICATION OF CANNABINOID MEDICINE TO BACK PAIN

Many patients report vaporizing or smoking an indica cannabis strain provides immediate and substantial pain relief. There is anecdotal evidence that smoking some sativa strains, the type that increases creativity and wakefulness may actually intensify perception of back pain, not the back pain itself. So, it is likely if you just tried a joint from a friend to see if it would help your back pain and it didn't, you might have used the wrong strain for back pain. Smoking or vaporizing an indica cannabis strain with CBD in it may be more effective at relieving pain than one without CBD.

To help relax painful, burning, tingling, or cramping back, neck, or legs, use a deep penetrating THC and/or CBD cream. Make sure you really rub it in where you are knotted or tight in the back, as opposed to applying it lightly like you do a body lotion. Using a heating pad on top of where you applied your lotion may help it penetrate more deeply. The sciatic nerve is deep in the back, and many low THC creams or creams without additional ingredients to increase bioavailability and penetration will not reach the nerve when applied locally. Look for the highest strength topical cannabis cream on the market, consult a caregiver who can make a specific formulation for you, or make one yourself by consulting a book on making cannabis topicals.

Finally, some patients prefer using cannabis transdermal patches, cannabis oil, cannabis oil pills, or cannabis edibles to treat their pain. These can all be safe and effective methods, but it may take some time to find a product that works best for you at the correct dosage.

RISKS OF TREATING A PATIENT WITH BACK PAIN WITH CANNABINOID MEDICINE

Many patients are already on opioid painkillers and may take some time to wean off them completely even if they want to switch to cannabis. Cannabis can be taken safely with most opioids, although those that are contradicted are highlighted below. In fact, one study found cannabis combined with opioids was more effective at reducing pain than opioids alone.[387]

If a patient is on any prescription medications that are contradicted with grapefruit, they should also avoid products with CBD in it or adjust their dosage under the care of their doctor. CBD can inhibit liver p450 enzymes in the same fashion as grapefruit does, increasing or (in rare cases) decreasing the amount of drug that is absorbed. Eating products with CBD or cannabis containing CBD with the specific opioids fentanyl, methadone, or oxycodone could result in an overdose or side effects such as respiratory depression or sedation. It is suggested that you reduce your dosage of opioids or CBD if you have adverse effects taking them and remember to go slow and talk to your doctor if possible. THC does not cause the same inhibition of p450 enzymes, so it's always an option to forgo CBD completely if you find it's not a fit with your current medication.

FIBROMYALGIA

Fibromyalgia is characterized by widespread musculoskeletal pain accompanied by fatigue, sleep, memory, and mood issues. It is often diagnosed by pressing on tender points throughout the body that result in pain upon light touching. Fibromyalgia flares occur when symptoms rapidly increase in severity or number; these flares may last for days or weeks and are often dependent on stress levels or triggers like poor diet.

Approximately 10 million patients in the United States have fibromyalgia, and 75-90% are women. While the cause of fibromyalgia is unknown, infections, physical or emotional trauma, and genetics appear to play a role in onset. Patients with lupus, osteoarthritis, and or rheumatoid arthritis are at higher risk of developing fibromyalgia.

In Canada, 30% of patients with fibromyalgia are on disability, whereas in the United States, the percentage is unclear because disability as well as a fibromyalgia diagnosis is harder for patients to obtain. In a survey conducted by the National Fibromyalgia Association in 2003, 99% of the respondents who were currently disabled because of fibromyalgia said that they would return to work immediately if they could find some relief for their pain.

Symptoms of fibromyalgia include muscle pain and tenderness, muscle spasms, joint pain, bone pain, neurological pain, pelvic pain, fatigue, sleep disturbances, headaches, anxiety or depression, gastrointestinal issues, and cognitive issues including memory problems.

Common treatments of fibromyalgia include anti-inflammatories such as Aleve (naproxen), Advil or Motrin (ibuprofen), aspirin, and meloxicam, pain relievers Tylenol (acetaminophen), morphine (MS-contin), and Percocet (oxycodone) and anti-anxiety medications including Valium (diazepam), Klonopin (clonazepam), Ativan (lorazepam) and Xanax (alprazolam). Anti-depressants including selective serotonin reuptake inhibitors (SSRIs) like Prozac (fluoxetine) and Zoloft (sertraline), selective norepinephrine inhibitors (SNRIs) like Cymbalta (duloxetine) and Savella (milnacipran), and tricyclic antidepressants like amitriptyline are also used.

Anti-seizure drug Lyrica (pregabalin) is most well-known for fibromyalgia because of the constant commercials played in the United States; Neurontin (gabapentin) is another anticonvulsant used to treat fibromyalgia. Finally, alternative therapies such as acupuncture, myofascial therapy, massage therapy, yoga, meditation, and cognitive therapy are also used to treat fibromyalgia.

ROLE OF THE ENDOCANNABINOID SYSTEM IN FIBROMYALGIA

Cannabis helps fibromyalgia by reducing neuropathic pain, pelvic pain, and other forms of pain. It reduces spasm, headaches, inflammation, and anxiety and stress that may trigger or worsen flares. It can improve mood and depression that often comes with having a painful chronic disease with no cure. Finally, cannabis may improve serotonin or other neurotransmitter imbalances in fibromyalgia.

No genetic causes of fibromyalgia have been found yet, and a blood test for diagnosis was only recently developed and not widely used. It is possible that mutations in genes that regulate the endocannabinoid system could be involved in its development, but no study has looked at that.

CLINICAL RESEARCH ON CANNABIS AND FIBROMYALGIA

There is limited clinical research on cannabis and fibromyalgia because of its Schedule 1 nature in the United States and limited funding on the medical benefits of cannabis. However, a survey by the National Pain Report found cannabis was more effective than standard treatments for fibromyalgia including Cymbalta, Lyrica, and Savella and fibromyalgia patients prefer it. No research has suggested harm from using cannabis in fibromyalgia patients.

Patients are already using cannabis, partly due to tightening restrictions on opioid use in the United States. The National Fibromyalgia and Chronic Pain Association completed a survey on the impact on patients of changing hydrocodone from Schedule 3 to Schedule 2. The survey found 17% of fibromyalgia patients who were no longer able to fill their hydrocodone prescription shifted to medical marijuana, and 13% moved to alcohol to treat pain, a much less desirable outcome.[388] Another study published in 2012 found 13% of fibromyalgia patients used cannabis, with 80% using smoked marijuana and 24% using prescription cannabinoids.[389]

In a pilot study of nine patients, THC in doses of 2.5-15 mg per day for three months significantly reduced subjective pain in the four patients that completed the study.[390] In a study of 40 patients with fibromyalgia, four weeks of 1 mg of nabilone, a synthetic THC-like drug that binds strongly to the CB1 receptor improved insomnia but have little impact on pain, mood or quality of life.[391] 28 fibromyalgia patients using cannabis had significantly reduced pain and stiffness and increased feeling of well-being, relaxation, and sleepiness two hours after use in another study.[392] Finally, a survey of fibromyalgia patients in Israel found 50% of patients stopped using all prescriptions medications for fibromyalgia when they began using cannabis, and there were significant improvements in all quality of life and symptom scores on the Revised Fibromyalgia Impact Questionnaire (FIQR).[393]

APPLICATION OF CANNABINOID MEDICINE TO FIBROMYALGIA

Because cannabis as a treatment for fibromyalgia has not been thoroughly researched, especially in terms of cannabinoids such as CBD and THCA, it is difficult to recommend dosages and cannabinoid ratios for fibromyalgia patients. However, from working with fibromyalgia patients, and because I am a fibromyalgia patient myself, I do have personal experience to share. To help relax painful, burning, tingling, or cramping arms, legs, back, neck, and feet, I use a deep penetrating THC cream that works for about three hours before re-application. To control pelvic pain, I use a suppository containing THC and CBD once a week.

I normally do not vape cannabis containing only THC during the day because I find I cannot provide the intense focus needed for scientific research, science writing or editing. Comedy writing, music, art, and dance seem amenable to using cannabis and creating, making sure books are properly formatted and referenced is not, at least for me. If I do choose to vape cannabis during the day to treat breakthrough pain, it is from a strain with high CBD and little THC, or one with a 1:1 CBD to THC ratio to provide balanced and long-lasting pain relief. Many patients can tolerate THC during the day, and some indica cannabis strains or hybrid sativa and indica strains can provide pain relief without causing sleepiness.

In addition to cannabis, I use a combination of dietary supplements and alternative therapies to control my fibromyalgia and other conditions despite living a stress-filled non-stop life. I make sure to take B vitamins, lysine (which limits viral replication, important for fibromyalgia patients who often have multiple viral infections), co-enzyme Q10, NAC, vitamin D, ashwagandha, 5-HTP, and melatonin at night. I also fit in a massage when I can fit it in or afford it; I know that massage and chiropractors are a luxury for many people. I alternate between taking Epsom salt baths and CBD or CBD and THC bath bomb hot baths each night to relieve pain and relax muscles.

RISKS OF TREATING A PATIENT WITH FIBROMYALGIA WITH CANNABINOID MEDICINE

There are several risks of treating a patient with cannabis or CBD products if they have fibromyalgia. First, if a patient is on any prescription medications that are contradicted with grapefruit, they should also avoid products with CBD in it or adjust their dosage under the care of their doctor. CBD can inhibit liver p450 enzymes in the same fashion as grapefruit does, increasing or (in rare cases) decreasing the amount of drug that is absorbed. Taking CBD or cannabis containing CBD with Zoloft may cause an overdose or side effects such as nausea, mood swings, agitation, itchy skin and dizziness, particularly in patients such starting Zoloft. CBD may also interact with Prozac, BuSpar, Valium, and Halcion.

For those patients who choose to take THC products, advise them to keep the THC dosage low, to not mix it with alcohol or other drugs, and to not consume it in a new place or with new people.[277]

CHAPTER 11

Women's Health and the Endocannabinoid System

"More human studies are needed to more fully understand the effects of marijuana dosing and chronicity on gonadotropin and ovarian hormone regulation, fertility, pregnancy maintenance, parturition and lactation." – Lisa Brents, Ph.D.

Women's health is an area of medicine neglected by both mainstream medicine and the cannabis industry until recently. Diseases impacting women receive less research funding from the National Institute of Health (NIH), less medications are developed for those diseases, and women are less likely to be diagnosed and treated for diseases that predominantly impact women. Case in point: there are many kinds of drugs to treat sexual dysfunction in men but none in women.

Cannabis and women's health is a passion of mine due to the benefits cannabis has brought me and clients I've worked with. It's the reason why I founded IMPACT Network, the first and only 501c3 nonprofit institute dedicated to clinical research, education, and advocacy on cannabis for women's health. 1 in 8 women will develop invasive breast cancer in her lifetime; cannabis can help. 84% of women have period pain; cannabis can replace Midol. 18% of women have migraine headaches and women are three times more likely to get them than men; cannabis is more effective than most treatments for migraine. 18% of women have anxiety and are twice as likely as men to develop it; CBD is a safe and effective treatment for it that doesn't cause sexual dysfunction. Menopause impacts all women; cannabis can help treat symptoms and prevent bone loss.

There are many conditions involving women's health that cannabis can effectively treat, however, inclusion of all of them would require a series, not a single book, and some have already been covered in previous chapters. This chapter will outline the involvement of endocannabinoid deficiency and the mechanism of cannabis treatment for the following conditions involving impacting women: pelvic pain, endometriosis, and menopause.

PELVIC PAIN

Pelvic pain is pain and/or cramps located in the abdomen and pelvis, and may be related to reproductive, urinary, digestive, or musculoskeletal issues. Women that have suffered from physical or sexual abuse also have an increased risk for chronic pelvic pain. I will be going over cannabis for endometriosis, a condition that underlies a significant proportion of pelvic pain cases, in the next section.

Pelvic pain can be acute or chronic (lasting more than 6 months), can be mild or severe, and be localized or radiate to the back, buttocks, and/or thighs. It can be sharp and stabbing or dull. Pelvic pain may only happen after certain activities, such as after sexual activity, after urination, or only at certain times, like right before the menstrual period starts or during ovulation.

Acute pelvic pain related to menstruation is called dysmenorrhea. Dysmenorrhea is reported by 84% of women, with 43% reporting pain with every period.[394] Severe dysmenorrhea is serious, resulting in work sick days that impact both employee and employer. Severe dysmenorrhea is often undertreated and poorly managed due to its cyclical nature.

Chronic pelvic pain lasting 6 months or more impact about 25% of women. It costs the American healthcare system over $900 million dollars a year, so chronic pelvic pain isn't a condition that should be ignored.[395] Chronic pelvic pain is misunderstood and undertreated, leaving women with additional issues like depression, anxiety, substance abuse, and sexual dysfunction. Chronic pelvic pain can cause work absences, disability, and harm relationships.

Common treatments for pelvic pain include medications, physical therapy, and surgery. Medications used are OTC, such as aspirin, ibuprofen (Advil), and acetaminophen (Tylenol), prescription muscle relaxants including gabapentin and baclofen, prescription anti-inflammatories including meloxicam, celecoxib (Celebrex), piroxicam (Feldene), diclofenac (Voltaren), etodolac (Lodine), and indomethacin (Indocin), and prescription opiates like oxycodone and morphine (MS-Contin) as a last resort for severe pelvic pain. Antidepressants are also prescribed:

- Selective serotonin reuptake Inhibitors (SSRIs) including Prozac, Paxil, Zoloft, Celexa and Lexapro.
- Serotonin-norepinephrine reuptake inhibitors (SNRIs) including Cymbalta and Effexor.
- Norepinephrine-dopamine reuptake inhibitors (NDRIs)

including Wellbutrin.

- Tricyclic antidepressants including amitriptyline and Vivactil.
- Atypical antidepressants and monoamine oxidase inhibitors (MAOIs) such as Parnate.

Hormonal therapies including hormonal birth control pills, patches, injections, implants and IUDs are also used to treat chronic pelvic pain. Antibiotics for STDs or pelvic inflammatory disease, including ofloxacin, metronidazole, ceftriaxone and doxycycline, are used when the source of pelvic pain is bacterial. Pelvic floor therapy is a specialized form of pelvic floor therapy which includes massaging, stretching, lengthening, and relaxing pelvic muscles. Surgery is used as a last resort to remove fibroids, endometriosis, and adhesions, to cut or destroy nerves that relay pelvic pain, or to perform a hysterectomy – complete or partial removal of the uterus.

ROLE OF ENDOCANNABINOID SYSTEM IN PELVIC PAIN

All components of the endocannabinoid system are found in reproductive organs and other organs that may contribute to pelvic pain. Cannabis has been used patients to self-medicate for pain and muscle spasms for thousands of years. CB1 receptors in the brain mediate anti-nociceptive effects of cannabis. Particular brain regions involved include the periaqueductal gray (PAG), thalamus, medulla, and amygdala. Cannabinoids also suppress the processing of pain in spinal dorsal horn. Mice that have the FAAH gene knocked out have high levels of anandamide and show reduced response to pain.[396] Blocking CB1 receptors with drugs causes hypersensitivity to pain, called hyperalgesia.

The placebo effect is also mediated by the endocannabinoid system in addition to the opioid system.[397] A single nucleotide polymorphism, or SNP, in the FAAH gene, which codes for the enzyme that breaks down anandamide, is associated with increased pain relief from placebo immediately and 24 hours after administration.[398]

There may be a link between mutations in genes that control the endocannabinoid system and perception of pain. SNPs in FAAH are also associated with decreased pain sensitivity when exposed to cold and decreased need for post-operative oxycodone pain relief in women with breast cancer.[381] However, no association between CNR1 SNPs and premenstrual dysphoric disorder (PMDD) in women was found.[399]

CLINICAL RESEARCH ON CANNABIS AND PELVIC PAIN

3.5% of patient's in HelloMD's 2016 survey of medical marijuana patients are using cannabis to treat symptoms of premenstrual syndrome, commonly abbreviated as PMS.[257] There have been no clinical trials of cannabis or CBD products in prevention or treatment of pelvic pain in women. A survey of men with chronic pelvic pain in Canada found more than 50% of men with the syndrome used cannabis for their pain and 61% found an improvement in symptoms.[400]

There have been clinical trials on a drug that manipulates the endocannabinoid system for relief of pelvic pain. Fatty amide hydrolase, abbreviated as FAAH, is the enzyme that breaks down anandamide. If you inhibit the activity of FAAH, you can prolong the activity of anandamide at the synapse and boost endocannabinoid function. Increased anandamide levels means more signaling at the

CB1 and CB2 receptors, providing pain relief.

One pharmaceutical company, Astellas Pharma, has developed a drug tentatively called ASP3652. ASP3652 inhibits FAAH, but cannot cross the blood-brain-barrier. Thus, ASP3652 inhibits FAAH only in the peripheral nervous system, not in the brain, reducing THC-like side effects normally seen with activation of CB1 receptors in the brain.

Phase 2 trials found 300 mg of ASP3652 twice a day was needed to boost anandamide blood levels to their peak values. Astellas Pharmaceutical's main goal is to develop this drug for chronic pelvic pain disorders.

APPLICATION OF CANNABINOID MEDICINE TO PELVIC PAIN

Cannabinoid therapy can be a safe alternative to medications for pelvic pain. Cannabis has less side effects than painkillers, hormonal treatments, or antidepressants, and no risk of overdose or death. In some instances, antidepressant use can increase the risk of suicide, and that has not been reported with cannabis use.

Some patients with mutations in the FAAH gene are actually at increased risk for opioid-induced respiratory depression and/or refractory postoperative nausea and vomiting (PONV), meaning that opiates and/or surgery are unsafe and cannabis is the wiser choice .[401]

Cannabis medicine is also a great alternative to taking OTC painkillers like Tylenol or prescription painkillers with acetaminophen added. Acetaminophen depletes the body of glutathione, a master antioxidant that recycles other antioxidants and is a cofactor for many biological processes. Glutathione deficiency increases oxidative stress, accumulation of toxins and heavy metals, and inability to repair DNA, perpetuating the cycle of pain.

Smoking or vaporizing “indica” strains of cannabis may provide immediate relief of pelvic pain symptoms and spasms. Indica strains may be more sedating for patients than “sativa” strains, so a hybrid strain of indica and sativa may be suggested for daytime use for pelvic pain and indica strain for nighttime use.

Taking CBD and/or THC orally in the form of pills, tinctures, or edibles can also help with pelvic pain, however due to metabolism through the liver, pain relief and level of sedation can be unpredictable, and correct dosage is highly personal. Oral administration of THC and CBD make take anywhere from 30 minutes to 2 hours to take effect, which can be too long for someone in severe pelvic pain.

Sublingual administration of cannabinoids, that is under the tongue, can take effect within 10 minutes and bypasses the liver, providing a quicker and more consistent pain relief profile than oral cannabinoid administration. Dosage is customized by the patient due to lack of dosage guidelines for this condition.

Topicals containing THC and/or CBD may be helpful for patients with pelvic pain and cramps. Simply have the patient rub the topical on their abdomen, avoiding their labia, and their lower back and combined with a heating pad, this may be enough to relieve pain without introducing THC into the bloodstream. This is especially helpful for patients that cannot have THC in their blood due to employer drug testing. Unfortunately, topicals do not work for a small percentage of patients, perhaps due to issues with skin penetrability.

Vaginal suppositories containing a combination of CBD and THC are an effective way to treat severe pelvic pain and cramps. Foria Relief is a product on the market containing 60 mg of THC and 10 mg of CBD in a cocoa butter base. Other product makers are coming out with cannabinoid vaginal suppositories, and these products can be made at home by caregivers using organic cannabis and organic coconut oil.

Pain and spasm relief is found within 30 minutes using a cannabinoid vaginal suppository, and because the cannabinoids are absorbed through the vaginal wall, first pass metabolism through the liver is avoided. This increases bioavailability of the cannabinoids and prevents a "high" feeling from the THC because it only being used by your body locally in your reproductive system.

RISKS OF TREATING A PATIENT WITH PELVIC PAIN WITH CANNABINOID MEDICINE

There are several risks of treating a patient with cannabis or CBD products if they have pelvic pain. First off, if a patient is on any prescription medications that are contradicted with grapefruit, they should also avoid products with CBD in it or adjust their dosage under the care of their doctor. CBD can inhibit liver p450 enzymes in the same fashion as grapefruit does, increasing or (in rare cases) decreasing the amount of drug that is absorbed. Taking CBD or cannabis containing CBD orally with opiate pain relievers fentanyl, oxycodone, or methadone may cause respiratory depression or overdose.

CBD may also interact with the antidepressants Zoloft and Prozac and the muscle relaxant Valium, increasing their side effects. CBD may also interact with hormonal birth control that contains either estradiol or ethinylestradiol, increasing risk of blood clots and breast cancer. The CBD drug interactions will not occur using routes of administration that avoid the liver, such as smoking, sublingual, and vaginal administration.

Finally, if a patient is currently using Effexor XR (also known as venlafaxine), combining Effexor XR with cannabis can reduce the effectiveness of the antidepressant as well as increase the risk of cannabis use disorder due to increasing severity of marijuana withdrawal.[329-330] If a patient is currently on Effexor XR and would like to try CBD or cannabis products, it is recommended that he or she switches to a different antidepressant first to reduce addiction risk.

ENDOMETRIOSIS

Endometriosis occurs when the tissue that lines the inside of the uterus, called the endometrium, grows outside the uterus. Endometriosis impacts 10% of all women, a total of 176 million women worldwide. Diagnosis of endometriosis may take up to a decade, often because women and doctors are uneducated about the disease, it mimics many other diseases, and diagnosis requires surgery.

Symptoms can range from no pain at all, to pain and heavy bleeding only during menstrual periods and disabling pain 24/7. Severity of pain is not related to the four stages of endometriosis. There is no clear cause of endometriosis, although there is increased risk if you have an autoimmune disorder, and there is no permanent cure.

Endometriosis can be found growing in the ovaries, bowels or pelvis, but occasionally grows in the lungs, brain and other areas. Endometriosis sheds similarly to uterine lining, causing bleeding and pain in organs during the menstrual period. Severe endometriosis can cause adhesions and scar tissue. Organs can attach to each other or the spine, causing severe pain and reducing mobility permanently.

Symptoms of endometriosis include:

- Dysmenorrhea (painful periods)
- Chronic back, abdominal, and/or pelvic pain, especially during menstrual period
- Pain during or after sex
- Pain with urination or bowel movements, especially during menstrual period
- Excessive heavy bleeding during period
- Bleeding between periods
- Nausea and bloating, especially during period
- Constipation and/or diarrhea, especially during period
- Fatigue
- Infertility

Common treatments of endometriosis include medications to slow the growth of the endometrium and surgery to remove endometriosis:

- Hormonal Birth Control: including pills, patches, and vaginal rings with estrogen, often continuously without allowing for periods.
- Progestin therapy: including Mirena, an IUD releasing the hormone, a hormone implant, or a hormone injection (Depo-Provera).
- Danazol is a drug that blocks ovarian-stimulating hormones, preventing menstruation.
- Lupron is an injection of a gonadotropin-releasing hormone agonists that blocks the production of ovarian-stimulating hormones, causing temporary menopause. It was originally used as chemotherapy to treat prostate cancer.
- Laparoscopic surgery is used to diagnose endometriosis as well as perform excision surgery to remove tissue.
- Painkillers are also used with little efficacy:
    - OTC: ibuprofen and naproxen.
    - Prescription: opiates should be avoided due to abuse liability.
- Finally, hysterectomy to remove the uterus, cervix, and ovaries is often done as a last resort, but still does not relieve symptoms for many women.

ROLE OF ENDOCANNABINOID SYSTEM IN ENDOMETRIOSIS

Interestingly endometriosis is often comorbid with gastrointestinal and immune disorders, two classes of disorders strongly linked to endocannabinoid system dysfunction.[402] The endocannabinoid system regulates migration of cells, and since endometriosis is abnormal migration of endometrial tissue, it is clear the endocannabinoid system is involved in the progression of this disease.

Many components of the endocannabinoid system are found in endometrial tissue and their levels are regulated by the menstrual cycle in rodent models of the disease. These include cannabinoid receptors type 1 and type 2 (CB1 and CB2), atypical cannabinoid receptors GPR18, N-acyl phosphatidylethanolamine phospholipase D (NAPE-PLD), an enzyme that synthesizes endocannabinoids, and fatty acid amide hydrolase (FAAH), an enzyme that breaks down endocannabinoids.

Endometriosis is linked to endocannabinoid dysfunction. Blood levels of endocannabinoids anandamide and 2-AG were elevated in women with endometriosis as compared to healthy women.[403] This is not healthy, but a response to decreased CB1 receptor expression in endometrial cells of women with endometriosis.[403-404] In fact, women with moderate-to-high pain symptoms had higher levels of anandamide than those with low-moderate pain symptoms. CB2 receptor, TRPV receptor and FAAH expression was normal in endometrial cells of women with endometriosis compared to healthy women. Reduced ECS function leads to growth of endometriosis throughout the body and more pain, and endometriosis pain is mediated through the CB1 receptor.[405]

Activating CB1 receptors on endometrial cells in endometriosis appear to have positive and negative effects. CB1 receptor activation appears to reduce growth of endometriosis lesions but encourage their migration. Human endometriosis cells proliferated (divided and grew) less when stimulated with a synthetic cannabinoid called WIN 55212-2.[406] Rodent studies of endometriosis found animals had more pain when treated with AM251, a drug that inhibits the cannabinoid receptors, and less pain when treated with WIN 55212-2.[405]

THC activates atypical cannabinoid receptors GPR18 and increases migration of endometrial cells, while CBD prevented the THC-induced migration.[122] This means administering THC and CBD together should reduce proliferation while not promoting migration of endometriosis cells. This is particularly interesting considering vaginal suppositories exist on the market that contain both CBD and THC.

Treating endometriosis is not all about the cannabinoids. Beta-caryophyllene, abbreviated BCP, is a terpene found in cannabis as well as many spices including black pepper, cloves, and copaiba. BCP activates CB2 receptors, which are found mainly in the immune system and brain, as well as the female reproductive system.[407] BCP reduced the growth of endometriosis in rodents by 50%.[408] Bayer Pharmaceuticals owns a patent, published in 2012, on synthetic CB2 agonists for treatment and prevention of endometriosis. Perhaps a CB2 drug for endometriosis will be introduced into their R&D pipeline in the future.

WHY IS THE ENDOCANNABINOID SYSTEM DISRUPTED IN WOMEN WITH ENDOMETRIOSIS?

No research has been performed to discover whether or not women with endometriosis have mutations in endocannabinoid system genes. However, environmental influences may be an easier cause to unravel.

Environmental toxins such as dioxins and PCBs have been linked to endocannabinoid dysfunction. 90% of human exposure to dioxins is through food, specifically meat, fish and dairy. Dioxin exposure almost completely wipes out levels of CB1 receptors in endometrial tissue from healthy women, similar to the levels found in endometrial tissue from women with endometriosis.[404] Women with endometriosis were found to have higher levels of dioxins in their fat tissue than healthy women.[409]

As women are subjected to pollution in the air, water, grass, and food as well as BPA in water bottles and receipts, it's no wonder why so many women in developed countries now have severe endometriosis. Future research may link more toxins to endometriosis risk as well as endocannabinoid deficiency.

CLINICAL RESEARCH ON CANNABIS AND ENDOMETRIOSIS

Cannabis reduces inflammation, which may be the root cause of endometriosis symptoms. Cannabis also reduces pain, spasms, nausea and vomiting, both from the disease and from side effects of medications taken for the disease. Cannabis may also reduce progression of endometriosis to advanced stages.

There have been no clinical trials of cannabis or CBD products in prevention or treatment of endometriosis in women, but synthetic drugs that target the endocannabinoid system are in development. An interesting study on atypical cannabinoid PEA in Europe showed promised for endometriosis pelvic pain. A pill containing 400 mg of PEA and 40 mg of transpolydatin, a pro-drug for the anti-oxidant resveratrol, taken twice a day for 90 days reduced pelvic pain related to endometriosis significantly after 30 days, although treatment with selective COX-2 inhibitor celecoxib (Celebrex) was more effective at pain relief than PEA/transpolydatin. .[410-411] 400 mg of PEA and 40 mg of transpolydatin once a day for 10 days also reduced pelvic pain.[412] Unfortunately PEA is hard to find in the American market, hopefully this will change in the future.

Future research should ask the following questions:

- Are women who smoke cannabis less likely to develop endometriosis?
- Do women that use cannabis experience less pain and decreased endometriosis growth?
- Are oral or transvaginal cannabis products the best way to treat endometriosis?
- Are mutations in endocannabinoid genes associated with endometriosis?
- Is there a non-invasive diagnostic test for endometriosis that can be developed using endocannabinoid system biomarkers?

APPLICATION OF CANNABINOID MEDICINE TO ENDOMETRIOSIS

Cannabinoid therapy can be a safe alternative to hormone replacement therapy, especially for women who cannot take it due to breast or ovarian cancer risk or lack of health insurance. It also has less side effects than estrogen replacement therapy or antidepressants, and no risk of overdose or death. In some instances, antidepressant use can increase the risk of suicide, and that has not been reported with cannabis use.

Juicing raw cannabis may reduce pain and inflammation associated with endometriosis, without the high experienced with THC. That's because raw cannabis has THCA and/or CBDA, the non-psychoactive raw acid forms of THC and CBD. For patients without access to raw cannabis juice, THCA tinctures or pills will have a similar effect.
All methods for using cannabis for pelvic pain apply for using cannabis for endometriosis. I highly suggest vaginal suppositories for their ability to stop the progression of endometriosis over merely masking the symptoms of the disease.

Future research on safety and efficacy of cannabinoid vaginal suppositories that should be performed:

- Bioavailability of THC and CBD via vaginal suppository
- Impact on vaginal suppositories on vaginal pH
- Impact of carriers, for example coconut oil versus cocoa butter
- Bioavailability of contaminants including pesticides or solvents through the vaginal wall
- Schedule of dosing required to maintain steady state levels of cannabinoids – daily or every couple of days?
- Efficacy toward pelvic pain and endometriosis

Finally, women with endometriosis are also strongly encouraged to avoid chemicals in their food, hair and beauty products, and environment in addition to using cannabis medicine. A vegan or vegetarian diet, along with organic fruits and vegetables, can support cannabis treatment due to low exposure to toxins.

RISKS OF TREATING A PATIENT WITH ENDOMETRIOSIS WITH CANNABINOID MEDICINE

There are several risks of treating a patient with cannabis or CBD products if they have endometriosis. CBD is a potent inhibitor of CYP3A4 and CYP2C9, two p450 liver enzymes that break down drugs including estrogen found in hormonal birth control.[413] Ethinyloestradiol is 30% metabolized by CYP3A4 and CYP2C9 enzymes, with the rest broken down by other processes or excreted in the urine.[414] CBD has been found to cause drug interactions through its inhibition of p450 liver enzymes. By inhibiting the breakdown of these other drugs, CBD can raise the blood level of concurrently administered drugs like epilepsy drugs, antipsychotics, and blood thinners. Thus, CBD is contraindicated with these drugs and can produce dangerous side effects.[415]

CBD could raise blood levels of estrogen and cause potential health risks such as blood clots in the legs or lungs, breast cancer, headaches, excess vaginal bleeding, and nausea and vomiting. It's important that women using estrogen-based birth control switch to progesterone-based or non-hormonal birth control, or perhaps switch to THC instead of CBD use.

In addition, is very important that women with endometriosis on hormonal treatments do not smoke, and this also means smoke cannabis. Smoking increases the risk of deadly blood clots, which is already elevated from hormone therapy. Vaporizing cannabis is better than smoking cannabis in a joint, pipe, or bong because it doesn't burn the cannabis. Smoking cannabis releases toxins similar to cigarettes, can cause lung irritation and often disintegrates cannabinoids with healing properties. Vaporizing cannabis heats the air around the cannabis, releasing a range of cannabinoids, each with unique health benefit.

MENOPAUSE

Menopause is the natural end of the menstrual cycle in women, and is defined as 12 months after the last menstrual period. The average age of menopause in American women is 51. By 2020, there will be more than 50 million American women in menopause, and most women are living a third or more of their lifespan after menopause. As life expectancy increases around the globe, so does the number of postmenopausal women. In 1998 there were 477 million postmenopausal women globally; in 2025 there will be 1.1 billion. That's right, by 2025 there will be 1.1 billion endocannabinoid deficient women worldwide.

Menopause can happen prematurely, that is, before women enter their 40s, due to genetics, illness, or medical procedures. In fact, many of the conditions women treat with cannabis are linked to premature menopause due to the illness or the traditional treatment, making cannabis a more appropriate treatment for women. These include epilepsy and cancer.

Symptoms of menopause include:

- Irregular periods
- Mood swings
- Hot flashes during the day
- Night sweats that prevent sleep

- Trouble concentrating
- Vaginal dryness
- Decreased sex drive
- Muscle loss
- Slowed metabolism
- Weight gain
- Urinary incontinence
- Thinning hair
- Dry skin

Common treatments of menopause include hormone therapy and medications. Hormone replacement therapy (HRT) is a combination of estrogen and progesterone, while estrogen replacement therapy (ERT) is only estrogen and is for women who have had a hysterectomy. Some women cannot use HRT or ERT because of previous history of breast cancer or blood clots. For these women, low doses of antidepressants are prescribed, including SNRIs Cymbalta and Effexor and NDRI Wellbutrin. Gabapentin (neurontin) is prescribed for hot flashes in for women who can't take hormones or have severe migraine.

Osteoporosis is a condition associated with menopause that can be prevented or treated with medication. These medications include bisphosphonates such as Fosamax, Actonel, Boniva, and Zoledronic acid, Evista, an estrogen receptor modulator that is also a breast cancer drug, and Forteo, a parathyroid hormone.

Holistic strategies for treating symptoms of menopause include taking 20-40 mg of black cohosh herb twice a day, avoiding caffeine and alcohol, following a healthy diet, having a good sleep schedule, doing regular exercise, quitting smoking, performing Kegel exercises to strengthen the pelvic muscles, and using vaginal lubricants to fight dryness.

ROLE OF ENDOCANNABINOID SYSTEM IN MENOPAUSE

The endocannabinoid system's role in menopause and postmenopausal health is an area of medicine lacking in research. One day genetic studies will see if mutations in endocannabinoid system genes are correlated with early or premature menopause. Because the reproductive system contains cannabinoid receptors that interact with estrogen, endocannabinoids directly influence the menstrual cycle and menopause.

Effects of aging on the endocannabinoid system are more pronounced in women than in men. Reduction in endocannabinoids signaling may be responsible for some of the negative symptoms we associate with menopause, like hot flashes. This is not surprising as estrogen levels are linked to endocannabinoid levels, and both peak at ovulation, something that does not occur in menopausal and postmenopausal women.[182] Fatty acid amide hydrolase (FAAH), the enzyme that breaks down the endocannabinoid anandamide and controls it levels, is regulated by both estrogen and progesterone.[416-417] In fact, activation of estrogen receptors and cannabinoid receptors on the same cells often synergize to produce greater effects than the combination of both by themselves.[418]

Estrogen recruits the endocannabinoid system to regulate emotional response and relieves anxiety and depression through its actions on the brain in areas like the hippocampus.[419] Lowered levels of estrogen during and after menopause means less activation of the endocannabinoid system, and poor ability to respond to stress and elevate mood accordingly.

Traditional treatments for menopause have focused on modulating neurotransmitters like serotonin or hormones like estrogen and progesterone. One class of neurotransmitters, endocannabinoids, are a novel therapeutic target. Endocannabinoids like anandamide and 2-AG regulate the pre-synaptic release of all other neurotransmitters. This means treating a patient with a treatment that stimulates cannabinoid receptors or boosts endogenous endocannabinoids may regulate serotonin, replacing the need for a traditional antidepressant.

The endocannabinoid system regulates the bone loss seen after menopause. Cannabinoid receptor type 2 (CB2) are found on bone cells, called osteoblasts. A common mutation in the CNR2 gene that codes CB2 in humans, resulting in fewer CB2 receptors, is associated with decreased lumbar spine bone mineral density (BMD) and increased risk of osteoporosis after menopause.[107,420]

CLINICAL RESEARCH ON CANNABIS AND MENOPAUSE

2% of patient's in HelloMD's 2016 survey of medical marijuana patients are using cannabis to treat symptoms of menopause.[257] A 2016 study found three months of medical marijuana treatment reduced self-reported symptoms of depression, reduced sleep disturbance, and improved quality of life, which may be relevant to relieving symptoms of menopause.[334]

There have been no clinical trials of cannabis or CBD products in prevention or treatment of menopause. However, Astellas

Pharmaceuticals has completed a Phase 2 clinical trial of drug ASP3652 in post-menopausal women. ASP3652 may be able to treat symptoms of menopause or osteoporosis in women without the typical psychoactive effective seen with oral THC treatment. However, however no results have been published yet as to the safety or efficacy of ASP3652 in post-menopausal women.

APPLICATION OF CANNABINOID MEDICINE TO MENOPAUSE

Cannabinoid therapy can be a safe alternative to hormone replacement therapy, especially for women who cannot take it due to breast or ovarian cancer risk or lack of health insurance. It also has less side effects than estrogen replacement therapy or antidepressants, and no risk of overdose or death. In some instances, antidepressant use can increase the risk of suicide, and that has not been reported with cannabis use.

Hormone replacement therapy (HRT) used to be the gold standard for treating menopause and post-menopausal symptoms. However, a study called the Women's Health Initiative (WHI) identified the dangers of HRT including increasing the risk of breast cancer, heart disease, blood clots, and stroke.[421] The study found HRT to be so dangerous that it was stopped early. Estrogen replacement therapy (ERT) increases the risk of blood clots and stroke but not breast cancer or heart disease according to the WHI study. Finally, increased risk of these serious conditions associated with HRT or ERT are long-term, and were present 3 years after the therapies were discontinued.

Cannabinoid therapy can also be a safe alternative to medications for osteoporosis. Side effects are the main reason patients quit osteoporosis drugs, and these include abnormal heart rhythms, flu-like illness, nausea, vomiting, and bone pain. Cannabis does not cause these side effects and in fact reduces pain. Trans-caryophyllene, a terpene related to BCP that also activates CB2 receptors, has been found to enhance the formation of bone and maintenance of bone mass in a recent study looking at osteoblasts.[422] Thus, trans-caryophyllene is protective against osteoporosis, and cannabis strains containing BCP or trans-caryophyllene may be helpful for menopause.

Smoking sativa cannabis strains can be helpful for fatigue during the day, as they can increase energy, creativity, and communication. Indica strains may be helpful at night, help patients go to and stay asleep. Using strains that have some CBD in them may be helpful to balance amotivational effects of THC as well as lower abuse potential.[335-336] Finally, cannabinoid vaginal suppositories maybe helpful in replacing hormone therapy and reducing vaginal dryness.

RISKS OF TREATING A PATIENT WITH MENOPAUSE WITH CANNABINOID MEDICINE

There are some risks of treating a patient with cannabis or CBD products if they have menopause, especially if they are using HRT. CBD is a potent inhibitor of CYP3A4 and CYP2C9, two p450 liver enzymes that break down drugs including estrogen found in hormonal birth control.[413] Ethinyloestradiol is 30% metabolized by CYP3A4 and CYP2C9 enzymes, with the rest broken down by other processes or excreted in the urine.[414] CBD could raise blood levels of estrogen and cause potential health risks such as blood clots in the legs or lungs, breast cancer, headaches, excess vaginal bleeding, and nausea and vomiting. It's important that women using HRT for menopause talk to their doctor about coming off of it, or perhaps switch to THC instead of CBD use.

In addition, is very important that women on HRT do not smoke, and this also means smoke cannabis. Smoking increases this risk of deadly blood clots, which is already elevated from hormone therapy. Vaporizing cannabis is better than smoking cannabis in a joint, pipe, or bong because it doesn't burn the cannabis. Smoking cannabis releases toxins similar to cigarettes, can cause lung irritation and often disintegrates cannabinoids with healing properties. Vaporizing cannabis heats the air around the cannabis, releasing a range of cannabinoids, each with unique health benefit.

CBD may also induce short-term memory deficits in some patients, which may be a serious concern in older patients. Recent animal research suggests this may be offset by taking caffeine in addition to CBD.[325]

CHAPTER 12

Other Conditions and the Endocannabinoid System

"Further research of these compounds could provide opportunities to treat a large number of clinical disorders where suppressing the immune response is actually beneficial"
– Prakash Nagarkatti, Ph.D.

There are many more conditions rooted in endocannabinoid deficiency, including those that impact the gastrointestinal system, the brain, the skin, and the immune system. This book unfortunately cannot go into depth into each one or else it would be a series of three or more books. This chapter will provide an overview of the role endocannabinoid deficiency plays in the autoimmune disorder lupus, skin conditions, hair conditions, and even creativity.

LUPUS

Lupus is a chronic autoimmune disease in which your body can't tell the difference between viruses, germs and bacteria and your body's own healthy tissue. This leads to your immune system creating antibodies that attack and destroy healthy tissue, leading to inflammation, pain and damage to body parts. Lupus is characterized by flares, where symptoms worsen, and remissions, when symptoms improve. Unlike HIV or AIDS, where the immune system is underactive, the immune system is overactive in lupus.

2 million Americans live with lupus, and most are women between the age of 15-45. The most severe cases of lupus are found in Asians and African-Americans. The most common type of lupus is system lupus erythematosus, which attacks several body organs. Drug-induced lupus is caused by using one of over 400 legal prescription drugs, including those used to treat Crohn's disease. Other types of lupus include cutaneous lupus, which mainly attacks skin and forms a butterfly-shaped rash across the nose, lupus nephritis, which attacks the kidneys, and neonatal lupus, which occurs in babies born to mothers with lupus.

Symptoms of lupus include pain all over but focused in hands, fingers, wrists, and knees, skin rashes, mouth sores, fatigue, mood changes, swelling of hands and feet, nausea, vomiting, depression, anxiety, seizures, fevers, weight loss, chest pain, hair loss, ulcers, swollen lymph nodes, blood clots, anemia and abnormal heart rate.

Common treatments of lupus include NSAIDs such as Aleve (naproxen) and Advil or Motrin (ibuprofen), anti-malaria drug Plaquenil (hydroxycholoroquinine), corticosteroids including A-Methapred and Medrol (methylprednisolone), immune system suppressants including Imuran or Azasan (azathioprine), CellCept (mycophenolate mofetil), and Trexall (methotrexate), and biologics Benlysta (belimumab) and Rituxan (rituximab). Alternative therapies are also used to treat lupus including acupuncture, meditation, and exercise.

ROLE OF THE ENDOCANNABINOID SYSTEM IN LUPUS

How the endocannabinoid system is disrupted in lupus is an area of medicine lacking in research. One day genetic studies will see if mutations in ECS genes are correlated with lupus. Because the immune system contains CB2 receptors, endocannabinoids directly influence the immune system.

Increased levels of follicle-stimulating hormone (FSH) in patients with lupus can have negative consequences on the endocannabinoid system. FAAH, the enzyme that breaks down anandamide, was identified as the sole endocannabinoid target of FSH and it increases its activity through multiple pathways.[423] Chronic increases in levels of FSH may stimulate FAAH gene expression and thus lower levels of anandamide, causing endocannabinoid deficiency.

Women with lupus are also more like to undergo premature menopause because inflammation caused by the disease can harm the ovaries. Premature menopause may reduce endocannabinoid system function, as outlined in Chapter 4 under causes of endocannabinoid deficiency.

APPLICATION OF CANNABINOID MEDICINE TO LUPUS

Pain and inflammation are two major symptoms of lupus, and cannabis helps relieve both without nasty side effects that prescription medications have. Cannabis increases levels of anti-inflammatory protein interleukin-10 and decreases levels of pro-inflammatory protein interleukin-2. Cannabis also suppresses the immune system by activating myeloid-derived suppressor cells (MDSCs).[424] MDSCs may help dampen the hyperactive immune system found in lupus. Cannabis also helps treat symptoms of nausea and abdominal cramping that are often severe side effects of commonly prescribed drug for lupus, such as Plaquenil and corticosteroids.

THCA is a non-psychoactive cannabinoid that relieves pain and inflammation and has shown promise in lupus patients. CBD is another non-psychoactive cannabinoid that can be taken with THCA and/or THC to treat lupus. Cannabinoids like THCV and CBD can stimulate bone growth and may offset the risk of osteoporosis seen with long-term corticosteroid use in lupus patients. Because cannabis is personalized medicine and the field is young, it may take some time for patients to discover the products, cannabinoid ratios, and dosages that works best for them.

RISKS OF TREATING A PATIENT WITH LUPUS WITH CANNABINOID MEDICINE

If a patient is on any prescription medications that are contradicted with grapefruit, they should also avoid products with CBD in it or adjust their dosage under the care of their doctor. CBD can inhibit liver p450 enzymes in the same fashion as grapefruit does, increasing or (in rare cases) decreasing the amount of drug that is absorbed. Taking CBD or cannabis containing CBD with methylprednisolone may cause hyperglycemia or other unwanted effects, and dosage may need to be reduced or the patient should be switched to prednisone, an alternative steroid not metabolized by CYP3A4.

SKIN AND HAIR CONDITIONS

CB1, CB2 and TRPV1 cannabinoid receptors are present in the skin, where they sense pain, touch, itch and temperature and regulate skin cell growth, oil production, hair production, and inflammation.[425] Few cannabinoid receptors are found deep in the skin and most are found near the surface. Endocannabinoid deficiency can result in skin that is cancerous, dry and itchy, or has hives, rashes, acne or has too little or too much hair. Interestingly, UV light activates CB1 and CB2 receptors in the skin and may play a role in development of skin cancer.[426]

ACNE

Acne is caused by bacteria, combined with dirt and oil, and reduced shedding of skin cells. Many of us have struggled with in our teenage years and may still deal with in our adult years. 85% of young adults have some form of acne, 15-30% have it severe enough to seek medical treatment, and 2-7% continue to struggle with it their entire lives or are left with disfiguring acne scars.

Current prescription and OTC acne treatments available are either expensive, ineffective, or consist of harsh chemicals with intolerable side effects. Stimulation of CB2 receptors in skin increases oil production, while CBD does the opposite, shutting down oil production and reducing acne.[427] Topical CBD application holds promise as a treatment for acne as it reduces inflammation and pathogen growth and reduces both proliferation of cells that secrete oil and total oil secreted on the face.[428] Because it does not dry out skin like Vitamin A-derived drug Accutane, CBD is a superior topical treatment. Unfortunately, CBD is often misunderstood legally and by society, and there may be significant hurdles in treating teenage acne with topical

CBD products.

ITCHY OR DRY SKIN

Pruritus, or itch, is a common skin issue with multiple causes including dermatitis. Activation of TRPV1 receptors in the skin causes inflammation and are linked to atopic dermatitis and allergic contact dermatitis.[429-430] TRPV1 antagonists could be therapeutic targets for dermatitis.

THC and anandamide stimulate CB2 receptors in skin to increase oil production, which can reduce dryness of skin.[427] Anandamide applied topically for three weeks is highly effective at reducing itchy skin, also known as pruritus and CB1 agonists applied topically relieve pain.[431-432] Eczema, characterized by itchy, dry and scaling skin, is also treated by topical treatment with endocannabinoids anandamide and PEA for 2 weeks and was found to be superior to traditional treatments like lactic acid or urea.[433]

PSORIASIS

2% of Americans have psoriasis, a skin condition characterized by overgrowth of skin cells called keratinocytes. Symptoms of psoriasis include red patches of skin covered by thick, silvery scales, dry cracked and possibly bleeding skin, itchy, burning or sore skin, and swollen and stiff joints. Psoriasis symptoms are often episodic and triggered by stress, illness or poor diet, with flares of worsening symptoms lasting weeks or months.

Cannabinoids CBD, CBG and CBN were found to be effective in reducing overgrowth of keratinocytes and may be a therapeutic target for psoriasis.[434] Anecdotally, patients with psoriasis have found relief from topical CBD cream or cream containing a 1:1 ratio of CBD:THC. Patients with psoriasis should not smoke cannabis because smoking cigarettes increases the severity of the disease and it is not clear yet whether toxins from burning and inhaling cannabis do the same thing. Eating cannabis edibles or using tinctures could be safer options for psoriasis patients.

UNWANTED BODY HAIR

THC and anandamide applied topically inhibit hair growth, due to activation of CB1 receptors in the hair follicles.[435] This could be of great use to women try to slow hair growth in their lip, armpits, legs or bikini area. Obviously, cannabis cream alone cannot stop growth of hair, but could be useful if used daily to prolong time in between shaving or waxing appointments.

ALOPECIA

Cannabinoids may treat alopecia, also known as baldness. Male pattern baldness impacts over 35 million men in the United States, and over 50 percent of men over 50 have some hair loss. CBD applied topically to the scalp or even orally could inhibit CB1 receptors on hair follicles and stimulate hair growth.[435] It is promising that oral treatment with inhibitors of CB1 receptors also stimulates hair growth. Alopecia may also be caused by high levels of prostaglandin D2 on the scalp; cannabinoids may reduce levels of this prostaglandin and inflammation at the hair follicle.[436]

RISKS OF TREATING A PATIENT WITH SKIN CONDITIONS WITH CANNABINOID MEDICINE

Using cannabis or CBD topical products for treatment of skin conditions is the least risky way to use cannabis, as patients will not test positive for THC in a drug test, CBD and THC will not enter the bloodstream and interact with other drugs, and side effects such as sleepiness or appetite increase are not seen with topicals.

If a patient is on any prescription medications that are contradicted with grapefruit, they should also avoid taking products orally with CBD in it or adjust their dosage under the care of their doctor. CBD can inhibit liver p450 enzymes in the same fashion as grapefruit does, increasing or (in rare cases) decreasing the amount of drug that is absorbed. Taking CBD or cannabis containing CBD orally with the erectile dysfunction drug Viagra (sildenafil) may cause unwanted side effects such as low blood pressure.

CREATIVITY

Cannabis can help musicians, artists, actors, dancers, writers and all creators enhance their creativity and improve their art by heightening their senses. Cannabis creates a sense of wonder, allowing creators to appreciate their surroundings and transform it into art. Cannabis also boosts hyper-priming, connecting two unrelated things and causing an “Aha!” moment.[437]

People who are more creative has more baseline brain activity in a region called the frontal lobe, and when they are performing creative tasks, they show more activation in that region than noncreative people.[438] Cannabis increases brain activity in the frontal lobe, suggesting it boosts creativity.[439-441] If you are a long-term cannabis user, it is best to do creative tasks while using cannabis and not during withdrawal of over 2 days because cannabis withdrawal can hamper frontal lobe activity and thus creativity.[442]

Finally, cannabis can relieve stress and self-criticism, helping a creator fully immerse themselves in a project or brainstorming without pausing to edit every 5 seconds. Cannabis enhances “flow,” a state necessary for happiness. High doses of THC, or the equivalent of 3 joints, can hamper brainstorming, but a low dose or equivalent of one joint can improve creative thinking skills.[443]

PART FOUR

The Vitamin Weed 4-Step Plan

WHAT IS THE VITAMIN WEED 4-STEP PLAN?

Cannabis and its derivative products like CBD oil can be quite expensive, and using them before your body is ready can be a big waste of money. One can compare it to spending tons of money of vitamins your body doesn't absorb, only to pee the majority of them out. Most people live such an unhealthy lifestyle that their body is unable to respond properly to cannabinoids when treated with them. Others have medical conditions or genetic mutations that prevent the endocannabinoid system from being fully functional.

The *Vitamin Weed 4-Step Plan* to reverse endocannabinoid deficiency helps save you time and money by preparing your body for cannabinoid therapy, restoring endocannabinoid system function, and then helping you maintain optimal levels of "Vitamin Weed."

STEP 1: ELIMINATE

As I mentioned in Chapter 3, there are numerous factors that can cause your endocannabinoid deficiency. Some of these you don't have control over, like your genes, but you have the power to change other factors like medication or food. Some things will be simple swaps, others will be changes that depend on visits with your doctor and research. The more factors you can eliminate, the less cannabis you will need and the more money you will save. As a bonus, getting rid of lifestyle factors that harm your endocannabinoid system will make you look and feel healthier without even adding cannabis.

STEP 2: PRIME

Once you have removed the factors shutting your endocannabinoid system down, it will take some time for it boost production of endocannabinoids and their receptors. You can speed this process along by "priming" receptors and unblocking the genes that make them by adding things to your diet that boost endocannabinoid function.

STEP 3: STRESS MANAGEMENT

As I mentioned in Chapter 3, chronic stress from emotional or physical sources can wreak havoc on your endocannabinoid system. When you are stressed out, your body downregulates cannabinoid receptors and its downstream signaling. This means you will become endocannabinoid deficient even if you are supplementing your body with high levels of phytocannabinoids or have reduced factors that harm your endocannabinoid system. It would be a shame for you to make the lifestyle changes in Step 1 and Step 2, and then spend money on cannabinoid products in Step 4, only to see no results! Step 3 is the most important step for maintaining a healthy endocannabinoid system for life.

STEP 4: VITAMIN WEED

If you live in a state or country where cannabis is not legal or for personal reasons just cannot partake, it is possible for you to skip Step 4 and still treat endocannabinoid deficiency. If you have access to cannabis or CBD products, I encourage you to incorporate Step 4 into your life because there is a difference between just restoring a deficiency and living at your maximum quality of life. Adding cannabinoid products will improve all aspects of your health, happiness, and relationships.

CHAPTER 13

The Vitamin Weed 4-Step Plan

Step 1: Eliminate

Patients often ask me why cannabis or CBD treatment isn't working for them? After reviewing the medications they are on, both prescription and OTC, diet, and lifestyle, it becomes pretty clear why cannabis wasn't working for them. They had destroyed their endocannabinoid system.

Cannabinoids are keys that fit into locks, called receptors. It doesn't matter how many keys you have if you have no locks to put them in. In this chapter, I'll review how to eliminate foods, toxins, medications, and drugs that shut down your endocannabinoid system from responding.

There are several ways things you put in your body can harm your endocannabinoid system:

1. They can block production of endocannabinoids including anandamide and 2-AG.
2. They can boost production of enzymes that break down endocannabinoids including FAAH or MAGL.
3. They can increase activity of enzymes like COX-2 to shift

production of endocannabinoid precursors from endocannabinoids to pro-inflammatory prostaglandins.

4. They can stop production of cannabinoid receptors.
5. They can prevent cannabinoids from being absorbed and binding to cannabinoid receptors.
6. They can block cannabinoid receptors.

FOOD

The food you eat can cause the most damage to your endocannabinoid system and overall cellular health. This section will cover the benefits of eliminating excitotoxins like MSG, GI irritants like dairy, sugar, and caffeine from your diet.

EXCITOTOXINS

Excitotoxins are chemicals that overstimulate neurons. They over activate glutamate receptors, causing them to fire rapidly until they become unresponsive and die. Once you lose those brain cells, they don't come back. Excitotoxins also increase free radical levels that causes additional cell death. Interestingly, excitotoxicity causes excess calcium to come into neurons, and causes arachidonic acid to turn into inflammatory prostaglandin instead of the endocannabinoid 2-AG. Exposure to excitoxins thus may cause temporary endocannabinoid deficiency.

SIGNS YOU MAY BE SENSITIVE TO EXCITOTOXINS AFTER EATING

Migraine	Hives	Diarrhea	Chest Pain
Rapid Heartbeat	Rash	Runny Nose	Headache
Sweating	Shortness of Breath	Nausea	Joint Pain
Heartburn	Insomnia	Weakness	Flushing
Fatigue	Drowsiness	Warm Tingling in Limbs	Breathing Difficulty
Depression	Facial Pressure	Hyperactivity	Seizures

Excitotoxins can be tolerated in very small doses by healthy people, but most Americans consume high doses of excitotoxins daily. Sadly, excitotoxins can cross the placenta and harm the brains of unborn children when pregnant mothers consume the chemicals. Young children with developing brains are highly sensitive to excitotoxins. Excitotoxins are especially dangerous in any amounts for patients with brain disorders or other chronic illnesses. In fact, excitotoxins can stimulate seizures, migraines, or flare-ups of pain in sensitive people. Patients with both fibromyalgia and irritable bowel syndrome had symptoms improve on an excitotoxin elimination diet, while symptoms returned when challenged with the excitotoxin MSG.[444]

ELIMINATE EXCITOTOXINS FROM YOUR DIET IF YOU HAVE THESE CONDITIONS

Migraine/Headache	Epilepsy	Autism
Fibromyalgia	Irritable Bowel Syndrome (IBS)	ADHD/ADD
Ulcerative Colitis	Traumatic Brain Injury (TBI)	Stroke
Crohn's disease	Alzheimer's disease	Parkinson's disease
Hypertension	Diabetes/Hypoglycemia	Amyotrophic Lateral Sclerosis (ALS)
Multiple Sclerosis (MS)	On a Weight-Loss Diet	New to Exercising

Why are we eating excitotoxins in the first place? Most of these excitotoxins are added to food for flavoring rather than adding nutritional value or active as a preservative. The cheap food we eat tastes so bad the makers have to add chemicals that cause brain damage to make it palatable to our taste buds. Sadly, these excitotoxins are all FDA-approved, which means the US government approved our daily brain damage so businesses can profit.

Think you are safe from excitotoxins? Chronic consumption of excitotoxins while healthy may worsen your brain's ability to repair itself when an unforeseen medical condition like brain injury, stroke, brain tumors, or degenerative disease occurs. 90% of migraines may be due to consumption of excitotoxins. Finally, we consume excitotoxins on a daily basis, and often multiple excitotoxins in the same meal. This leads to massive amounts of glutamate release which harm our brain and body.

MSG

Monosodium glutamate, also known as MSG, was originally isolated from the Japanese seaweed *kombu*. Many consumers are aware of MSG and choose to avoid foods with MSG on the label. Food makers have gotten around this by calling MSG other names on the label, and the FDA has done nothing to regulate this blatant deceptive practice.

25% of the global population reacts negatively to MSG, according to NOMSG. Adverse reactions to MSG include migraine, headache, nausea, vomiting, pain, stomach upset, diarrhea, asthma attack, shortness of breath, rash, runny nose, flushing, anxiety, panic attack, increased heart rate, mood swings, confusion, bags under the eyes, and mouth lesions.

The easiest way to avoid MSG is to shop at grocery stores that ban foods with MSG and eat at restaurants that also ban it. MSG-free grocery stores include: Trader Joes, Natural Grocers, and Whole Foods. Other names that monosodium glutamate or MSG go by on food labels: glutamic acid, sodium hydrogen glutamate, glutamate, monopotassium glutamate, yeast extract, autolyzed yeast, yeast food, yeast nutrient, hydrolyzed protein, hydrolyzed vegetable protein, hydrolyzed animal protein, hydrolyzed plant protein, soy protein isolate, soy protein concentrate, whey protein, whey protein concentrate, whey protein isolate, autolyzed plant protein, hydrolyzed oat flour, textured protein, caseinate, sodium caseinate, calcium caseinate, natural flavors, flavoring, natural flavorings, natural beef flavor, natural chicken flavor, malt flavoring, chicken flavoring, seasoning, spices, kombu extract, broth, bouillon, stock, and enzymes. It is important to know that food with these terms on the label do not necessarily contain MSG, but it usually does. If you are buying your food from a standard or ethnic grocery store, it most likely has MSG.

The fifth taste bud, called "umami," is activated by the natural amino acid glutamic acid as well as MSG. Cheese, milk, seaweed, peas, and meat have high levels of glutamic acid, but it should be made clear that these foods do not naturally contain MSG. Glutamic acid is a natural form of glutamate that can exacerbate excitotoxicity if you are consuming other excitotoxins. If you are sensitive to MSG or have a medical condition that requires avoiding excitotoxins, try eliminating one or more of these foods and see if it improves your condition.

ASPARTAME

Aspartame is a no-calorie sugar alternative marketed as Equal, NutraSweet, and Spoonful. It is found in over 6000 products including diet sodas and diet foods. Aspartame is broken down into aspartate, also called aspartic acid, once eaten and becomes an excitatory amino acid, similar to glutamate. Aspartate crosses the blood-brain barrier, and in excess concentrations, can cause excitoxicity and brain cell death.[445]

Aspartame is also broken down into phenylalanine, an amino acid that is the precursor for the neurotransmitters norepinephrine, epinephrine, and dopamine, as well as methanol. Methanol is further broken down into formaldehyde and then into formate. While levels of methanol produced by eating aspartame products are minimal compared to drinking citrus juice or alcohol, in excess consumption or in patients with neurological conditions, the methanol accumulation could be a problem.

If you are looking to incorporate CBD or cannabis into your wellness plan, put products with aspartame in them on your naughty list!

CYSTEINE

L-cysteine is an excitatory amino acid that causes neuron death via glutamate receptor excitotoxicity.[446] However, cysteine is also a building block for glutathione, a master antioxidant that can counter the effects of cytotoxicity. Thus, most people likely do not need to avoid L-cysteine. Foods rich in cysteine that could be avoided if you are extremely sensitive to excitotoxins include soy, sunflower seeds, beef, lamb, chicken, turkey, oats, eggs, dairy, legumes, and whole grains. Most of these foods could be avoided on a vegan or vegetarian diet.

CASEIN

Casein, or caseinate is found in protein powders, shakes and bars, yogurt, soup, gravy, meat products, ice cream, baked goods, coffee creamers, pasta, spreads, and cheese products. There are several forms of casein, the best being natural casein, cheese casein, or milk protein concentrate (MPC). Casein is rich in glutamate, but more natural forms of casein digest so slowly as to not cause excitotoxicity. Avoid chemical acid casein or lactic acid casein, which likely has excitoxins in it due to the manufacturing process and its ability to break down faster than natural casein.

GELATIN

Pure gelatin is not an excitotoxin, but gelatin often contains MSG, which is an excitotoxin. Avoid Jell-O, and even gummy bears with CBD or THC in them because they likely have MSG as well as artificial food coloring that will impair your wellness plan progress.

L-BOAA

L-beta-oxalyl-amino-alanine (L-BOAA), also known as oxayldiaminopropionic acid (ODAP) is a structural analogue of the neurotransmitter glutamate found in the legume Lathyrus sativus. Eating too much of this grass pea can cause a neurodegenerative condition called neurolathyrism, which is characterized by lower-body paralysis.[447] This pea is food staple in India, Bangladesh, Nepal and Ethiopia, where epidemics of neurolathyrism occur during famines. It is not commonly eaten in other countries. If you are consuming this legume, cease if you'd like to follow the *Vitamin Weed 4-Step Plan*.

DOMOIC ACID

Domoic acid (DA), an analogue of glutamate, is found in high levels in shellfish, sardines and anchovies. It is produced by algae, where it eaten by the marine life aforementioned, and then eaten by otters, sea lions, crabs, and humans. Humans that consume seafood with abnormally high levels of domoic acid can suffer short-term memory loss, seizures and even death, but this is very, very rare. The syndrome associated with domoic acid exposure is called Amnesic Shellfish Poisoning (ASP).

Because domoic acid is highly stable, it can damage the kidneys at a concentration 100 times lower than the concentration required to cause brain damage. People who are sensitive to MSG and other neurotoxins should likely avoid shellfish to avoid accumulating domoic acid in the kidney or brain.

GLUTAMATE

Avoid natural foods high in glutamate, they too in excess quantities or in combination with excitotoxins can trigger excitoxicity. These foods include peas, tomatoes, mushrooms, walnuts, grape juice, wheat gluten, broccoli, soy, potatoes, and parmesan and Roquefort cheeses.

GI IRRITANTS

The gut is your second brain. When your gut is chronically inflamed, you won't absorb nutrients from food and the rest of your body will fall apart. Living a Western lifestyle puts you at greater risk for leaky gut syndrome, a real medical condition that most doctors know nothing about. Years of poor diet choices, stress, and OTC and prescription medications including NSAIDs can easily lead to leaky gut.

Leaky gut occurs when the lining of the gut is damaged, and toxins and undigested food are absorbed back into the bloodstream. This causes a cycle of sickness that is almost impossible to break free from.

CONDITIONS POSSIBLY LINKED TO LEAKY GUT SYNDROME

Migraine/Headache	Arthritis	Autism
Fibromyalgia	Irritable Bowel Syndrome (IBS)	Fatigue
Thyroid Issues	Heart Disease	Diabetes
Multiple Sclerosis (MS)	Inability to Lose Weight	

If you are concerned you may have leaky gut, ask your doctor to run two blood tests: zonulin and lipopolysaccharides (LPS). Elevation of either protein indicates the gut has been breached and things that should not come back out of your gut are back in your bloodstream. Avoid the foods below to start the slow process of healing your gut and preparing for adding cannabinoids to accelerate that process.

CARAGEENAN

Carageenan, derived from MSG, is an excitotoxin many health conscious organic food consumers are unwittingly exposed to on a daily basis. Carageenan is extracted from red seaweed and used widely in the food industry. Carageenan is often found in almond, brown rice, and coconut milk as well as creamers and toothpastes as a thickener.

Carageenan causes an immune response in the digestive tract, causing inflammation, bleeding, and potentially even gastrointestinal cancer and diabetes. Carageenan causes flares of diseases that impact the GI tract, including ulcerative colitis, IBS, and colon cancer. When our gut is inflamed, our brain suffers, as 95% of our serotonin is produced in the gut. Avoid products with carrageenan to have a healthy brain and gut and create an environment where cannabinoids have a better chance of healing your body.

GLUTEN

Gluten is a protein found in wheat, rye, barley and triticale that acts as the glue that holds foods together. Going on a gluten-free diet has become trendy and even tried by patients looking to lose weight, but is giving up bread really necessary for good health?

About 1 in 133 Americans suffer from an autoimmune disorder called Celiac disease, and exposure to gluten causes damage to the small intestine. Celiac is diagnosed through celiac disease antibodies found in the blood, and then confirmed with a biopsy of the small intestine. The treatment for Celiac disease is a 100% gluten-free life, which means not even cooking with the same equipment that was previously used to prepare foods with gluten in the them.

1 in 20 Americans are estimated to be merely sensitive to gluten, and suffer symptoms such as fatigue, bloating, gas, stomach ache, diarrhea, nausea, migraine headache, joint pain, anxiety, or acne after eating foods with gluten in them. Others have no true gluten-sensitivity, but benefit from the reduction in processed foods and sugars that come from adhering to a gluten-free diet.

Anyone with an autoimmune disorder or symptoms of endocannabinoid deficiency would benefit from reducing or eliminating gluten from their diet. If, after 3 months on a gluten-free diet, you do not have improvement in symptoms, try adding back foods one by one to ensure that they don't cause symptom flares.

FOODS TO ELIMINATE CONTAINING GLUTEN (OR SUBSTIUTE WITH GLUTEN-FREE VERSIONS)

Bread	Soy Sauce	Flour Tortillas	Candy Bars
Baked Goods	Teriyaki Sauce	Pancakes	Malt Vinegar
Pasta	Croutons	Waffles	Energy Bars
Cereal	Beer	Stuffing	Omelets at Restaurants
Soups	Pizza	Gravy	Vegetarian Burgers
Salad Dressings	Noodles	French Fries	Processed Lunch Meat

Certain vitamins, supplements, OTC medications, and prescription drugs may also contain gluten. Even skin creams, shampoos and conditioners and toothpastes can contain gluten. Check the label or call the manufacturer to be sure that the product is gluten-free.

DAIRY

Lactose intolerance occurs when your body can't break down lactose, the form of sugar found in milk and dairy products. Lactose intolerance is usually hereditary, but often doesn't start until teen or adult years. Symptoms include bloating, gas, cramps, diarrhea, vomiting, and stomach pain.

While there is no treatment for lactose intolerance, avoiding dairy products of taking lactase products to help you digest dairy lactose will eliminate the symptoms outlined above. Milk and other dairy products also contain casein, which was outlined above has being excitotoxic and also promotes inflammation in the bodies. Even if you aren't lactose intolerant, avoiding dairy may help reduce many symptoms often linked to autoimmune disease.

SUCRALOSE

Sucralose is a no-calorie sugar alternative marketed as Splenda. Sucralose is found in hundreds of products, including diet sodas and teas, protein powders, and candies. Sucralose is to be avoided due to its role in disrupting healthy hormone regulation.

Sucralose may kill as much as 50% of healthy bacteria in your gut.[448] Sucralose may also cause issues in glucose and insulin control in diabetics.[448] New research suggests sucralose releases dioxins known as chloropropanols when heated or baked, which is not safe because sucralose is used in baking and cooking. Dioxins are endocrine disruptors which have numerous negative health effects. Finally, sucralose may be linked to cancer.

NIGHTSHADES

Nightshades are a family of vegetables which includes tomatoes, potatoes, eggplant, goji berries, and peppers. It also includes tobacco, which means people sensitive to nightshades should avoid smoking. Nightshades contain alkaloids which inhibit the activity of cholinesterase, increasing levels of the neurotransmitter acetylcholine. Consumption of nightshades are often associated with pain and inflammation in people sensitive to them or patients with autoimmune disorders or chronic pain.

An accumulation of cholinesterase inhibitors, whether from nightshades, caffeine, vodka, and pesticides from produce, can lead to numerous negative symptoms including pain, muscle spasms, muscle tenderness, headache, and stiff joints. It may take up to 3 months of abstaining from nightshades to see reduction in inflammation and pain, especially for patients with arthritis.

ELIMINATE NIGHTSHADES FROM YOUR DIET IF YOU HAVE THESE CONDITIONS

Food Allergies	Celiac disease	Gluten Sensitivity
Ulcerative Colitis	Crohn's disease	Lyme disease
Fibromyalgia	Irritable Bowel Syndrome (IBS)	Lupus
Multiple Sclerosis (MS)	Arthritis	Diabetes

SUGAR

All sugar is not the same. Types of sugar include sucrose, fructose, glucose, lactose, maltose, and galactose. Glucose is produced in the body by the breakdown of carbohydrates in the body and is the main source of energy for cells. Lactose is a sugar found in milk and dairy products. Galactose is found in beets, dairy products, and some gums. Maltose is found in cooked sweet potatoes, some breakfast cereals, breads, beers, and malted milkshakes, and is broken down into glucose in order to be used by the body. Sucrose is a sugar broken down into glucose and fructose.

Fructose is a sugar found in processed foods that contain high-fructose corn syrup, corn syrup solids, honey, molasses, fruit juices, maple syrup, and agave nectar. Fructose is also found in sugar alcohols including sorbitol, maltitol, mannitol, xylitol, erythritol, isomalt, lactitol, and hydrogenated starch hydrolysates. These sugar alcohols are often found in diet foods and drinks as well as candies and gums.

Most fruits, as well as table sugar, are half sucrose and half fructose. Fruits that are disproportionally high in fructose include apples, pears, pomegranates, grapes, blueberries, tomatoes, lychees, plum, and persimmon. Bananas, mangoes, grapefruit, pineapples, kiwis, mandarin oranges, raspberries and cherries also contain high amounts of fructose.

Fructose is only metabolized in the liver, and this is bad for people with liver issues because fructose not broken down by the liver gets turned into fat. Some people are fructose-intolerant and benefit greatly from a low-fructose diet. Others actually have a rare condition called hereditary fructose intolerance and require a fructose-free diet.

In any case, lowering your fructose could help you lose weight, reduce inflammation, and lower your risk of type 2 diabetes and cardiovascular disease. Reducing fructose intake can also help reduce your cancer risk, as fructose activates the 12-LOX pathway that helps cancer cells spread throughout the body.

CANDIDA

Many people suffer from candida overgrowth throughout the body, which is the same fungus that causes yeast infections in women. How do you get candida in the first place? Antibiotic treatment can wipe out health bacteria that normally keep candida from overgrowing, and a high-sugar diet can also cause candida to flourish.

Candida infection causes major disturbances in your gut flora, causing GI upset as well as negatively influencing your mood. Symptoms of candida infection include recurring yeast infections, fungal infections on the nails and skin, fatigue, digestive issues, thrush on the tongue, sinus infections, depression, brain fog, joint pain, weakened immune system, and food allergies or intolerances.

Candida produces acetaldehyde and other toxins including ammonia and uric acid. High levels of acetaldehyde, classified as a carcinogen, causes issues like DNA damage, nerve damage and reduced oxygen to the brain, further exacerbating health issues. Acetaldehyde is found in bread, coffee, and ripe fruit. It is also produced by metabolism of alcohol, where it a contributor to hangovers. It's best to avoid anything that contains or produces acetaldehyde if you suspect you have a candida infection.

To reduce growth of candida, a reduced or even strict no-sugar diet is advised. Avoiding all sugars stated in the previous section is a great start.

CAFFEINE

Caffeine is the commonly used drug in the world, and most people won't get to work without a cup of coffee. But there is clearly some people that use too much coffee, whether its downing energy drinks, or layering soda with coffee with energy drinks throughout the day. More than 500 mg of caffeine a day can lead to insomnia, irritability, nervousness, fast heartbeat, muscle tremors and an upset stomach. Recently teenagers have even died from overconsumption of caffeine.

Reducing your caffeine intake is easy. Just reduce or cut out coffee, energy drink, soda and tea out of your diet. In the next chapter I'll introduce healthy alternatives to caffeine so you don't further add to your fatigue.

ENVIRONMENTAL TOXINS

The air you breathe outdoors and indoors, the water you drink and bathe in, your clothing, furniture, beauty products and cleaning products are huge determinants of your health. Thankfully, besides air pollution, you can control most environmental toxins. This section will cover the benefits of eliminating environmental toxins including pesticides, endocrine disruptors, and substances of abuse.

PESTICIDES

Pesticides are found in our food, our lawns, and the cotton in our clothes and tampons. Purchasing organic, GMO-free foods and tampons can limit your pesticide exposure, but these chemicals are everywhere in our environment and nearly unavoidable.

ROUNDUP

The most harmful pesticide to your health is glyphosate, marketed as Roundup and produced by Monsanto. Plants are genetic modified (GMO) in order to withstand being treated with Roundup. Technically GMO foods are not what is unsafe for humans to consume, it's the glyphosate that's sprayed on it.

Glyphosate has been linked to kidney and liver issues, cancer, reproductive problems and many other issues in peer-review scientific journals, yet is still legal to use in the United States due to the fact that Roundup is a 5 billion dollar a year brand. The World Health Organization (WHO) has classified glyphosate as a class 2A probable human carcinogen.

Foods that tend to have the most glyphosate sprayed on them are corn, corn oil, corn syrup, soy, wheat, and oats. Unfortunately, this means avoiding almost all processed foods, breads, pastas, baked foods, tofu, and sauces. Many people that feel they are gluten-sensitive or possibly suffering from Celiac disease may in fact just be sensitive to glyphosate sprayed on wheat.

Glyphosate works by inhibiting the shikimate pathway, which is present in our gut bacteria but not our body's cells. By killing gut bacteria, glyphosate puts us at risk for obesity, autism, GI disorders, and mood disorders. Ingesting pesticides may be particularly bad for children, impairing brain development, and potentially leading to behavioral or learning issues.

THE DIRTY DOZEN

Sadly, trying to eat healthy by increasing your fruit and vegetable intake could backfire because you're actually eating more pesticides, which are often neurotoxins. The Environmental Working Group (EWG) analyzed tests run by the U.S. Department of Agriculture (USDA) on 48 types of produce and found 70% were contaminated with pesticides. The USDA found a total of 178 different pesticides and pesticide breakdown products on produce samples.

In order to reduce pesticide exposure, you should buy organic produce. People who often or always buy organic produce have lower levels of insecticides in their urine, even when they ate more produce than people who rarely or never bought organic produce. However, organic produce is more expensive and most people don't have the luxury to purchase all their food organic. To make your dollar stretch further, focus on purchasing the following "Dirty Dozen" in organic section, as these produce have the highest number and concentration of pesticides as determined by the EWG.

THE DIRTY DOZEN: BUY ORGANIC PRODUCE TO AVOID PESTICIDES

Strawberries	Spinach	Nectarines	Apples
Peaches	Pears	Cherries	Grapes
Celery	Tomatoes	Sweet Bell Peppers	Potatoes

You'll note tomatoes, potatoes, and sweet bell peppers on the above "Dirty Dozen" list are also nightshades which can cause pain and inflammation. It's best to avoid them altogether instead of buying organic nightshades.

To remove about 75-80% pesticides from "regular" produce, wash them in cold water, and makes sure you get in the nooks and crannies, where pesticide residue may build up. To remove almost 100% of pesticides, you'll need to wash with a 2% solution of salt water instead. Keep a spray bottle next to the sink and make washing your produce a ritual if it's not part of your life already.

ENDOCRINE DISRUPTORS

Endocrine disruptors are chemicals that mimic sex and thyroid hormones and disrupt our endocrine signaling, causing harm to our reproductive, immune, and nervous systems. Endocrine disruptors can also bind to hormone receptors and prevent natural hormones from binding or prevent natural hormones from being made or broken down. Endocrine disruptors can cause even greater harm to the developing fetus and the rapidly growing brain of children.

Endocrine disruptors have been linked to endometriosis, infertility, obesity, birth defects, and even cancer. It's estimated that exposure to endocrine disruptors in the United States cost the country over $300 billion a year in healthcare and lost productivity costs.[450] Endocrine disruptors are everywhere, from the ink on receipts to tins of food to water bottles to fragrances. Limiting exposure to endocrine disruptors will allow your body to start healing and be receptive to cannabis treatment.

THE DIRTY DOZEN ENDOCRINE DISRUPTORS

BPA	Dioxin	Atrazine	Phthalates
Perchlorate	Fire Retardants	Lead	Arsenic
Mercury	Perfluorinated Chemicals	Organophosphate Pesticides	Glycol Ethers

Broken down below is what these endocrine disruptors are and how to avoid them. Ways to avoid coming into contact with endocrine disruptors in general include:

1) Washing your hands with a soap that does not have fragrance or anti-bacterial properties.

2) Avoiding lotions, sunscreens, and other beauty products with parabens, synthetic fragrances and other toxic chemicals. Look for organic or chemical-free formulations.

3) Avoid air fresheners, laundry detergents with fragrance, and cleaning products with fragrance.

BPA

Bisphenol A (BPA) is used to make plastics, ink on receipts, and canned food containers. 93% of Americans have BPA in their bodies, and much of it is stored in fat. BPA-Free plastics made with BPA alternatives like bisphenol S (BPS) were unfortunately found to also be endocrine disruptors. Sadly, plastics made from hemp could completely substitute for endocrine disrupting plastics, but the United

States makes it extremely difficult for farmers to cultivate and sell hemp. To avoid BPA and BPS, drink out of glass or steel reusable water containers, don't touch receipts and tell your cashier to throw them out, and avoid foods in plastic or can containers.

DIOXIN

Environmental toxins such as dioxins and PCBs have been linked to endocannabinoid dysfunction. 90% of human exposure to dioxins is through food, specifically meat, fish and dairy as well as breakdown of the artificial sweetener sucralose. Dioxin exposure almost completely wipes out levels of CB1 receptors in endometrial tissue from healthy women, similar to the levels found in endometrial tissue from women with endometriosis.[404] Women with endometriosis were found to have higher levels of dioxins in their fat tissue than healthy women.[409]

As women are subjected to pollution in the air, water, grass, and food as well as BPA in water bottles and receipts, it's no wonder why so many women in developed countries now have severe endometriosis. Future research may link more toxins to endometriosis risk as well as endocannabinoid deficiency. If you suffer from pelvic pain, consider cutting all exposure to dioxins, even if that means going vegan, eating no sucralose, and not using water bottles.

ATRAZINE

Atrazine is a pesticide used on corn and found in the US drinking water. It's such a strong endocrine disruptor it can turn male frogs into female frogs. In order to avoid Atrazine, get a water filter certified to remove atrazine (not all do), and avoid eating corn and corn syrup, as most of it is GMO and contaminated with atrazine and Roundup.

PHTHALATES

Phthalates are used in fragrances and beauty products to make them longer wearing; they are also used to make plastics soft. Phthalates disrupt the thyroid and cause testicular harm. To avoid phthalates, don't use plastic food containers, plastic wrap, vinyl flooring, fragrance, or beauty products with fragrance.

PERCHLORATE

Perchlorate is made during processing of rocket fuel, and is found in our drinking water. It blocks iodine in the body, which causes thyroid dysfunction. To avoid perchlorate, get a reverse osmosis filter. Brita filters are not enough to remove perchlorate if you live in a town with high amounts in the water.

FIRE RETARDANTS

Fire retardants such as polybrominated biphenyl ethers (PBDEs) were originally used on furniture, carpet and even children's clothing to prevent fires. Sadly, the chemicals have been shown to not be effective at preventing fires, but are still used. Fire retardants cause $268 billion in healthcare spending per year and are virtually impossible to avoid. It is found in breast milk of all mothers, which is linked to reduction in IQ of children. To attempt to reduce exposure, use a vacuum with a HEPA filter, buy furniture made after January 2015 that state the furniture has no added flame-retardant chemicals, and replace old carpets and furniture.

LEAD

Lead is found in paint manufactured before 1978 as well as the drinking water. Lead can cause brain damage and lowered IQ in children exposed to it, but even in adults, kidney, nervous system, and GI tract issues can happen. To avoid lead exposure, don't live in old buildings that contain lead paint, and if you do, vacuum frequently and do not remove the pain yourself. Use a certified water filter to reduce exposure from drinking water.

ARSENIC

Arsenic is a heavy metal found in apples and the drinking water. High levels can cause bladder, lung and skin cancer, as well as interfere with how your body breaks down sugars for energy. To avoid arsenic, get a certified water filter, and rinse rise and pastas before cooking.

MERCURY

Mercury is a heavy metal produced from burning coal, and is present in the air and water. It causes disruption of the menstrual cycle and fertility in women. To avoid mercury, be picky about the fish you eat, especially if you are pregnant or breastfeeding. Buy wild-caught Alaskan salmon over other types that can be very high in mercury.

PERFLUORINATED CHEMICALS

Perfluorinated chemicals (PFCs) are used on Teflon pots and pans, nonstick cookware, microwave popcorn bags and fast food containers. 99% of Americans have PFCs in their bloodstream, and this is linked to kidney disease, thyroid disease, high cholesterol, low sperm count, and low birth weight in children. To avoid exposure to PFCS, make homemade popcorn instead of microwave popcorn and don't buy nonstick cookware. Avoid eating fast-food to avoid PFCs and for many more health reasons.

ORGANOPHOSPHATE PESTICIDES

Organophosphate pesticides are commonly used and are neurotoxins to both insects and humans. To avoid, buy organic fruits and vegetables.

GLYCOL ETHERS

Glycol ethers are found in cleaning products, brake fluid, paint, and beauty products. Glycol ethers can cause birth defects, impair fertility, reduce testicle size, and cause asthma. To avoid exposure to glycol ethers, use organic, nontoxic cleaning and beauty products.

DRUGS

Alcohol and substance use and abuse can cause inflammation and damage to your brain and other organs. The worst side effect of substance use is overdose and death. If your body is always inflamed and dehydrated in a hangover state, you are not creating an environment for cannabis treatment to be successful. At best, cannabis might bring you back to a non-hangover state, but it won't lift you all the way to healthy.

Cannabis can be a great alternative to alcohol and other recreational drugs, and can also help protect the brain, liver and other organs from damage while using those substances. For example, CBD or cannabis use might protect the brain from the neurotoxicity of methamphetamine use. Using alcohol and cannabis together can cause alcohol to be more intoxicating, so be careful and don't over consume.

MEDICATIONS

You're taught that prescription or OTC medications are used to make you healthy, but in reality, they often harm your endocannabinoid system and your health. This section will focus on harms of Tylenol, a common painkiller almost every American has used at some time in their life, and alternatives to hormonal birth control, which most American women of child-bearing age have also used during their life.

ACETAMINOPHEN

Sold by the brand name Tylenol, the OTC drug acetaminophen is generally thought of a harmless drug that reduces fever and pain. In fact, 79% of Americans regularly take acetaminophen.[451] However, a side effect of Tylenol is that it depletes the body of glutathione, which it requires to be metabolized in the liver.[452] A metabolite of Tylenol, N-acetyl-benzoquinoneimine (NAPQI), also requires glutathione to be metabolized. When glutathione runs out, liver and brain damage occur. Unfortunately, most of the population is glutathione deficient to begin with, so we are all suffering from the effects of Tylenol.

Acetaminophen use, especially in infants and young children, has been associated with autism, asthma, and attention deficit disorder

(ADHD).[453-455] Acetaminophen is classified as safe for pregnant women to use, but it is possible that its use is responsible for the rise in neurodevelopmental disorders in the United States. More than 35% of pregnant women in the United States use acetaminophen.[456] This means most of our population is deficient in glutathione from the fetal stage.

Why is glutathione so important? It's the master antioxidant your body naturally produces, and levels are correlated with health status and age.[457] Glutathione is a cofactor for many biological processes, including recycling other antioxidants including vitamin C, vitamin E, and alpha lipoic acid (ALA). The sulfur group in the chemical structure of glutathione sticks to toxins like heavy metals and carries them into the bile and out of your body.

Glutathione deficiency leads to increased oxidative stress, accumulation of toxins and heavy metals, inability to repair DNA, reduced supply of oxygen and energy to cells, and eventual cell death. Many diseases are characterized by low glutathione, yet the drugs prescribed to treat the chronic illnesses further deplete glutathione, causing the disease symptoms to worsen over time instead of getting better. Patients suffering from chronic diseases as well as alcoholics have low levels of glutathione, so taking Tylenol will deplete their glutathione reserves. Once liver glutathione is used up, NAPQI becomes toxic, binding to mitochondrial proteins and cause liver cells to die.[458]

Even healthy people are always fighting a losing battle with glutathione. Glutathione production decreased at an average rate of 10% per decade after age 20.[459] Couple that with exposure to environmental toxins like pollution and cigarette smoke, stress, and western diet, and it's clear most people are deficient in glutathione. Some people are also genetically prone to glutathione deficiency via mutations in GSTT1, GSTM1, GSTM2, GSTP1, MTHFR or C677T genes, and others have epigenetic changes that have silenced these critical genes.

Symptoms of glutathione deficiency include headaches, fatigue, dizziness, frequent colds, rashes, joint pain, brain fog, dry skin, depression, sleep disorders, and declining health. Supplementation with factors that increase glutathione cause drastic changes in people who are severely deficient in the antioxidant. Healthy people will not have as dramatic changes, but will notice an increase in energy or mental performance when their limited are tested in terms of physical or mental exercise. Chapter 14 on Priming Your Endocannabinoid System will guide you in increasing glutathione in the body.

Factors that decrease your glutathione levels besides Tylenol:

- prescription drugs
- alcohol
- synthetic food dyes (red #40, yellow #4, yellow #5, etc.)
- pesticide residue on foods
- heavy metal exposure (lead, mercury, copper, cadmium, etc.)
- indoor air pollutants (scented detergents and fabric softeners, air fresheners, chemical cleaners)
- aspartame
- nitrates and other chemical food preservatives
- fumes from acetone, gasoline, and paint remover

As a side note, Tylenol does not just relieve physical pain, it also blunts our response to emotional pain. While this may not matter for occasional users of Tylenol, chronic users of Tylenol or prescription painkillers that have acetaminophen like Vicodin or Percocet could become emotionally flat.[460] In fact, MRI studies have shown acetaminophen reduces activity in several brain areas including the insula, cingulate cortex, prefrontal cortex, and thalamus.[460-461] It may even be possible that prescription painkillers containing acetaminophen are more likely to be abused because of its effects on mood. Combined with its negative effects on glutathione, it's best to avoid acetaminophen.

HORMONAL BIRTH CONTROL

Hormonal birth control is associated with hormonal imbalance and endocannabinoid deficiency. While the choice of pregnancy prevention is a deeply personal one and you should use the method that works best for you, it may be time to consider a non-hormonal method for numerous health reasons, including avoidance of side effects including nausea, weight gain, mood changes, swollen breasts, and risks for deadly blood clots. Alternatives to hormonal birth control include IUDs, male or female sterilization, barrier methods, or fertility awareness-based methods.

IUD

Intrauterine devices (IUDs) are more commonly used in developing nations than industrialized nations, but this is due to the pharmaceutical industry pushing hormonal birth control as opposed to it being an ineffective or undesirable form of pregnancy prevention.

The IUD comes in two flavors in the United States: hormonal and copper. The hormonal IUD is to be avoided and goes by the brand names Mirena and Skyla. The copper IUD goes by the name ParaGard and is effective for 12 years. The copper IUD is effective in women that have never been pregnant, contrary to the public opinion.

While the upfront cost and discomfort of insertion are negatives, the benefits of having pregnancy prevention for 12 years without additional thought or payment makes it an ideal form of birth control for young women. It can be removed at any time, making it an ideal method for women that do not know when they want to start a family.

BARRIER METHODS

Barrier methods include male and female condoms, cervical caps, sponges, and spermicide. These methods are less effective that hormonal birth control and IUDs, as they require you have one on hand when you decide to have sex, as well as proper placement in the heat of the moment. Even when used properly, these methods can simply fail due to mechanical reasons (aka the condom breaks). They are one of the only methods to protect against sexually transmitted diseases (STDs) when they work.

STERILIZATION

Sterilization is a permanent or semi-permanent method of birth control and is the most commonly used birth control method in the United States. Female sterilization, also known as tubal ligation, is performed more frequently than male sterilization, also known as vasectomy. Female sterilization is nearly 100% effective but usually irreversible.

During female sterilization, the fallopian tubes are closed or a piece is removed. A new procedure called Essure puts an insert into the fallopian tubes, causing tissue to grow around them and block the tubes. A benefit of Essure is that general anesthesia and a surgical setting is not needed. 50% of female sterilizations are performed shortly after childbirth or abortion.

Male sterilization, commonly known as a vasectomy, is a simple, painless procedure that can be performed in an outpatient setting. There is very little bleeding, no stiches, and no general anesthesia is required. Vasectomy is highly effective and less than 1% of men with a vasectomy will cause a pregnancy. A vasectomy takes three months to be 100% reliable, so backup forms of birth control should be used for three months after the procedure.

Male sterilization is cheaper and safer than traditional female sterilization. Another advantage is that vasectomy can be reversed, as opposed to female sterilization.

FERTILITY AWARENESS METHODS

Fertility awareness methods (FAM) are also known as natural family planning. Only 1-3% of women use FAM according to the CDC, but 1 in 5 women would consider it as an option if either they or their doctor were educated were about it.[462] FAM methods include Billings Ovulation Method, the Creighton Model, the Symptothermal Method, Standard Days Methods, and Two Days Method. FAM is not to be confused with the rhythm method, which predicts fertile days solely on length of cycles and is notoriously inaccurate.

FAM used to be labor intensive, requiring daily tracking of

temperature and vaginal secretions. However, new digital health apps like Kindara, Glow, and Ovuline have made this process easy and connected women to a community that are passionate about their health as they are. These apps have some of the highest number of subscribers of all health apps. When used consistently, unintended pregnancy is under 2%.

Another benefit of FAM is that it helps women get in touch with their fertility and empowers them. It also helps them understand how their body works so that when it is time to have children, they do not have the same infertility problems as women that have spent decades shutting down their fertility with hormonal birth control.

CHAPTER 14

The Vitamin Weed 4-Step Plan

Step 2: Prime

Now that you've stopped putting things inside your body that stop your endocannabinoid system from working, it's time to give your endocannabinoid system a tune-up. Let's prime those cannabinoid receptors to receive the phytocannabinoids you'll be adding to your diet in Step 4.

In this chapter, I'll review how to add foods and dietary supplements that boost your endocannabinoid system and substitute prescription and OTC drugs with alternatives that don't impair your system.

There are several ways things you put in your body can boost your endocannabinoid system:

1. They can boost production of endocannabinoids including anandamide and 2-AG.
2. They can block production of enzymes that break down endocannabinoids including FAAH or MAGL.
3. They can decrease activity of enzymes like COX-2 to shift production of endocannabinoid precursors from pro-inflammatory prostaglandins to endocannabinoids.

4. They can boost production of cannabinoid receptors.
5. They can boost absorption and bioavailability of cannabinoids.
6. They can inhibit p450 liver enzymes that break down cannabinoids so they stay in your body longer.

GLUTATHIONE

Cannabis will have an easier job of healing you if you are not deficient in glutathione. Glutathione is a master antioxidant made by the liver and is a possible biomarker for how long you will live. Glutathione is important in many bodily processes, from killing cancer cells through apoptosis, to detoxifying fat, to neutralizing free radicals, to building proteins, to binding to drugs to help them break down, to promoting immune cell function.

Raising your glutathione levels are especially important if you have smoked or plan to smoke marijuana. Chronic marijuana smokers have reduced levels of glutathione in their lungs, likely the results of oxidative stress caused by toxins produced by burning and not vaping cannabis.[463] Glutathione levels are also depleted with diabetes, radiation therapy for cancer, exposure to heavy metals, chronic stress, infections, injuries, and aging.

WAYS TO TAKE OTC AND PRESCRIPTION GLUTATHIONE

Glutathione is available in several prescription forms, such as intramuscular shot, IV drip, inhaler, and oral pill depending on the condition it is prescribed for. Glutathione is prescribed for heavy metal poisoning, to prevent toxicity of chemotherapy in cancer patients, glaucoma, liver disease, asthma, Alzheimer's disease, male infertility, and much more. If you have a chronic disease, it might be a good idea to talk to your healthcare provider about your glutathione levels and way to increase them.

Taking OTC oral glutathione supplements is not effective at raising glutathione levels because it is broken down in the digestive tract. There are multiple ways to boost glutathione without a prescription, but don't try all of them at once. Excessively high glutathione levels can actually tell your body to produce less, so when you stop supplementing with glutathione your levels are worse than when you started.

SUPPLEMENTS TO BOOST GLUTATHIONE

If you have had a long history of acetaminophen use, or continue to use it, you should start take N-Acetylcysteine (NAC) supplements to repair the liver and brain toxicity it caused and increase your glutathione levels.[464] It is pretty unethical that Tylenol is formulated without NAC, but this a time where you have to be proactive about your health instead of expecting a drug manufacturer to do the right thing.

Melatonin supplementation taken before bed can raise glutathione in the brain, liver, muscle, and blood, repairing your body while you sleep.[465] Melatonin supplementation is especially important in older patients that make less melatonin than in their younger years. For those that cannot swallow pills easily, tart cherry juice is one of the few foods that contains melatonin.

Selenium is a mineral that helps the body recycle and produce glutathione.[466] Vitamin C and Vitamin E are also important for recycling glutathione, and all three are usually found in standard multivitamins.

Milk thistle detoxifies the liver and regenerates injured liver cells. The active ingredient in milk thistle is silymarin, which prevents breakdown of glutathione.[467] Milk thistle can interfere with hormonal birth control methods, so be sure to use a backup method to prevent accidental pregnancy or just avoid if you are a woman. Make sure to use low doses of milk thistle and to not use for an extended amount of time; it can become toxic.

FOODS CONTAINING GLUTATHIONE

Many foods containing the building blocks of glutathione. While adding these foods won't be as effective as taking a NAC supplement, they do support a healthy antioxidant system and have additional health benefits beyond glutathione.

Sulfur-rich foods provide the sulfur group that is so important to glutathione. Sulfur-rich foods include onions, garlic, and cruciferous vegetables including broccoli, cauliflower, kale, cabbage, and watercress. Foods rich in the amino acid cysteine also build glutathione. Cysteine is found in dairy products, eggs, red meat, poultry, fish, whole grains, and beans. Other foods that boost glutathione include watermelon, spinach and Brussel sprouts.

Raw milk contains multiple precursors to glutathione, including lactoferrin, beta-lactalbumin and serum albumin. Pasteurized milk, which is what is sold in grocery stores, does not contains these ingredients because the heat and mechanical stress of pasteurization breaks them down. Raw milk is illegal in many states, so finding a source may be difficult unless you live near a farm.

ANTI-CANDIDA DIET

Candida albicans is a fungus living in your mouth and gut where it helps your body break down and absorb nutrients. It is also responsible for vaginal yeast infections, leaky gut, and candidiasis, a condition in which candida grows like wild throughout the body. If your body is weakened by a Candida infection, it may be hard to reap the benefits of cannabis treatment.

Risk factors of candida overgrowth including eating a high sugar and/or carbohydrate diet, drinking alcohol regularly, eating a lot of fermented foods like kimchi, komubcha and pickles, experiencing chronic stress, using hormonal contraceptives, having diabetes, having a weakened immune system, and taking antibiotics that destroy your natural gut and vaginal flora. Symptoms of candida overgrowth include gas, bloating, joint pain, bad breath, fatigue, craving sweets like ice cream or candy, brain fog, lack of sex drive, weak immune system, white coating on the tongue (thrush), sinus issues, athlete's foot, vaginal yeast infections, and urinary tract infections. Candida overgrowth can be diagnosed by a comprehensive stool test or by a urine Organix Dybsbiosis test, which looks for elevated levels of a waste product of candida called D-arabinitol.

FOODS TO EAT TO STARVE CANDIDA OVERGROWTH

Avocado	Artichoke	Garlic	Almond
Lemon	Asparagus	Kale	Coconut
Lime	Broccoli	Onion	Flax Seed
Olive	Cabbage	Rutabaga	Hazelnut
Anchovies	Celery	Spinach	Sunflower Seed
Chicken	Cucumber	Tomato	Yogurt
Egg	Eggplant	Zucchini	Olive Oil
Salmon	Herbal Tea	Sauerkraut	Sesame Oil
Sardines	Quinoa	Buckwheat	Ginger
Turkey	Millet	Oat Bran	Cinnamon

WAYS TO TREAT CANDIDA

Eliminating all sugars and carbohydrates from your diet including fruits, alcohol, rice, bread, and pasta for one week to one month or longer depending on the severity of your infection is the best long-term solution to killing a systemic candida infection. Adding the foods in the above table can further discourage candida from living in your body. Once your symptoms of candida infection are gone or minimal, you can start adding probiotics or fermented vegetables to regrow healthy flora in your gut.

Visiting a doctor and getting a candida infection confirmed by stool or urine test will result in prescription anti-fungal drugs being prescribed like fluconazole, itraconazole, posaconazole, nystatin, clotrimazole, or amphotericin B. It is up to you whether you would like to use those medications in conjunction with the anti-candida diet and natural approaches including cannabis or go all-natural.

BENEFIT OF CANNABIS TO KILL CANDIDA

Cannabis is anti-fungal, and can be used in a variety of ways to tackle a resistant candida infection or prevent a recurrence of candida. Anecdotally, women that suffer from recurrent vaginal yeast infections prior to using cannabis have reduced frequency and severity of infections, with many having completely eliminated infections. Cannabis cream can be applied to feet, under breasts, and other areas that candida has overgrown. Cannabis suppositories, preferably made with coconut oil instead of cocoa butter to preserve a proper vaginal pH and flora, can kill vaginal yeast infections. Rectal cannabis suppositories can also help kill candida in the GI tract. If you make your own suppositories at home, you can also add 2 drops of lavender, clove, oregano, or myrrh essential oil to boost candida die off.

Cannabis oil, capsules, tinctures, and edibles could reduce candida growth. It's important to eat sugar-free edibles, otherwise the sugar will actually feed the candida and counteract the effects of THC and other compounds in cannabis. Finally, smoking cannabis is likely not enough to kill candida, and toxins in smoke may actually contribute to inflammation that promotes an environment for candida to thrive.

CBC is the second most common cannabinoid in strains of cannabis that contain THC but little CBD. CBC is effective against candida.[468] CBC isolate, capsules, or tinctures containing only CBC are not on the market yet, but a CBC transdermal cream is available from Mary's

Medicinals. This could be applied topically to fight yeast.

DIETARY PHYTOCANNABINOIDS

When someone says phytocannabinoids, or plant-derived cannabinoids, we immediately think of THC or CBD, cannabinoids from cannabis or hemp. But there are dietary phytocannabinoids found in many other plants beside cannabis. Some of these phytocannabinoids directly activate CB1 or CB2 receptors, some inhibit FAAH and raise anandamide levels, and most have additional benefits including being antioxidants or activating estrogen receptors. In this chapter we will cover phytocannabinoids from chocolate, black pepper, carrots, echinacea, soy, and other rarer sources.

BETA-CARYOPHYLLENE

The terpene beta-caryophyllene (BCP) is a dietary phytocannabinoid that activates CB2 receptors and does not activate CB1 receptors, avoiding any psychoactivity if taken.[469] It is found in many spices including oregano, cinnamon, ginger, basil, rosemary, hops, cloves, white pepper, and black pepper as well as cannabis and hemp, where it makes up to 35% of the plant. It is estimated that the average person eats between 10 and 200 mg of BCP a day.

SOURCES OF BETA-CARYOPHYLLENE

Plant	% BCP in Essential Oil
West African Pepper (black) West African Pepper (white)	57.59 51.75
Copaiba	50
Cannabis	3-37.5 depending on strain
Malabathrum	25.3
Basil	4-19.8
Cloves	1.7-19.5
Hops	5.1-14.5

Cannabis strains to smoke that are high in BCP content include Sour Diesel, Skywalker OG, Rockstar, OG Kush, Bubba Kush, and Chemdawg. A fun fact: BCP is broken down into caryophyllene oxide, and that compound is what drug-sniffing police dogs used to identify cannabis in states where it was or still is illegal.

Full-spectrum cannabis or hemp oils, tinctures, and pills should also contain significant amounts of BCP, while CBD isolate or THC isolate products will not. Copaiba oil, also known as copa oil, is available as a somewhat pricey BCP supplement online and through Doterra. BCP is "generally regarded as safe" (GRAS) by the FDA and is allowed as a dietary supplement or food ingredient in the United States. Due to BCP's antibacterial properties it is used as a food preservative and additive.

HOW BCP WORKS

BCP has other actions besides CB2 receptors, making it nearly as "dirty" of a drug as CBD, which has nearly 10 mechanisms of action. BCP activates PPAR receptors, which explains its additional immune and anti-inflammatory actions.[407] BCP's activation of both CB2 receptors and PPAR receptors is important for improvement of symptoms in a mouse model of ulcerative colitis.[470] BCP also activates the mu-opioid receptor, involved in pain relief.[471-472] BCP does not have any action on GABA, NMDA, or serotonin receptors.[473]

BENEFITS OF USING BCP

BCP has strong anti-bacterial and anti-viral properties against a multitude of microbes as well as kills parasites.[407] It is also a stronger anti-oxidant than Vitamin C or Vitamin E.[474] BCP can also reduce liver and kidney damage.[407] BCP also can boost the power of chemotherapy to kill cancer cells. BCP helps move paclitaxel (Taxol), a drug used to treat breast, ovarian and lung cancer, across the cell membrane to cause apoptosis.[475]

BCP either by itself or in combination with fatty acid docashexaenoic acid (DHA) is an effective and long-lasting pain reliever that does not develop tolerance.[476-477] In fact, BCP may be highly effective in treating long-term severe chronic pain, without the side effects of addiction, sleepiness, or liver damage.

Beta-caryophyllene selectively activates CB2 receptors instead of CB1 receptors and decreases drug-seeking behaviors.[337] CB2 receptors are found on dopamine neurons in the ventral tegmental area and nucleus accumbens, regulating cocaine, alcohol, opioid, and nicotine addiction.[478] Black pepper extracts containing BCP have also been marketed to reduce the "high" from cannabis products.

Through activation of CB2 receptors, BCP decreases seizure activity in epilepsy, but the complete mechanism is unknown.[407] BCP works through the CB2 receptor to reduce dopamine neuron damage in a mouse model of Parkinson's disease.[479] BCP has even been shown to extend lifespan in worms, with the hope that it does the same in humans.[480]

POSSIBLE RISKS OF USING BCP

BCP inhibits nicotinic acetylcholine receptors (alpha-7-nAChRs) involved in long-term memory in the hippocampus, as well as present in the spleen and lymph nodes.[407] Interestingly, anandamide also inhibits alpha-7 receptors.[481] Because alpha-7 receptors activation improves cognitive function and inhibiting them worsens it, taking BCP or products that contain it may initially cause focus or memory problems. This has been reported with CBD oil use, which also contains BCP. However, other alpha-7 antagonists such as the Alzheimer's drug memantine show that initial cognitive issues are remedied by long-term use of the drug as the brain readjusts to the drug.

The take home here is if you do experience cognitive issues when first taking BCP, note if they go away after 1, 2 or 3 weeks of use. If they are still there after 4 weeks, discontinue use. In general, the benefits of taking BCP outweigh the risk, and BCP will boost the positive effects of adding cannabis or CBD to your health regimen.

PALMITOYLETHANOLAMIDE

PEA is an endocannabinoid that activates cannabinoid receptors that are not CB1 and CB2, including TPRV1, GPR55 and PPAR-alpha receptors.[482] PEA boosts anandamide activity and contributes to the entourage effect. PEA is also found in several foods, including egg yolk, peanut oil, and soybean lecithin (which is often used in cannabis edibles).

Dietary PEA is of limited use by itself because it is rapidly metabolized in the body and large doses taken regularly are required. It is more effective for pain relief in conjunction with cannabinoids, acetaminophen, or tramadol.[483-484] Local injection of PEA, dissolved in corn oil, in areas of musculoskeletal pain can increase tissue levels of PEA and reduce pain and inflammation more effectively.[485]

While not made in the United States, PEA is manufactured as PeaPure, PeaVera and Normast in several European countries. PEA is produced by almost every living thing, and there are over 350 research studies dating back 50 years. PEA has been studied in over 40 clinical trials with over 6,000 patients using it safely.

BENEFITS OF USING PEA

A pill containing 400 mg of PEA and 40 mg of transpolydatin, a pro-drug for the anti-oxidant resveratrol, taken twice a day for 90 days reduced pelvic pain related to endometriosis significantly after 30 days, although treatment with selective COX-2 inhibitor celecoxib (Celebrex) was more effective at pain relief than PEA/transpolydatin.[68,410,411] 400 mg of PEA and 40 mg of transpolydatin once a day for 10 days also reduced pelvic pain.[412]

Two week treatment with 300 mg of PEA (Normast) twice a day is more effective at reducing TMJ pain than 600 mg three times a day of NSAID ibuprofen.[67] Treatment with 300 mg of PEA (Normast) twice daily significantly reduced diabetic neuropathic pain and the effects persisted one month after treatment was discontinued.[486] Treatment with 400 mg of PEA three times a day (PeaPure) reduced severe neuropathic pain in combination with topical pain relief.[487]

PEA can be very safe and effective for fibromyalgia and neuropathic pain. PEA may reduce glutamate excitoxicity associated with chronic illness like fibromyalgia or dietary excitoxins like monosodium glutamate (MSG) and aspartame. PEA is reported to have minimal side effects and lack of adverse interactions when taken with other drugs for neuropathic pain including pregabalin (Lyrica), gabapentin, tramadol, amitriptyline and duloxetine.[488] PEA powder can also be taken sublingually to reduce metabolism through the liver and enhance pain relief.

PEA may be a new therapeutic for neuroinflammation. It increases the number of CB2 receptors on microglia, which are glial cells that are the first form of immune defense in the brain.[482] PEA is also a COX-2 inhibitor, which causes reduction in both inflammation and pain and prevents anandamide from being broken down into an inflammatory prostaglandin.[489]

CHOCOLATE

RAW CACAO

Raw cacao, or unheated chocolate, is a rich source of anandamide, PEA (described later in this chapter) and antioxidants like Vitamin C in food.[177] It also contains the mild stimulant theobromine, endocannabinoid precursors omega-6 fatty acids, magnesium, zinc, and arginin.[490]

Raw cacao stimulates your serotonin system. It contains tryptophan, the amino acid that serotonin is built from, as well as serotonin itself. It even contains monoamine oxidase inhibitors (MAOIs), which inhibit the breakdown of serotonin and are even prescribed as antidepressants.

DARK CHOCOLATE

Anandamide, as well as two other NAEs, OEA and LEA, were discovered in dark chocolate by neuroscientist Daniele Piomelli in 1996.[11] The amount of anandamide in dark chocolate is too small to produce a THC-like effect in humans, especially when the majority of the cannabinoids are broken down in the gastrointestinal tract by FAAH or NAAA.[177] It is possible that eating dark chocolate in combination with THC use could potentiate the effects of the chocolate cannabinoids.

Dark chocolate is rich in antioxidants, boosts the release of pain-relieving endorphins, and even stimulates the release of feel good neurotransmitter serotonin due to tryptophan in dark chocolate. It also contains theobromine, which is a weaker stimulant than caffeine and increases alertness. So whether or not the endocannabinoids present ever make it from your gut to your brain, dark chocolate could activate cannabinoid and serotonin receptors, making you relaxed.

CARROTS

Carrots contains falcarinol, a polyacetylene compound that interacts with both CB1 and CB2 receptors. Polyacetylenes are being investigated for their potential to improve human health through anti-cancer, anti-bacterial, anti-fungal, anti-inflammatory, and serotonin-promoting activities.[491] Falcarinol may be protective against some cancers, and inhibits breast cancer resistance protein (BCRP/ABCG2), which causes some forms of breast cancer to stop responding to chemotherapy.[492-494]

Cooking carrots actually releases more falcarinol than eating them raw or drinking carrot juice. Carrots combine great with raw cannabis juice to cover up the bitter taste of the raw cannabis and may amplify its anti-cancer effects. Falcarinol is also found in red ginseng and parsley to lesser extent than carrots.

POTENTIAL RISKS OF USING FALCARINOL

One thing to be careful of is that falcarinol acts as an inverse agonist at the CB1 receptor, blocking anandamide, and causing inflammation in human skin if applied topically.[495-496] So don't apply skin creams or topicals with carrots in them, especially if you have skin issues like eczema. Stick to eating carrots.

ECHINACEA

Echinacea contains N-alkylamides that bind the CB2 receptor and PPAR-gamma, inhibit FAAH, and have anti-inflammatory properties.[497-499] It is possible for oral supplementation with echinacea to provide high enough blood levels of these N-alkylamides to have anti-inflammatory benefits.[500] Echinacea has anti-bacterial, anti-fungal and antiviral properties. It reduces duration of colds by one and half days as well as reduces risk of catching a cold in the first place by 58%.[501]

DIM

3,3′-diindolylmethane (DIM) is a fatty acid and metabolite of indole-3-carbinol that is a weak activator of the CB2 receptor.[502] DIM modulates immune response with potent anticancer activity, especially for prostate cancer prevention and treatment.[503-504] DIM can be produced in the body by eating cabbage, turnips, Brussel sprouts, mustard, or cruciferous vegetables including broccoli, cauliflower, kale, cabbage, and kohlrabi. You can also buy DIM or its precursor indole-3-carbinol as a dietary supplement.

POTENTIAL RISKS OF TAKING DIM

A very recent study found DIM binds to the pro-inflammatory orphan G protein-coupled receptor GPR84.[505] Drugs blocking GPR84 are in trials to treat the GI tract disorder ulcerative colitis as well as acid reflux, which means that activation of GPR84 by eating foods that convert to DIM may flare these conditions. If you have stomach issues, you most likely already avoid DIM-containing foods like cabbage.

In any case, DIM is a tool in your tool box, especially if you are at risk for cancer, have cancer or are a cancer survivor. When taken at peak dose of 1000 mg indole-3-carbinol, DIM only stays in your blood stream for 2 hours and is cleared rapidly.[506]

RUE

The medicinal herb *Ruta graveolens* is commonly called rue, common rue, ruta grav, or herb of grace. Rue is not to be confused with goat's rue or meadow rue. While it originated from the Balkan Peninsula, rue is now grown around the world.

BENEFITS OF USING RUE

Rue is commonly used as a medicinal herb to treat soreness in bones, joints, tendons, and cartilage as well as sprains or broken bones. Rue's herbal connection to bone healing makes sense because rutamarin, a chemical found in the plant, binds weakly to CB2 receptors, which would stimulate bone growth and repair. Rue also contains the isoflavone quercetin, a weak inhibitor of FAAH, and the terpene limonene. Rue is also used to treat muscle spasms, cramps, and epilepsy, and rutamarin has been shown to relieve spasms in research studies.[507]

Rutamarin helps glucose transporter 4 (GLUT4) come inside the cell in response to the hormone insulin.[508] Rutamarin can help treat symptoms of type 2 diabetes, where GLUT4 function is impaired, and rue has been used in folk medicine for that purpose.

Rutamarin's other biological functions may be related to its function as cannabinoid. Rutamarin also has anticancer properties, as it inhibits the growth of several tumor cell lines.[509] Finally, rutamarin is a potent antiviral drug that inhibits human topoisomerase II (Topo II), a protein that viruses use to replicate.[510] HU-331, a research drug synthesized from CBD, also inhibits Top II and has anti-cancer properties, showing similarities to rutamarin.[511] Rue has also been used topically to treat varicose veins, relieve back pain, and even eyestrain.

HOW TO TAKE RUE

Rue can be used as a tea, a tincture or a topical cream. Do not take rue before meals or in large doses at one time. To prepare rue tea, add 1 tsp rue leaves to one cup of boiling water for 5 minutes, strain and sweeten with honey. Take only ½ a cup of rue tea a day.

POTENTIAL RISKS OF TAKING RUE

Taking rue is not without risks. Rue is not safe in large doses as it can damage the liver and can cause gastric pain, vomiting, and even death. It may also stimulate uterine contractions and result in abortion in pregnant women. Rue should not be taken if you are pregnant, breastfeeding, have liver disease, kidney or urinary tract problems. Taking rutamarin by itself as a dietary supplement may reduce these risks.

BLACK TRUFFLES

Black truffles, a rare and expensive type of mushroom, were recently discovered to contain anandamide but not 2-AG.[12] The older the black truffle is, the more anandamide it contains. Other species of truffles are currently being tested for the presence of anandamide.

How was this discovered? Human cells that produce melanin have a fully functioning endocannabinoid system, and it was likely that any living thing that contained melanin might have components of the endocannabinoid system.[512] Interestingly, black truffles don't contain cannabinoid receptors, suggesting anandamide production is to attract animals to eat the truffles and disperse their spores, rather than for the truffles themselves. Humans are not the only animals that eat black truffles. Pigs, meerkats, grizzly bears, chacma baboons, and a marsupial called the long-footed potoroo also eat anandamide in the form of black truffles.

FAAH INHIBITORS

Fatty acid amide hydrolase (FAAH) inhibitors prevent the breakdown of anandamide, boosting its levels at CB1 and CB2 receptors. There are several plant-based and synthetic FAAH inhibitors that can boost your anandamide levels and prime your endocannabinoid system for cannabis use. This section will cover isoflavones and NSAIDs.

ISOFLAVONES

A natural class of chemicals called isoflavones have shown to be effective in inhibiting FAAH. Isoflavones have a long half-life and only need to be taken once daily when taken long-term.[89] Soy isoflavones decrease levels of oxidative DNA damage in humans.[513]

BIOCHANIN-A

Biochanin-A is a flavonoid that is found naturally in several food including soy, peanuts, alfalfa sprouts, red clover, chickpeas, and other legumes. Biochanin A is also a phytoestrogen, meaning it is a plant-derived chemical that has properties similar to the hormone estrogen. It inhibits growth and signaling of HER-2+ breast cancer cells, a form that is particularly aggressive.[514]

Biochanin-A is a natural inhibitor of FAAH, as well as an agonist of PPARα, but does not have any effect on FAAH-2, CB1 or CB2.[515] Biochanin-A does not cause effects by itself, but potentiates the behavioral effects of anandamide.[515] Biochanin-A was shown to be a more potent inhibitor of FAAH than genistein, another isoflavone described below in this chapter. The effects of biochanin-A on FAAH inhibition appear to be limited to the body, as it does not alter brain levels of anandamide, but does increase the behavioral effects of anandamide.

Biochanin-A has neuroprotective properties. It reduces neuropathic pain in a mouse model of diabetes.[516] It also protects dopamine neurons against damage and death in a rat model of Parkinson's disease.[517]

KAEMPFEROL

Kaempferol is an isoflavone found in tea, broccoli, apples, strawberries, beans, endives, and tobacco leaves.[518-519] The average dietary intake of kaempferol by adults is 5 mg/day.[520] Consumption of a bowl of endive soup, containing 8.65 mg of kaempferol, results in blood levels of 0.1 μm, while black tea containing 15 mg of kaempferol raised blood levels to 0.05 μm.[521-522]

HOW KAEMPFEROL WORKS

Kaempferol inhibits FAAH as well as activates anti-inflammatory PPARγ receptors.[523-524] It has antioxidant, anti-viral and anti-bacterial properties, and may boost the effectiveness of antibiotics.[525] Finally, high intake of kaempferol in the diet is associated with reduced risk of type 2 diabetes.[525]

ANTI-CANCER EFFECTS OF KAEMPFEROL

Kaempferol is powerful against multiple forms of cancer. Kaempferol increases apoptosis of breast cancer cells as well as inhibits estrogen receptor signaling to reduce growth of breast cancer tumors.[526-527] Kaempferol also reduces metastasis of ovarian cancer cells.[519] Intake of flavanols are associated with reduced risk of pancreatic cancer in smokers, with kaempferol having the largest risk reduction.[528] Finally, kaempferol is also effective in reducing gastric cancer risk, reducing growth of leukemia cells, and increasing apoptosis of lung cancer cells.[525,529,530]

QUERCETIN

The isoflavone quercetin is a weak inhibitor of FAAH, and the average adult intake is 16 mg/day.[520,523] Black tea containing 49 mg of quercetin raised blood levels to 0.1 μm.[522] Oral combination of kaempferol and quercetin reduce pain and is anti-inflammatory in rodents.[531]

DAIDZEIN

Daidzein (7-hydroxy-3-(4-hydroxyphenyl)-4H-chromen-4-one) is an isoflavone found in soybeans and legumes.[532] It can also be purchased as a supplement online. Daidzein is less effective at inhibiting FAAH than genistein, described later in this chapter.[515] Daidzein has anti-inflammatory and antimicrobial properties.[533] Finally, daidzein can increase apoptosis of breast cancer cells as well as boost efficacy of tamoxifen to prevent growth of breast cancer tumors.[534-535]

Only 30% of Caucasian adults compared to 50% of Asians have the ability to metabolize daidzein to equol, which is the most potent metabolite of soy.[536] This may be because they lack the gut bacteria that converts daidzein into equol.[537] Equol activates ER-beta receptors, and thus daidzein should be avoided in breast cancer patients, especially those more likely to be equol converters.[536]

GENISTEIN

Genistein is an isoflavone found in soy, fava beans, kudzu, lupin, psoralea and even coffee.[538] Genistein can also be purchased as a supplement online. Soy milk has 24 mg of genistein and 8.25 mg of daidzein in a serving.[539]

Genistein-containing kudzu is used to feed goats in the southern United States, suggesting goat meat may be a good source of genistein. Kudzu also contain isoflavones daidzein and puerarin, which has been studied as a treatment for Alzheimer's disease.[540] Kudzu is one of the 50 fundamental herbs in traditional Chinese medicine (TCM), where it is known as gé gēn. It is used anecdotally to treat migraines, cluster headaches, tinnitus, vertigo, and diarrhea, and is known as a remedy for alcohol hangover.

HOW GENISTEIN WORKS

Genistein not only inhibits FAAH, but also reduces anandamide uptake into the cel.[533] Blood levels of the isoflavones genistein and daidzein in Asians reached 2-4 μM.[541] This suggests consuming enough isoflavones in food to inhibit FAAH in the body is a possible goal. Only a small amount of genistein crosses the blood-brain barrier.[549]

Genistein is the major isoflavone found in soybeans. As an inhibitor of protein tyrosine kinase, it inhibits synthesis of glycosaminoglycans (GAGs)-long chains of sugar carbohydrates in cells that build bone and connective tissue.[542] Genistein also inhibits transcription of transcription factor EB (TFEB).[543]

BENEFITS OF TAKING GENISTEIN

Soy isoflavones genistein and daidzein in soybean reduce cholesterol levels.[544] Genistein also reduced symptoms of menopause such as hot flashes, sleep disturbance, headaches, pain, dizziness, tiredness, and vaginal dryness .[545-547] Genistein synergizes with anticancer drugs such as tamoxifen, adriamycin and docetaxel, altering major pathways associated with apoptosis, cell cycle, angiogenesis, and metastasis.[548]

Patients with Sanfilippo syndrome, a rare disease characterized by a deficit in GAG breakdown, show marked improvement in symptoms when treated with oral genistein for a year that lasted for several years after treatment.[542,550,551]

ISOFLAVONE DEFICIENCY IN WESTERN COUNTRIES

Consumption of soy products is much higher in Asian countries compared to Western countries, ranging from 20-50 grams daily compared to less than 4 mg milligram daily in the United States.[552-55] The average postmenopausal Caucasian woman eats 39 μg of daidzein, 70 μg of genistein, 31 μg of formononetin, and 31 μg of biochanin-A, making total phytoestrogen intake less than 1 mg daily compared to 20-80 mg of phytoestrogens for Asians.[552] Menopausal symptoms such as hot flashes are greatly reduced in Asians, with 10-

25% experiencing versus 58-93% of Western women.[555] Consumption of soy products likely plays a role in reduced symptoms of menopause in Asian women.

Gut bacteria can convert genistein into 5-hydroxy-equo.[537] Because only 30% of Caucasians compared to 50% of Asians have the ability to metabolize it via gut bacteria, Caucasians likely suffer from 5-hydroxyl-equol deficiency as well.[536] Finally, intake of soy isoflavones only boosts bone density in postmenopausal women and not in premenopausal women.[556-557]

DANGERS OF ISOFLAVONE EXPOSURE IN INFANTS

In the United States, only 25% of infant formula is soy based, and levels of isoflavones are 500 times higher in infant fed soy formula versus formula made from cow's milk.[558] The daily exposure of infants to estrogenic isoflavones in soy formula is 10 times higher based on body weight than the dose that has hormonal effects in adults eating soy foods.[559] This may explain the association between autistic behaviors and soy formula use.[560-561]

FORMONONETIN

Formononetin is an isoflavone, phytoestrogen, and weak inhibitor of FAAH. It is found naturally in astragalus root, red clover as well as legumes including green beans, lima beans, and soy.[561] Formononetin is a main ingredient in "Huang-qi," a popular traditional Chinese medicine.[562]

Formononetin can be useful for both menopausal women and sport injuries, as it can prevent development of osteoporosis and regenerate bone.[563-564] Formononetin is also antimicrobial and is highly effective against Candida yeast.[565] Finally, formononetin can alleviate symptoms of retinal neuropathy in a rodent model.[562]

NSAIDS

Non-steroidal anti-inflammatory drugs (NSAIDs) are an effective and cheap but possibly risky way to boost levels of endocannabinoids in your brain and body. All NSAIDs inhibit COX-1 and COX-2 enzymes to different degrees, with the added bonus of inhibiting FAAH from breaking down anandamide (AEA).[566] NSAIDs also prevent AEA and 2-AG as well as their precursor arachidonic acid (AA) from being turned into inflammatory prostaglandins by inhibiting COX-2. While NSAIDs can boost endocannabinoid levels by themselves, when combined with cannabinoid treatment, they synergize to produce even bigger effects than expected from simply adding the effects of taking either NSAIDs or cannabinoid treatment alone. When you take an NSAID, you can take a smaller dose or THC, CBD, or cannabis and have the same amount of relief from pain, spams, or nausea.

RISKS OF NSAIDS

People who take NSAIDs daily for long periods of time may have a higher risk of heart attack or stroke. Talk to your doctor about the safety of taking NSAIDs, especially if you have a personal or family history of smoking, high cholesterol, heart attack, stroke, heart disease, diabetes, or high blood pressure. Do not take NSAIDs if you use the anticoagulants or blood thinners such as warfarin (Coumadin).

Most NSAIDs are acidic and cause damage to the GI tract. Long-term use of NSAIDs can cause heartburn, ulcers, abdominal pain, diarrhea, pulmonary embolisms, and other unpleasant side effects including death.[567] NSAIDs also reduces the immune response and should not be used after vaccination.[568]

OTHER WAYS TO BOOST ENDOCANNABINOID SYSTEM FUNCTION

The final way to prime your endocannabinoid system for optimal function is to increase levels of beneficial endocannabinoids. This section will cover COX-2 inhibitors and diet, drug and lifestyle changes that boost endocannabinoid production.

COX-2 INHIBITION

Cyclooxygenase-2 (COX-2) is the enzyme that breaks down arachidonic acid, anandamide, and 2-AG into inflammatory and pain-causing prostaglandins. COX-2 is not present in every cell in the body but is upregulated in many types of cancer cells including non-melanoma skin cancers. This is why COX-2 inhibition is a target for cancer treatment and prevention.

RISKS

Prescription COX-2 inhibitor are so powerful that their side effect profiles are deadly. Celebrex (celecoxib) is a prescription NSAID that was 30 times more selective at inhibiting COX-2 than COX-1 and was in clinical trials for prostate, colon, and breast cancer treatment and prevention. However, Celebrex was found to cause heart attacks, stroke, and death as well as serious GI bleeding and perforation in patients. Celebrex now carries a “black box” warning of cardiovascular and gastrointestinal risk but was not removed from the market. An earlier COX-2 inhibitor Vioxx (rofecoxib) was removed from the market in 2004 due to cardiovascular risks. It is not suggested to take Celebrex to enhance your endocannabinoid system as the risks are too great.

CBDA

Cannabidiolic acid (CBDA), the raw acidic precursor of CBD, is a selective COX-2 inhibitor and NSAID. CBDA is found in raw hemp or certain strains of raw cannabis juice. It's also found in capsules and tinctures that have not been decarboxylated into CBD.

CBDA is nine times more selective at inhibiting COX-2 than COX-1. Similar to Celebrex, CBDA inhibits migration of human breast cancer cells.[297] Little research on raw cannabinoids including CBDA has occurred, so it unclear whether CBDA has anti-cancer effects on other forms of cancer and what the mechanism is.

GUINEENSINE

ENTOURAGE EFFECT

The entourage effect, which is when terpenes, cannabinoids, and other chemicals in the cannabis plant synergize to increase health benefits, is a key concept for boosting your endocannabinoid system. It applies whether you take a whole-plant cannabis or hemp oil, or you combine terpenes and dietary phytocannabinoids from different sources.

Black pepper has its own entourage effect, as beta-caryophyllene isn't the only terpene found in the plant. Limonene, beta-pinene, myrcene, and many other terpenes co-exist, as well as piperine (Bioperine), which boosts bioavailability of many chemicals in the body and supplements.

HOW IT WORKS

Guineensine is a *N*-isobutylamide found in several types of pepper including black pepper and is used in traditional Chinese medicine. It is the most potent reuptake inhibitor of anandamide and 2-AG found in food, which means that it boosts levels of both cannabinoids.[569-570] Guineensine does not inhibit FAAH, but rather inhibits FAAH-like anandamide transporter (FLAT) that brings anandamide into the cell for breakdown.[571] Guineensine relieves neuropathic pain through its inhibition of FLAT.[571]

Guineensine is also a monoamine oxidase inhibitor (MAOi), which means it prevents breakdown of dopamine, norepinephrine and serotonin and may have antidepressant properties.[572] Guineensine also inhibits cholesterol acyltransferase (ACAT), which means it may prevent or treat atherosclerosis caused by the buildup of cholesterol.[573] Guineensine is a potent anti-inflammatory and adding black pepper to your diet will boost the performance of any cannabinoid you take.[574]

BETA-MYRCENE

Beta-myrcene is a terpene found in mangos, hops, bay leaves, lemongrass, eucalyptus, and many other plants. Wild thyme oil contains about 40% myrcene, while cannabis oils contain between 30-65% myrcene depending on the strain. Myrcene is present in many cosmetics, soaps, and is a common food flavoring. Myrcene reduces inflammation, spasms, insomnia and pain.

HOW IT WORKS

Myrcene helps other chemicals cross the blood-brain barrier more easily so they have greater effects on the brain instead of the body. Myrcene also increases the maximum saturation level of the CB1 receptor. This would boost the effectiveness of endocannabinoids or phytocannabinoids because weaker chemicals that activate the CB1 receptor would not be able to bind. Finally, myrcene relieves pain by causing release of endorphins that activate opioid receptors.[575]

RISKS

Myrcene can increase the psychoactivity of THC or other cannabinoids in cannabis; this may make a user more sleepy or inactive, a phenomenon associated with "couch-lock." Some CBD users claim they feel "high" after using even though there is no psychoactivity associated with CBD; this may be due to feeling sleepy or out of it from myrcene present in the oil or tincture. Strains such as White Widow, Jack Herer, and Himalayan Gold are particularly high in myrcene. Check the terpene content of your strain or product if you are sensitive to the effects of myrcene. Alternately, if you use cannabis to go to sleep, look for high myrcene levels.

BOOSTING CANNABINOID PRODUCTION

New research come out monthly unraveling the secrets of our

endocannabinoid system and the foods, drugs, and lifestyle changes that improve its function.

FOOD

Following a Mediterranean diet has anti-inflammatory and life-extending benefits, but it also boosts your endocannabinoid system. Increasing intake of olive oil boosts brain levels of anandamide and atypical endocannabinoid OEA without changing brain levels of 2-AG.[76] Cannabis tinctures made in olive oil may remedy endocannabinoid deficiency better than tinctures made with different carrier oils.

Flavonoids 7-hydroxyflavone and 3,7-dihydroxyflavone are antioxidants that inhibit FAAH.[523,576] Increasing intake of fatty acids in fish oil or arachidonic acid does not change levels of anandamide or any of the atypical endocannabinoids.[76] Increasing intake of safflower oil boosts atypical endocannabinoid LEA in the brain, intestine, and liver.[76]

PRESCRIPTION DRUGS

Chronic treatment with antidepressant drugs like Prozac boosts anandamide brain levels in the hippocampus and dorsal striatum of rodents and the effect persists for at least 10 days after the last treatment.[577]

LIFESTYLE

UVB light from the sun or indoor tanning can stimulate AEA and 2-AG production in your melanocytes.[512]

CHAPTER 15

The Vitamin Weed 4-Step Plan

Step 3: Stress Management

"That's the side effects [of marijuana]: hungry, happy, sleepy." - comedian Katt Williams

Now that your endocannabinoid system is running in tip-top shape, it's time to maintain it. Stress is the number one thing that can throw your endocannabinoid system out of whack and wipe out all your progress so far. Chronic stress is the mortal enemy of a healthy endocannabinoid system. But thankfully, cannabis is also a great stress reliever by itself and also enhances the methods of stress relief outlined later in this chapter.

There are three types of stress:

1) Acute Stress - a short-term event that can range from a nuisance like a fire alarm that won't go off to a traumatizing event like a robbery.

2) Episodic Stress - a short-term event that recurs in nature, like a long commute in traffic to work or deadlines at work.

3) Chronic Stress - acute or episodic stress that endures for not hours

or days, but weeks.

In this chapter, I'll review sources of stress, stress relievers, and help you choose a stress management program that will supercharge your endocannabinoid system.

SOURCES OF STRESS

It's important to identify the stressors in your life so you can manage your response to them. Otherwise, you might not know your blood is boiling and causing an internal cascade of responses resulting in eventual downregulation of your endocannabinoid system.

SLEEP DEPRIVATION

Your endocannabinoid system is burned out when you are sleep deprived. Getting quality sleep every night will help you see results with the *Vitamin Weed 4-Step Plan* faster. As a bonus, cannabis can also help you fall asleep and stay asleep easier, leading to more energy and focus during the day. Let's start off by finding out what your baseline quality of sleep is.

THE HOW RESTED DO I FEEL QUIZ

1. I sleep:

a. whenever I get a chance to nap.
b. tossing and turning all night.
c. better than my partner.
d. great.

2. I get up during the night:

a. multiple times.
b. after my partner's snoring wakes me up.
c. just once to go to the bathroom.
d. never.

3. I feel like _________ during the day:

a. a complete zombie.
b. I need 4 Starbucks lattes.
c. I never have enough energy to complete chores around the house.
d. a spring chicken.

4. I would change ____________ about my bed:

a. everything, from my mattress to my pillow, I am so uncomfortable.
b. my pillow, I can never find one that doesn't hurt my

neck.

c. the temperature of the room, it's never cool enough.

d. my sheets, I would go for a higher thread count.

5. I exercise ________:

a. right before bed.

b. in the afternoon.

c. never.

d. in the morning.

6. I eat these foods before bed:

a. soda containing caffeine.

b. spicy foods.

c. ice cream.

d. a cup of chamomile tea.

7. When it comes to sleep, I get:"

a. sleep? what's that? I am a zombie.

b. it varies each day. I snore, have insomnia, or some other sleep problem.

c. 5-6 hours daily, but I make up for it by sleeping on the weekends.

d. 7-8 hours of it daily. I feel pretty rested when I wake up.

8. I have the following conditions:

a. obstructive sleep apnea.

b. I sleep walk.

c. I snore a little.

d. none of the above.

9. These items are turned on in my bedroom:

a. lamps or overhead lighting

b. television or computer monitor and phone

c. my phone on or next to my bed

d. nothing.

10. My bedroom is painted:

a. red.

b. yellow.

c. primary or dark blue, green, or purple.

d. pastel blue, green, or purple.

ANSWER KEY

If you chose mostly As, your sleep habits are downright tragic. You probably feel like a zombie, and live every day tired, uninspired, and strung out on coffee or energy drinks. Your body has gotten used to this extreme state of physiological stress, and likely can't remember how to function normally. The good news: with a couple of small changes, you'll see the most rapid results in the quality of your life and health. The bad news: it's going to hurt (cue the caffeine or pill withdrawal headache) before it gets better.

If you chose mostly Bs, you are struggling with health, work, or family issues that make it extremely hard to get a good night's rest. You may not be in a position to make the big changes needed to give you the quality sleep you need every night. The good news: there are small changes you can make to get the best quality sleep in the limited amount of time you have. The bad news: your body will always be fighting an uphill battle against sleep deprivation, and you'll have to load up on extra supplements to fight oxidative stress.

If you chose mostly Cs, you know what good sleep hygiene is, and really try to make it work. Unfortunately, life's stresses like work, school and family keep getting in the way. Free time is your most valued possession but you're bankrupt right now. The good news: with some time-management skill training, you'll be able to set a consistent sleep schedule and maybe even add an extra half hour of sleep every day! The bad news: you'll have to learn to say no to someone, and start making yourself a priority.

If you chose mostly Ds, you get enough sleep, you just need to improve the quality of your sleep. Most people don't realize all the little things that are blocking their brain from getting deep sleep and letting their brain and body slip into repair mode. The good news: change will be painless. The bad news: you might not notice changes in your focus, creativity, or health immediately. Keep with the changes and with a month or more you'll feel like the best version of yourself.

There are some obvious reasons for sleep deprivation, like you simply aren't scheduling 7-8 hours a day because you're working long hours, just had a baby, or stay up all night watching TV. Drug or alcohol use, excessive caffeine use especially after noon, some mental health disorders including schizophrenia, some medical conditions like fibromyalgia, and some medications may also impact the length or quality of sleep. Sleep disorders, as outline below, are a big part of why many people suffer from poor sleep.

There are some obvious reasons for sleep deprivation, like you simply aren't scheduling 7-8 hours a day because you're working long hours, just had a baby, or stay up all night watching TV. Drug or alcohol use, excessive caffeine use especially after noon, some mental health disorders including schizophrenia, some medical conditions like fibromyalgia, and some medications may also impact the length or quality of sleep. Sleep disorders, as outline below, are a big part of why many people suffer from poor sleep.

SLEEP DISORDERS

Sleep disorders range in severity from simply frustrating to causing so much chronic sleep deprivation that the patient is suicidal. Treating sleep disorders with cannabis or in addition to cannabis is key to a healthy endocannabinoid system.

INSOMNIA

Insomnia is the most common and well-known sleep disorder. 95% of Americans have had at least one episode of insomnia during their life, caused by stress, medical conditions including back pain, or medications that interfere with sleep. Insomnia occurs when you cannot fall asleep, stay asleep, or maintain quality sleep despite your strong desire to sleep. It is also associated with daytime fatigue and lack of focus. Chronic insomnia is associated with development of substance abuse and mental health disorders. Approximately 30% of adults have chronic insomnia, but because most patients don't go the doctor for treatment, it is hard to get an exact number.

SLEEP APNEA

18 million American adults have sleep apnea, with approximately 3-7% of men and 2-5% of women suffering from obstructive sleep apnea. Sleep apnea has become more common over the years in the United States due to rising obesity rates, which contribute to airway blockage.

There are three types of sleep apnea:

1) Obstructive Sleep Apnea - when the upper airway is blocked multiple times during sleep, reducing or completely stopping the flow of air.

2) Central Sleep Apnea - when your brain doesn't send signals to breathe during sleep.

3) Complex Sleep Apnea Syndrome - a combination of the above two types of sleep apnea.

All three types of sleep apnea contribute to poor quality of sleep and lack of feeling refreshed upon waking. The time spent in specific sleep stages such as REM sleep stage may be shortened or completely eliminated as well.

RESTLESS LEG SYNDROME (RLS)

10% of Americans suffer from Restless Legs Syndrome. RLS make you feel like you have to move your legs constantly, partly due to feelings of itching, burning, tingling, crawling and other uncomfortable sensations that will not go away unless the limbs are moved. Symptoms are worst at night, and cause patients to have problems falling and staying asleep, similar to insomnia.

SHIFT WORK SLEEP DISORDER (SWSD)

20% of Americans working full-time work a shift outside of the traditional 9 am to 5 pm daytime shift. Working a night time or graveyard shift can shift the circadian rhythm, resulting in sleep issues similar to insomnia. Not every shift worker develops shift work sleep disorder, with only 10-40% of workers experiencing the condition.

PARASOMNIAS

Parasomnias include abnormal sleep behaviors including sleep walking, sleep talking, eating during sleep, having sex during sleep, being aggressive during sleep, being paralyzed during sleep and having severe nightmares or hallucinations. Parasomnias can occur while falling asleep or during any sleep stage. About 10% of Americans suffer from parasomnias, but they are more common in children than adults. Patients with parasomnias sometimes disrupt the sleep of those around them more than their own sleep, so the impact of having a parasomnia can range from none to severe.

NARCOLEPSY

About 3 million patients worldwide suffer from narcolepsy, a sleep disorder in which patients sudden fall asleep or have a strong urge to sleep. Patients with narcolepsy has severe daytime drowsiness, impacting their ability to work and function. Some patients may also fall over in a sleep attack due to cataplexy or loss of muscle tone. Narcolepsy attacks can be long sleep sessions or brief while driving or doing other monotonous tasks.

LIFE CHANGES

Work may be the biggest chronic stressor in our lives, but abrupt life changes like death of a spouse or chronic stress like an abusive relationship can be just as damaging to our physical and emotional health. More than one stressful life event may be happening at the same time, causing significant harm to health.

Stressful life events are ranked in impact from biggest to least by the Holmes and Rahe Stress Scale.[578]

Life Event	**Life Change Units**
Death of a spouse	100
Divorce	73
Marital separation	65
In jail	63
Death of a close family member	63
Personal injury or illness	53
Marriage	50
Fired from work	47
Marital reconciliation	45

Retirement	45
Change in health of family member	44
Pregnancy	40
Sexual difficulties	39
Gain a new family member	39
Business readjustment	39
Change in financial state	38
Death of a close friend	37
Major mortgage	31
Foreclosure of mortgage or loan	30
Change in responsibilities at work	29
Child leaving home	29
Trouble with in-laws	29
Outstanding personal achievement	28
Spouse starts or stops work	26
Begin or end school	26
Change in living conditions	25
Revision of personal habits	24
Trouble with boss	23
Change in working hours or conditions	20
Change in residence	20
Change in schools	20
Change in recreation	19
Change in church activities	19
Change in social activities	19
Minor mortgage or loan	17

Change in sleeping habits	16
Change in number of family reunions	15
Change in eating habits	15
Vacation	13
Christmas	12
Minor violation of law	11

WORK

Your job can be a source of purpose, pride and income, but for many people, it is actually their top source of chronic stress.[579] Long hours, unreasonable deadlines or targets, and low salary can make your job a nightmare. Lack of training, lack of breaks, lack of job security and noisy or unsafe working conditions can also contribute to work stress. Poor relationships with your boss, co-workers, trainees and clients or customers can also be stressful. A work culture that supports bullying, sexual harassment or misogyny is toxic and can even cause PTSD. Finally, simple things like not have any role in decision making or creative decisions can add up and cause chronic stress.

In the next section I'll outline how to reduce stress at work, maintain healthy relationships, and relieve stress at home when you are unable to change your work conditions.

STRESS RELIEVERS

Now that you have identified potential sources of stress in your life, you're on your way to preventing or managing them if unavoidable. Thankfully there are a variety of ways to manage stress. You can pick one and religiously practice it, or you can pick and choose from options and find your zen.

SLEEP

Getting 7-8 hours a night of solid sleep is one of the best ways to reduce both physical and emotional stress. There is a variety of ways you can do that, from time management, to lifestyle changes, to medication, to cannabis.

SLEEP HYGIENE

Get to bed the same time every day, even on the weekend, to establish a sleep schedule so your body will start to get sleepy without your help and you can wake up in the morning even without an alarm clock. Avoid napping during the day, especially during the afternoon. Exercise regularly to be able to get to sleep easily and stay asleep. But don't work out an hour or two before bed. Getting your heart rate up may prevent you from falling asleep.

Your bedroom should be five things to help you get to sleep at night: painted a calming color, pitch black, quiet, comfortable, and cool. Light blue, green, or lavender are great colors for bedroom walls, while red or yellow will keep you up. If you can't keep outside noise or inside noise (say from a snoring partner) down, try turning on a fan or putting in earplugs. In terms of comfort, make sure your mattress is replaced every 10 years, wash and replace your pillows regularly, get comfy high-thread count sheets, and keep your bedroom free from allergens by regularly vacuuming and changing sheets. Keep your bedroom between 60 and 67 degrees Fahrenheit to get to sleep quicker and prevent waking up in sweats.

Lighting in the bedroom is a complex subject in our technology addicted culture. Your bedroom should be pitch black, meaning no night lights, no TVs on, no curtains open (buy blackout curtains if possible), and no electronics on. Many computers, alarm clocks, and other electronics have small lights that may even blink, disrupting your sleep environment. Your cell phone is the worst offender, as it emits blue light that can seriously disrupt your sleep. Avoid using your cell phone or laptop for an hour before bed to get sleepy, and definitely don't use either device in bed if you want to get to sleep. Candy Crush is not going to help you fall asleep! If you can't shut off all the light sources in your bedroom, try an eye mask to block out the light. Also, try not to get up to go to the bathroom in the middle of the night, as turning on the bathroom light can be enough to breakdown the melatonin your brain naturally makes in the night to keep you asleep.

What you put in your body has a huge impact on your sleep. A glass of wine or other alcoholic drink may help you go to sleep, but later in the night, you may be more likely to get up in your sleep and have less deep sleep. Caffeine found in coffee, energy drinks, teas and sodas may keep you up if you drink a lot of it or drink after noon. Obviously other stimulants, such as Adderall and Ritalin or illegal drugs like cocaine can keep you up and disrupt your sleep and should be avoided. Even cannabis, which is a treatment for sleep disorders, can cause reduced deep sleep if used at the wrong dosage.

Big meals before bed, especially heavy on protein, fat or spices, can keep you up. If you have sleep issues, try a warm glass of milk, which contains tryptophan, a precursor to serotonin which helps promote sleep, or tart cherry juice, which contains melatonin. A banana before bed can also help you sleep because it contains natural muscle relaxants potassium and magnesium.

TRADITIONAL TREATMENTS FOR SLEEP DISORDERS

Sleep apnea can be treated by medications that open the airway during sleep or by nightly use of a continuous positive air pressure (CPAP) machine. Many patients dislike having a mask over their face, and discontinue use of a CPAP machine despite benefits. Significant weight loss can also treat or even eliminate obstructive sleep apnea in some patients. An alternative or complementary treatment for sleep apnea is using cannabis in various forms, which will be outlined in Step Four.

Insomnia can be treated with prescription or OTC medications, but that often leaves you with poor sleep quality, a groggy feeling waking up, and even the potential for abuse or addiction. Common medications include zolpidem (Ambien), dipenhydramine (Benadryl), and doxylamine succinate (Unisom). Natural supplements for insomnia include valerian root and melatonin, as well as topical application or inhalation of lavender oil. Cannabis can also be used to treat insomnia.

BENEFITS OF USING CANNABIS FOR SLEEP

THC in cannabis can reduce the amount it takes you to fall asleep whether you have insomnia or you are healthy.[580] It can also help you stay asleep, a problem that people with insomnia, chronic pain, or sleep apnea struggle with.[581] Is smoking cannabis the same as eating it? The answer is no, and no clinical trial has validated whether smoking cannabis improves or hurts sleep.

A recent study found 2.5 mg or 10 mg of THC taken as a pill one hour before bed was helpful to reduce symptoms of obstructive sleep apnea, although 10 mg was better. 10 mg of THC reduced both shallow and interrupted breathing, decreased subjective sleepiness, and increased treatment satisfaction. Patients that took 10 mg of THC each night reduced symptom severity by 33% compared to CPAP users.[582]

Cannabis has also been shown to be effective for sleep disturbances associated with PTSD, which may also translate to other mental health issues. A max dosage of 3 mg of synthetic THC analogue nabilone for seven weeks reduced frequency and intensity of nightmares in military personnel with PTSD in a small pilot study.[342] An average final dose of 4 mg of nabilone for an average length of 11 weeks decreased PTSD-associated insomnia, nightmares, PTSD symptoms, and chronic pain in prisoners.[343] Finally, in a pilot study of 10 patients with PTSD on stable medication, adding 5 mg of THC twice a day reduced frequency of nightmares and improved both sleep quality as well as frequency of nightmares.[344]

WHAT CANNABIS PRODUCTS TO USE

The strain you use to help you go to sleep is important, whether you eat an edible or smoke cannabis. Sativas will keep you up at night while indicas will help you get relaxed and sleepy. Always ask your budtender whether the product you are buying will help you go to sleep or keep you alert. Think of it like Dayquil and Nyquil. You don't want to take the wrong one at the wrong time.

What your edible is made with can also impact the quality of your sleep. A coffee flavored edible made with real coffee beans will keep you up at night, no matter what strain the cannabis in it is. Some people may also want to avoid edibles with chocolate at night.

For those who use or are interested in using CBD oil on a daily basis, take your dose during the morning or early afternoon because it increases alertness and can prevent you from going to sleep. CBD can also counteract the effects of THC, so don't use it as the same time you are smoking or eating a sleepy time strain of cannabis.

Finally, CBN is a cannabinoid that is very helpful for insomnia. There are now CBN pills and CBN patches on the market; CBN is also found in old cannabis after THC breaks down into CBN. Very little is required to induce sleep, with 2.5mg of CBN taken orally being effective anecdotally.

WHAT TO DO IF YOU CAN'T WAKE UP IN THE MORNING

Eating more than 20 mg of THC before bedtime will make it difficult for you to wake up the next day. If you still do not feel sleepy 2 hours after eating up to 20 mg of THC, try vaping cannabis to slighting increase your blood THC levels without causing a sleep hangover. If you wake up the next morning and feel like you are high or just can't get up, try using CBD oil to counteract the effects of THC and wake up. A cup of coffee, some breakfast, and a shower will also get you out the door. Finally, some patients find the supplement citicoline is effective when taken upon waking for issues related to grogginess or brain fog caused by an overnight dose of cannabis.

SEX

Fulfilling sex, whether with yourself or a partner, whether or not you reach orgasm, can be an incredible stress reliever. The unfortunate part is stress actually decrease libido, or interest in sex, because cortisol causes sex-hormone-binding globulin to bind with testosterone. The less sex you have, the less sex you want. Make an effort to work on your sexual health to manage stress and prevent a downward spiral.

SEX WITH YOURSELF

Self-love can be the best kind of love. Masturbation releases dopamine and oxytocin, making you feel good and increasing your sense of well-being. Masturbation to orgasm also activates your endocannabinoid system. It releases the endocannabinoid 2-AG in two studies, but doesn't change blood levels of anandamide.[583] Orgasm relaxes you, boosts your immune system, relieves anxiety and muscle tension, and much like meditation, provides a break from negative thoughts. It can help you get to sleep, which can reduce stress in of itself.

SEX WITH A PARTNER

Penetrative sex with a partner provides more health benefits than masturbation or other forms of sex. In one study, women had greater reduction in blood pressure, and more oxytocin release.[584] Daily sex for two weeks reduces cortisol more than just one session in two weeks and boosts new brain cell growth in the hippocampus.[585] Risky or unprotected sex, or sex with a partner that does not care about your needs or is abusive, will increase stress rather than release it. Continue on to the section about Healthy Relationships in this chapter to explore what the signs of unhealthy relationship are and what to do to leave or repair your relationship.

BENEFITS OF USING CANNABIS FOR INCREASING SEXUAL LIBIDO OR PERFORMANCE

Cannabis can increase your sex drive, remove inhibitions, enhance your sensitivity to touch, and help you feel closer to your partner. All these things add up to helping you orgasm, and cannabis may even strengthen and lengthen your orgasm. You can vape or smoke cannabis before sexual activity, but the effect will not last as long as an edible will. Take an edible 30 minutes to an hour before sexual activity so that it can "kick in." Since you want to feel the psychoactive effects of THC, you don't want to microdose, but you also don't want to eat so much THC you have a bad experience, feel sick, or fall asleep. The perfect dose is different for each person; we suggest you started at 10-20 mg of THC the first time you use cannabis to improve your bedroom activities. If at any time you don't feel good, drink water, relax, and know that the THC will wear off eventually, just like the buzz from alcohol does. Remember the dose you gave yourself, and go lower next time.

Another option for improving your sexual experience without having any head "buzz" is using a lubricant with cannabis in it that will only activate your clitoris and the tissue around it. Some lubricants contain THC only, some have CBD only, and some have a combination of the two. Note that cannabis lubricants when applied properly will not make the user high like smoking or eating cannabis can. CBD-only lubricants will not bring as strong orgasms or arousal as THC-containing lubricants, but this may be appropriate for women who already have a healthy libido. Many lubricants are made with coconut oil and are not safe to use with condoms, meaning they can break down the latex and increase risk of STD exposure or pregnancy. Cannabis lubricants are usually safe to eat, meaning that if they get into the mouth during oral sex, it is non-toxic but may get your partner high later on, similar to consuming an edible. Be sure to let your partner know you have used a cannabis lubricant, because you are exposing them to a drug containing topical and you should have their consent.

BENEFITS OF USING CANNABIS FOR PAINFUL SEX

About 1 in 10 women suffer from endometriosis, a condition which includes symptoms of pain during sex, long, heavy and painful menstrual periods, and infertility. Characterized by uterine tissue growing outside the uterus on the ovaries, pelvis, intestine, or even lungs, endometriosis can cause scar tissue and even organs attaching to each other. There is no cure for this disease, diagnosis can take up to a decade, and many women are denied pain management. Sadly, many women with endometriosis avoid sex because it can cause crippling pelvic pain for up to a week. Many patients often break up with their partner because it's just too hard to deal with them wanting sex when it hurts them.

Finally, there may be a solution to painful sex as well as a way to manage endometriosis. It's our good friend cannabis. Many women with endometriosis report marijuana use reduces the pain during and after sex. Smoke it, use it topically on your pelvis, back, or even girl parts (use Foria or another THC or CBD-infused lubricant for that, not regular cannabis cream), or eat it, and you and your partner will be happy. Cannabis suppositories can also help relax women and men that find sex uncomfortable or impossible. There are suppositories made for insertion into the vagina, and suppositories made for insertion into the rectum for anal sex, like Foria Explore.

CANNABIS DOES NOT CAUSE SEXUAL DYSFUNCTION OR INFERTILITY

Cannabis users in the United States have more frequent sexual intercourse, suggesting cannabis may be an aphrodisiac and not a performance killer.[586] Currently no research has demonstrated whether cannabis has a positive or negative effect on male erections, and it is clear different forms of consumption (smoking versus eating edibles) may have differing effects on duration of effects. For women, cannabis can cause dry mouth, dry eyes, and dry vagina. Vaginal dryness can be treated with regular or cannabis-infused lubricants and by drinking extra water.

For those of you trying to conceive, it's a myth that cannabis use in you or your partner will stop you from getting pregnant. The PRESTO study found 12% of women and 14% of men trying to conceive used cannabis, and did not have increased risk of infertility compared to those who did not use cannabis.[587]

MINDFULNESS

Mindfulness is a mental state of being in the present moment. By raising awareness of and controlling your thoughts, your breath, your muscles, and your stress levels, you become in full control of your body.

DEEP BREATHING

Just five minutes of deep breathing, starting through your nose, to your belly and then through your head, can reduce signs of stress. Deep breathing can slow your heart rate and lower blood pressure, reducing the stress hormone cortisol. There are even apps on your smartphone or smartwatch that can assist you in breathing in and out for 1, 5 or 10 minutes every couple of hours.

MEDITATION

Meditation is focusing your thoughts on a single activity, object, or thought, such as the sound of your breathing or walking a circular path. By tuning out extraneous thoughts, clarity and a calming sense of peace can be found. Benefits of meditation are bountiful. Five minutes of meditation can refresh you as much as an extra hour of sleep, although longer sessions of meditation will see bigger health benefits. Daily meditation can also be as effective as an antidepressant in relieving anxiety, depression, and pain. Meditation increases volume in the hippocampus, a brain area important for learning and memory, and decreases brain volume in the amygdala, an area important for fear and anxiety.

PROGRESSIVE MUSCLE RELAXATION (PMR)

PMR is a simple technique in which you relax your muscles in your body, group by group, until you achieve full body relaxation and stress reduction. You can do this at home, at your desk, or even in the car driving. Clinical research shows PMR reduces both self-reported stress and stress hormone levels.[588]

BIOFEEDBACK

Biofeedback is a technique that trains you to be aware of when your body is showing signs of stress and to relax yourself before it becomes harmful. Traditional biofeedback treatment for four weeks significant reduced levels of stress, anxiety, and depression in one clinical research study.[589] New equipment such as portable EEG headbands have made this method available outside of the doctor's office.

TIME MANAGEMENT

Feeling like we have no control over our lives because we are always running out of time is a huge source of stress. Being aware of what your priorities are, and making time for those things, is key to happiness. Often, we are busy, but not productive. Or, we don't know when to say know. Spend 10 minutes each morning planning your day, or 10 minutes at night planning the next day. Make sure you schedule 30-60 minutes each day for self-care, whether that's a yoga class, reading a book before bed, taking an Epsom salt bath, or watching a funny movie. Finally, try to schedule a solid 7-8 hours of sleep. It really is possible, especially if you cut out all the wasted time in your day, like reading junk emails or playing Candy Crush on your phone mindlessly.

BODY WORK

Body work is a great way to reduce stress, and can include methods that involve touch like massage, reflexology or chiropractic adjustment, or energy healing methods that do not involve touch like reiki. This section will focus on body work that involves touch. The buzz people feel when getting deep tissue massage or a chiropractic adjustment is due partly to endorphins, the body's natural opioid system, as well as the endocannabinoid system. Osteopathic manipulative treatment (OMT) in healthy patients boosts blood levels of anandamide by 168% without changing 2-AG levels and also boosted feeling of well-being and "high."[590]

MASSAGE

Massage is one of the best ways to relieve stress. Massage decreases cortisol and increases levels of dopamine and serotonin.[591] Massage decreases anxiety in patients with generalized anxiety disorder (GAD).[592] Even a simple 15 minute scalp massage is able to reduce cortisol levels, blood pressure, and heart rate.[593]

There are four main types of massage:

1) Swedish massage - the most well-known type of massage, this involves long kneading and circular strokes to gently massage your muscles.

2) Deep tissue massage - similar to Swedish massage, deep tissue applies more pressure in order to work on tendons, muscle tissue, and fascia, the protective layer surrounding muscles, bones and joints.

3) Sports massage - may be a combo of Swedish and Deep massage, with the goal of treating and preventing injuries from sports or workouts.

4) Thai massage - combines acupressure, Ayurveda, and assisted yoga positions to relax and stretch without the addition of massage lotions or oils.

Other types of massage include reflexology, pregnancy massage, hot stone massage, shiatsu massage, scalp massage, and aromatherapy massage. All forms of massage can be augmented by adding CBD or cannabis cream to help relax muscles and relieve pain. Ask your massage therapist if they are open to using a cannabis topical during your massage, and to let them know to wear gloves because they could absorb cannabis while applying it to you.

KNOT ROLLER

Using a knot roller on your back, legs, and arms can be an inexpensive home version of a massage. The fancy term for knot rolling is self-myofascial release (SMR), and it has been shown clinically to increase joint range of motion (ROM).[594] SMR is especially effective for fibromyalgia patients.

When you release painful contracted knots in your muscles, you reduce stress, anxiety, and pain and improve sleep. A knot roller can be firm with lots of big knobs, or more flexible and foam depending on your pain level and whether you can tolerate deep massage. Knot or foam rollers can also be used to modify yoga poses and make them easier. Short foam rollers for your feet or golf balls can help reduce tension in feet and even treat symptoms of plantar fasciitis, reducing pain and stress. Drink water after SMR, and if you feel sore, try using a CBD or cannabis topical to relieve pain and relax muscles.

ACUPUNCTURE

Acupuncture involves placing fine needles into points on meridians, or "energy highways" which run through the body and influence different organs. Acupuncture is based in Chinese medicine, and is focused on correcting imbalances in organs and energy blockages. Clinical research shows acupuncture works to improve sleep, reduce depression, and lower stress hormones just as well or better than traditional Western medicine.[595-596] Although acupuncture is painless and relaxing if you are severely averse to needles, you may want to avoid this stress buster.

EXERCISE

Exercise, no matter what the form, the length, or the intensity, is a great way to reduce stress and increase energy. Exercise can be low-impact like walking, yoga, or swimming, or high-intensity like running, kickboxing, riding a bicycle or playing soccer. Exercise does more than just decreases cortisol levels, it boosts your glutathione levels, keeping your cellular defense system healthy. Strapped for time? Strength training for just 20 minutes three times a week can be enough to boost glutathione levels.

YOGA

Yoga is a combination of mindfulness and exercise, making it a killer stress reliever. Different poses have different ways of relieving muscle tension and activate different organs. You can easily search on the internet yoga poses for stress relief to find easy poses to try. The benefits of yoga are biggest with regular practice, which can be as little as one or two sessions a week. In clinical studies, yoga has been found to lower cortisol and relieve depression.[597]

CARDIO

Regular cardio can increase heart health, induce weight loss, improve energy levels, and boost mood. It is important to note that low intensity exercise can cause mild physiological stress inside the body, but reduce emotional stress and overall cortisol levels.[598] Endurance exercise like marathon running, however, is very stressful to the body and not recommended as a way to reduce stress.

We've all heard of runner's high, that calm, euphoric feeling that comes over you after a long run or other workout. The runner's high was thought to come from a combination of dopamine as well as endorphins, your body's natural painkillers. Recently it was discovered that endocannabinoids, specifically anandamide, are the biggest component of runner's high.[599] It makes sense that using cannabis or CBD before or during exercise may augment that runner's high due to boosting anandamide and cannabinoid signaling.

BENEFITS OF USING CANNABIS FOR EXERCISE

CBD and cannabis use can reduce joint stiffness, headaches, and chronic pain from being an occasional, regular, or professional athlete. This can be from smoking it, eating it, or using it as a topical before and after a workout. CBD can protect against brain injury and chronic traumatic encephalopathy (CTE), a condition caused by repeated hits to the head in football, boxing, soccer, and other contact sports. Over 99% of NFL football players have CTE, and this has spurred an ongoing research study at John Hopkins University. Unfortunately, the NFL has still banned cannabis use.

In October of 2017, the World Anti-Doping Agency (WADA) removed CBD from its 2018 list of prohibited substances, but THC or cannabis products still remain on the list. WADA provides regulations for all sports and all countries, and removing the CBD ban means athletes like MMA fighters can use CBD to protect their brain and relieve pain without failing a drug test. Unfortunately, this has not changed rules for high school sports or other private entities, meaning check the rules about CBD or cannabis before you use if you are subject to drug testing.

Yoga can be practiced safely with cannabis use, and in fact, "ganja" yoga classes are popping up in Colorado, California and other states where marijuana has been legalized. It is possible that practicing yoga while high may increase the relaxing effects of yoga or may help practitioners hold poses for longer. Much like yoga, cannabis helps restore balance in the mind and body.

Cannabis may actual reduce perceived exertion during exercise, increasing length and intensity of workouts. Many athletes find cannabis makes workouts more enjoyable and they fly by. If you have a hard time getting motivated, smoking cannabis before working out may put you in the mindset to do so. There are thousands of people worldwide that have gotten into shape after starting to use cannabis and working out, even when they had chronic illnesses that caused pain and fatigue. Cannabis use is also associated with 3% reduction of body mass index (BMI), meaning you may lose weight just by using it, with or without exercise.[600] Interestingly, this is despite cannabis increasing appetite, meaning you might not have to starve on a restricted-calorie diet to get into shape.

One caveat to cannabis use and performance is that a recent study of male athletes found increased levels of inflammation marker CRP in athletes who use cannabis.[601] is possible that elevated CRP is related to toxins from smoking cannabis, and vaping or eating cannabis may be a healthier way to ingest cannabis without increasing inflammation. There are good takeaways from the study. Testosterone levels, oxygen use, muscle fatigue, and cortisol levels were not statistically different between cannabis users and non-users, suggesting cannabis has no negative impact on athletic performance.[601]

SELF-CARE

Self-care is emotional hygiene; it's taking time to reduce your stress and treat yourself as special. Self-care is all the rage with millennials, who spend twice as much on self-care activities like life coaching, diet plans, and bath bombs than boomers.

BATHS

Hot baths with magnesium-rich Epsom salts can relax muscles, reduce stress, and help you get to sleep after a long day. Cannabis is now being added to the mix, with CBD or THC-infused Epsom salts available in many states. There are also cannabis-infused bath bombs that also have muscle-relaxing and pain-relieving properties. Depending on the dosage of THC in bath bombs, you may experience some psychoactivity or high if you are a woman.

READING

Reading books, magazines, or online articles is relaxing and can help you fall asleep. Reading can also expand your mind, promote self-growth, and provide you with the knowledge to secure a better or less stressful job.

SAYING NO

Saying no is probably the biggest act of self-love you can perform. Although uncomfortable at first, the benefits of not overextending yourself or doing something you do not want to do will provide long-term stress relief. Work-life balance is also a must; feel comfortable setting boundaries like not checking email on the weekends.

TAKING CONTROL OF YOUR HEALTH

In these busy days, we have to prioritize our health and not skip annual doctor checkups, pap smears, and more. Many cancer survivors regret canceling or rescheduling appointments that if they had actually made the first time, would have diagnosed their cancer much earlier. If you don't feel good, don't self-diagnose or self-medicate by visiting Google. Cancer and other threats to our health often present as something innocuous, like a stomach ache that won't go away. Become aware of your body and take it in for a tune-up when something seems funny.

SELF-EXPRESSION

Self-expression is sharing your ideas, thoughts, and feelings through dance, art, music, writing, or other forms. No matter what the form, self-expression is speaking your truth and reduces stress. Cannabis is complementary to most forms of self-expression and can amplify both the art and the release of stress.

CREATIVITY

Cannabis can help musicians, artists, actors, dancers, writers and all creators enhance their creativity and improve their art by heightening their senses. Cannabis creates a sense of wonder, allowing creators to appreciate their surroundings and transform it into art. Cannabis also boosts hyper-priming, connecting two unrelated things and causing an "Aha!" moment.[437] Smoking sativa strains or eating edibles is more likely to boost creativity than smoking indica strains, which tend to reduce energy.

People who are more creative has more baseline brain activity in a region called the frontal lobe, and when they are performing creative tasks, they show more activation in that region than noncreative people.[438] Cannabis increases brain activity in the frontal lobe, suggesting it boosts creativity.[439-441] If you are a long-term cannabis user, it is best to do creative tasks while using cannabis and not during withdrawal of over 2 days because cannabis withdrawal can hamper frontal lobe activity and thus creativity.[442]

Finally, cannabis can relieve stress and self-criticism, helping a creator fully immerse themselves in a project or brainstorming without pausing to edit every 5 seconds. Cannabis enhances "flow," a state necessary for happiness. High doses of THC, or the equivalent of 3 joints, can hamper brainstorming, but a low dose or equivalent of one joint can improve creative thinking skills.[443]

DANCING

Dancing is a combination of exercise and self-expression, which can kill stress whether you are performing ballet, rocking out at a night club, or belly-dancing. There's no wrong way to dance, so just getting up for five minutes and dancing can boost your mood and lower your cortisol. For some people dancing is uncomfortable because it's not a part of their culture or they don't feel in touch with their bodies. Signing up for dance classes, or even watching dance videos on YouTube can help improve your coordination, boost self-image, and get you active.

MUSIC

Often when people are stressed out, they avoid listening to music. This can be harmful, as listening or playing music can reduce stress. Music lowers blood pressure, heart rate, and cortisol depending on the genre.[602] Heavy metal or high-tempo EDM music may not have the same stress relieving effect as say, Beethoven classical music. Not surprisingly, smoking cannabis is very popular for people attending concerts or writing music. Using cannabis in addition to hearing music can make music more pleasurable or boost creativity in writing.

OTHER FORMS

Maybe you're not a dancer or a musician. Even picking up an adult coloring book or app can provide an outlet for your stress and help you get into a meditative state. Puff and paint sessions where attendees use cannabis and all paint the same thing are very popular in states that have legalized medical marijuana. Other forms of self-expression are knitting, building furniture, personalizing clothing, and writing poetry. Just don't handle heavy machinery or sharp tools if you're using cannabis while you relax.

SHARING YOUR FEELINGS

Speaking your truth and sharing your emotions, whether to yourself, to friends and family, or to a therapist, can be the greatest stress reliever.

KEEPING A JOURNAL

Writing your feelings down or what happened each day in your diary or journal can be therapeutic and an inexpensive way to reduce your stress. Physically writing can be more stress relieving than typing into a Word document on your computer, but both methods are better than not journaling. Journaling can help you identify your fears, goals, and problems, which can help you make concrete steps in managing each of them. Writing negative thoughts about yourself or situations you are in, and then throwing those pages away, can help you release that negative baggage and prevent lasting harm from those thoughts.[603] Writing in a journal can also reduce stress because it is a substitute for potentially stressful activities, like spending hours on Facebook and negatively impacting your mood.

TALKING TO FRIENDS AND FAMILY

People with a strong circle of friends or family that they can turn to for support live longer.[604] Stress is what takes years off of your life, so it makes sense that friends and family support reduce stress and improve your health. They can also get you out of a bad mood, by taking you out of your home or situation and distracting with hobbies, events, or a trip to your favorite restaurant. Finally, asking friends for favors or help can removing the feeling of being helpless or being in an impossible situation.

It should be noted that talking to friends or family members that do not support your lifestyle, or are dealing with issues themselves, may not be stress relieving and actually increase your anxiety or depression. For example, friends with eating disorders or self-harming behavior may promote harmful behaviors instead of encouraging you to get help.

TALKING TO A THERAPIST

Sometimes talking with friends and family or journaling just isn't enough to deal with stress. If you are abusing drugs or alcohol, have depression or other mental illness that is preventing you from being able to relax or deploy coping mechanisms, or if you have chronic, disabling pain, talking with a therapist can help you manage these conditions as well as reduce your stress. A therapist may prescribe medications in addition to therapies such as cognitive behavioral therapy (CBT), where you reframe negative thought patterns that come about due to stress.

HUGS AND OTHER FORMS OF TOUCHING

The hormone oxytocin is released when we hug, reducing blood pressure and anxiety while improving memory and immune health.[605] Hugging strangers or people we dislike is not helpful, because the lack of trust actually increases anxiety. 10-20 seconds a day of hugging is all it takes to have chronic stress relief. Hand-holding for longer periods will augment the benefits of hugging. Cuddling, even with a pet, can also reduce stress.

LAUGHING

Laughing is one of the quickest, most effective and fun ways to relieve stress. Laughing reduces blood pressure, lowers cortisol, improves your immune system, increases your sense of well-being, and releases endorphins, one of your body's natural painkillers. In one clinical study, seniors watching *America's Funniest Home Videos* not only had reduced cortisol stress hormone levels at three time points measured, but have improved short-term memory.[606] Easy ways to get laughing including watching a funny TV show, movie, comedy set or YouTube video. You're 30 times more likely to laugh while with other people than alone. Finally, cannabis can enhance your sense of humor or get you giggling when you were previously in a funk.

BENEFITS OF USING CANNABIS FOR LAUGHING

Cannabis increases blood flow to two brain areas involved in laughter, the right frontal and left temporal lobes.[607] Cannabis also increases dopamine and serotonin, two neurotransmitters responsible for pleasure and elevated mood. Finally, cannabis amplifies emotions. It can make funny things seem funnier, and serious things feel more serious. Using cannabis responsibly in the right context, like using cannabis instead of drinking before a comedy show, can provide a fantastic release from stress.

WHAT CANNABIS PRODUCTS TO USE FOR LAUGHING

Smoking sativa strains, known for providing energy, euphoria, and creativity, are more likely to produce laughter than indica strains that may produce "couch lock" and sleepiness. Eating edibles as a dosage of 10 mg or more THC, no matter what the strain, is usually associated with increased euphoria. The drawback is that it can take 45 minutes to an hour for an edible to kick in, so, if you are ridiculously stressed or depressed, smoking is a better choice and will provide relief in less than 10 minutes.

HEALTHY RELATIONSHIPS

Healthy relationships come in all forms and lengths. The stronger your social network, and we're not talking the number of your Facebook friends, the less stressed out you will be and the longer you will live.

SPOUSE OR PARTNER

A healthy relationship is stress-relieving. Happily married couples have less stress and are less likely to suffer from depression, even if they were depressed before getting married.[608] A bad or worse, abusive relationship, can kill you, whether or not you or your partner is creating most of the discord in the relationship. Learning when to leave can be one the best things you can do for your health if the relationship is beyond repair.

Respecting your partner and understanding you cannot control your partner's thoughts or actions provide the foundation for a healthy relationship. Open communication, active listening, building trust, living with lack of judgement, and using alcohol or recreational drugs in moderation is also key to a long-lasting relationship. Make sure you don't depend on your partner to fulfil all your needs by maintaining relationships with your friends and family while in a new or old relationship, and take time to pursue hobbies or develop your career.

BENEFITS OF USING CANNABIS FOR RELATIONSHIPS

Researchers at the University of Buffalo found cannabis improves marriages instead of harms them.[609] The study looked at domestic violence between 634 couples over the first 9 years of marriage. Contributing factors including history of domestic violence the year before marriage, antisocial behavior, and marijuana use by either spouse were examined. Interestingly, couples in which both partners used cannabis had the lowest domestic abuse compared to those who were only neither used or only one partner used. The more frequently cannabis was used by either husband or wife, the less frequently the husband abused the wife. The more frequently the husband used cannabis, the less frequently the wife abused the husband.

One negative to marijuana use in marriage: a wife that uses cannabis is more likely to abuse their husband if they already were abusing their partner the year before they were married.[609] If you are in an abusive relationship, please seek help. If you are the abuser, please seek help. It's never too late to change.

FAMILY

The traits and benefits of a healthy family are similar to a healthy marriage. Communication with your parents, siblings, or children should be open, non-judgmental, and supportive. Unlike a romantic relationship, it may impossible to permanently end a relationship with an abusive parent or adult child without significant stigma or emotional trauma. However, being blood does not excuse someone from abusive behavior or boundary crossing. Speak up, seek therapy, and maintain distance when necessary. For some people, cutting the cord in a hostile family relationship removes one of the largest sources of stress in their life.

BOSS

Having a healthy relationship with your boss can cut the most significant source of stress in your life, your job. Ask for feedback, aim to make your boss look good, offer to help take things off his or her plate, know when you are hassling your boss with too many emails or walk-ins, and keep your boss informed of your progress. Set boundaries, and don't let your boss bully you. This should go without saying, but it is not healthy to date your boss, and if you are the boss, to date your employees. Look for another job to transition into if your romantic interests outweigh the impact on your current job.

CO-WORKERS

You may spend more time with your co-workers than your spouse. Be respectful, communicate issues, don't get overly drunk at work functions or happy hour, and don't Facebook friend everyone at your office to maintain work-life balance. Your work place may also have policies about dating co-workers; even if they don't, you may want to avoid the drama of having to work with an ex or a fling at your office every day.

CHAPTER 16

The Vitamin Weed 4-Step Plan

Step 4: Vitamin Weed

It's time to get to the grand finale. Now that your mind, body, and soul is recharged, and your endocannabinoid system is primed to receive cannabinoids, let's add *Vitamin Weed*. This chapter will provide an overview of ways to use cannabis, cannabinoids and terpenes found in cannabis products, drug interactions and risk of consuming cannabis products, and solutions to reasons why you can't use cannabis or why it hasn't worked for you. Combined with the information shared in the rest of the book, you're on your way to the healthiest and happiest version of you.

WHO USES CANNABIS?

100% of humans use cannabinoids, as we consume on average 200 mg of dietary phytocannabinoids found in spices and other foods. Cannabinoids are chemical substances found in many living things, including plants, some types of fungus, and in living animals including humans. Cannabinoids as a class of chemicals are not illegal, but some cannabinoids found in cannabis, such as THC, have been made illegal through misunderstanding and prohibition mindset. There are over 138 cannabinoids in cannabis alone.

A common misconception is that marijuana is the gateway drug, and people who use it are criminals or drug addicts. Most of the stigma associated with cannabis use is the fact that it is illegal. More than 45% of American adults report that they have used cannabis, according to a 2012 survey from SAMHSA. Cannabis use has doubled from 2001 to 2013, to 9.5% of American adults.[610] There has never been a better time to try cannabis, as stigma is lowering everyday as people come out of the cannabis closet.

Historically, cannabis has been consumed for over 5,000 years throughout the globe. Men make up 60% of cannabis users, but women are not an insignificant minority, making up 40% of users. If laws regarding child custody were not so harsh on mothers that use cannabis, it is likely that the proportion of male and female users would be nearly equal. Seniors are the demographic most rapidly increasing in cannabis use, most likely because it replaces many of their medications and gives them back quality of life that is not found on prescription medications.

PHYTOCANNABINOIDS

There are hundreds of phytocannabinoids found in the cannabis plant, each with a broad range of health benefits. We are learning more about some of these rarer cannabinoids like CBC or CBG every day and will continue to as cannabis legalization across the world makes it easier to isolate, sell, and study these cannabinoids. This section will group CBGA, THCA and its breakdown products, CBDA and breakdown product CBD, CBCA and its breakdown products, and

CBGVA and its breakdown product THCVA and its breakdown product THCV for ease of understanding the hierarchy of cannabinoid production.

CBGA

Cannabigerolic acid (CBGA) is similar to a stem cell; it's the cannabinoid produced in the cannabis plant from which all other cannabinoids are derived. CBGA itself is formed from olivetolic acid and geranyl pyrophosphate reacting. CBGA can turn into THCA, CBDA, or CBCA depending on what enzymes (THC-synthase, CBD-synthase, and CBC-synthase) are present in the cannabis plant. Industrial hemp plants tend to have more CBGA and CBDA than marijuana strains which convert most of its CBGA into THCA. There are no commercial products with CBGA, although decarboxylated hemp products contain CBG and there are now CBG isolate products on the market.

CBG

Cannabigerol (CBG) is created when CBGA is dried or heated (decarboxylated) in cannabis storage or by smoking. CBG was first discovered in 1964 in cannabis and is also found in the African plant *Helichrysum umbraculigerum*. Other rare and synthetic forms of CBG including cannabigerolic acid monomethyl ether (CBGAM), cannabigerol monomethyl ether (CBGM), and cannabinerolic acid (*trans* CBGA).[611]

CBG is non-psychoactive and can activate alpha-2 adrenergic receptors, and block CB1, CB2, and 5-HT1A serotonin receptors.[612] CBG shows great antibacterial activity against gram positive bacteria.[613] CBG improves symptoms of inflammatory bowel disease (IBD), inhibits growth of several types of cancer including colon, breast, liver, lung and ovarian cancer, and interacts with multiple TRP channels including TRPM8.[614-616] CBG also relieves intraocular pressure and may be a useful therapeutic for glaucoma.[617-618] Finally, CBG is neuroprotective and may be drug target for multiple sclerosis and Huntington's disease.[619-620]

CBG derived from the hemp plant is not a scheduled drug in the United States or via the UN Convention on Psychotropic Substances. CBG derived from cannabis strains containing THC is Schedule 1 and cannot be shipped over state lines.

THCA-DERIVED CANNABINOIDS

THCA

Tetrahydrocannabinolic acid (THCA) is created when THC-synthase converts CBGA into THCA. It was discovered in 1965 by Dr. Friedhelm Korte.[621] THCA does not convert in the body to THC and is not psychoactive.[622] There are three forms of THCA, tetrahydrocannabinolic acid A (THCA-A), tetrahydrocannabinolic acid B (THCA-B), and tetrahydrocannabinolic acid-C_4 (THCA-C_4).

THCA show very weak activation at CB1 and CB2 receptors and its clinical efficacy may not be through these receptors.[622] THCA does not appears to not cross the blood-brain-barrier, and its activities are likely on receptors located only in the body, not the brain.[624-625] THCA increases appetite and is a potent inhibitor of nausea and vomiting and, more so than THC, and this response appears to be mediated through CB1 receptors in the body and not the brain.[626-627]

THCA inhibits both COX-1 and COX-2 enzymes, which mediates its anti-inflammatory and pain-relieving actions.[628] It activates atypical cannabinoids receptors TRPA1 and TRPV2 and blocks TRPV1 and TRPM8 receptors.[629] THCA inhibits both DGL and MGL, the enzymes that make and breakdown 2-AG, but has no influence on FAAH, the enzyme that breaks down anandamide.[629]

THCA is effective in reducing proliferation of both prostate cancer cells and breast cancer cells.[300,630] THCA may also protect dopamine neurons against cell death in a model of Parkinson's disease.[631] Finally, THCA has gained interested as both a treatment for seizures in epilepsy as well autism, lupus, fibromyalgia, and arthritis.[632-633]

THCA has many benefits in comparison to its psychoactive child THC. THC is a double-edged sword, stimulating both pro-inflammatory and anti-inflammatory pathways. THCA appears to have only anti-inflammatory actions, which makes it superior to THC. THCA is known to inhibit levels of pro-inflammatory tumor necrosis factor alpha (TNF-alpha) and activity of pro-inflammatory phosphatidylcholine specific phospholipase C (PC-PLC), while THC stimulates both proteins.

THCA is not shelf stable and converted easily to CBNA upon exposure to air and light at room temperature after just one day in a study of cannabis tea.[634] For optimal preservation of THCA raw cannabis juice must be flash-frozen. THCA stays longer as THCA instead of converting to THC when it is in olive oil compared to alcohol tinctures, and when it is kept in the fridge instead of on the shelf at room temperature.[635-636] THCA is more water soluble than THC, which is fat soluble.

Be wary of crystalline THCA advertised to be above 90% or higher purity, as it likely is not pure and has degraded to a significant amount of THC in processing or sitting on the shelf. Also know that raw cannabis juice in your fridge may degrade slightly into psychoactive THC over one or more days. Keep your THCA tinctures in the fridge to prevent them from turning into THC. And finally, perhaps the best way to consume THCA is by preparing fresh cannabis tea (boil water and put cannabis in it, don't boil the cannabis).

CBNA

Cannabinolic acid (CBNA) is created when THCA is aged through exposure to oxygen, heat and UV light. CBNA is non-psychoactive and unstable. Little is known about it, whereas more is known about the cannabinoid it converts to after decarboxylation, cannabinol (CBN).

Δ^9-THC

Delta-9-tetrahydrocannabinol (THC) is created when THC-synthase converts CBGA into THCA, and that THCA is dried or heated, a process called decarboxylation. The structure of THC was identified in 1964 by Dr. Raphael Mechoulam.[637] There are several rare forms of THC known including tetrahydrocannabinol-C_4 (THC-C_4), tetrahydrocannabiorcolic acid (THCOA), and tetrahydrocannabiorcol (THCO).[611]

THC binds to both CB1 and CB2 receptors and has actions that increase levels of endocannabinoids. THC binds to fatty acid binding proteins (FABPs), preventing anandamide from being transported into the cell and broken down.[638] This boosts anandamide levels. The psychoactivity of THC is linked to its actions on CB1 receptors, whereas its binding to CB2 receptors, mainly found on immune system cells, doesn't cause psychoactivity.

Despite its reputation for pain relief, THC can be both powerfully pro-inflammatory and anti-inflammatory. It is still much more powerful of a pain reliever than CBD, which only has anti-inflammatory effects. Because THC binds to CB2 receptors on immune cells, it can suppress the immune system with chronic use. CB2 receptors are present in the skin, and topical application of creams with THC are used to reduce pain and rashes.

Bioavailability of THC, and thus effects including how "high" a user feels, varies widely between users and smoking sessions. Regular smokers of cannabis absorb 50-70% more THC than novices because they know how to inhale cannabis smoke more efficiently. When THC is smoked, it is absorbed directly in the lungs, where it is distributed to other tissues and very little remains in the blood to be metabolized in the liver. Peak blood levels of THC are obtained 10 minutes after smoking a joint contain15 mg THC, and THC is almost undetectable after three hours.[639]

11-hydroxy-delta-9-tetrahydrocannabinol (11-OH-THC) is a metabolite that forms when THC undergoes first-pass metabolism in the liver. Levels of 11-OH-THC are over 10 times higher when you eat an edible containing THC versus when you smoke cannabis containing THC because ingredients broken down in the GI tract are taken through the bloodstream to the liver before being circulated through the body. When THC is eaten, blood levels of THC and 11-OH-THC are relatively stable from one to eight hours.[640] 11-OH-THC crosses the blood-brain-barrier more easily than THC, is 3-7 times more active at CB1 receptors, and is about four times more psychoactive than THC.[640-641] 11-OH-THC is further metabolized into 11-carboxy-delta-9-tetrahydrocannabinol (11-COOH-THC), which is not psychoactive.[641]

CBN

Cannabinol (CBN) is created when THC degrades during cannabis storage through exposure to oxygen, heat and UV light or when CBNA is decarboxylated. CBN was first named in 1896 and its chemical structure was identified in 194.[642-643] There are several rare forms of CBN including cannabinol methyl ether (CBNM), cannabinol-C_4 (CBN-C_4), cannabivarin (CBV), cannabinol-C_2 (CBN-C_2), and cannabinol-C_1 (CBN-C_1).[611] Interestingly, CBN is the only cannabinoid that can be detected in the air outside or in house dust because THC, CBC, and CBG are all degraded by air and light.[644]

CBN is a weak activator of CB1 receptors and binds more strongly to CB2 receptors, but weaker than THC does.[645-646] In terms of pain relief, CBN is equivalent to Tylenol whereas THC provides pain relief more similar to morphine.[647] Anecdotally, CBN is used as a sleep aid, alone or in combination with THC. CBN was recently found to bind to DNA, which means it may have efficacy as an antiviral, anticancer, or antibiotic drug.[648]

There has been little clinical research on CBN. One clinical trial in 1975 of 5 men tested effects of the following oral doses: 50 mg CBN, 25 mg THC, 12.5 mg THC + 25 mg CBN, and 25 mg + 50 mg CBN.[649] Blood pressure and body temperature did not change with THC, CBN, or any combination of the two. CBN did not increase heart rate while THC did and combining CBN with THC did not produce a further increase in heart rate. THC slowed perception of time while CBN did not, but the combination of the two produced both overestimates and underestimates of time. THC caused patients to feel dizzy, drunk, drowsy and drugged, while CBN alone did not, but the combination of both caused a bigger impact than THC alone.

A final note is that cannabis from the Federal government (NIDA) used for clinical research contains 11-23 times the CBN content and only 27% of the THC that cannabis sold in dispensaries to the general public.[650] This may be due to NIDA providing old or improperly stored cannabis to researchers and makes clinical research with the cannabis provided irrelevant to actual public health.

Δ^8-THC

Delta-8-tetrahydrocannabinol (Δ^8-THC) is created when THC is degraded in storage. Δ^8-THC was discovered in 1977 and has one alternative form known called delta-8-tetrahydrocannabinolic acid (Δ^8-THCA).[611] Δ^8-THC binds to CB1 receptors and CB2 receptors but is less psychoactive than THC. Δ^8-THC was tolerated and effective to stop vomiting in children with cancer, and increased appetite at low doses more strongly than Δ^9-THC.[651-652] Δ^8-THC is described by the National Cancer Institute as a cannabinoid that is neuroprotective, appetite stimulation, pain relieving, anxiety relieving, and anti-nausea.[653]

CBDA-DERIVED CANNABINOIDS

CBDA

Cannabidiolic acid (CBDA) is created when CBD-synthase converts CBGA into CBDA. Unlike CBD, which mainly works by increasing levels of anandamide and blocks other substances from binding to CB1 and CB2 receptors, CBDA does not interact with typical components of the endocannabinoid system.

CBDA is a selective cyclooxygenase-2 (COX-2) inhibitor. COX-2 inhibitors are a form of non-steroidal anti-inflammatory drugs (NSAIDs) that inhibit only COX-2, an enzyme responsible for inflammation and pain. Traditional NSAIDs, like aspirin, ibuprofen and naproxen, block both COX-1 and COX-2. In fact, aspirin is 170 times more potent in inhibiting COX-1 than COX-2. COX-1 inhibition has the side effects of stomach upset, bleeding and ulcers.

The only selective COX-2 inhibitor on the market, Celebrex, is available by prescription only, and has common side effects of nausea, abdominal pain, headache, diarrhea, flatulence and insomnia. CBDA is 9 times more potent in inhibiting COX-2 than COX-1, while prescription drug Celebrex is 30 times more potent inhibiting COX-2 than COX-1. Raw cannabis juice offers COX-2 inhibition without the side effects of Celebrex due to the entourage effect of multiple cannabinoids as well lower efficacy of COX-2 inhibition.

Indeed, CBDA is an effective treatment for acute nausea in chemotherapy patients, partly because like CBDA, it activates serotonin receptor subtype 5-HT1A.[654] CBDA is also an effective treatment for anticipatory nausea (AN), which occurs when someone vomits in response to a context, visual or smell before he or she is actually nauseous. AN develops in 29% of patients receiving chemotherapy. Raw cannabis juice may also be a solution to the nausea and vomiting that pregnant women experience as "morning sickness."

Several types of cancer cells, including human breast cancer cells, overexpress COX-2. Over a decade of scientific research suggests COX-2 inhibitors prevent and treat cancer, including colon cancer, breast cancer, and neuroblastomas (brain cancer). The National Cancer Institute (NCI) is now running clinical trials to confirm this activity in humans with selective COX-2 inhibitor Celebrex. A recent study found CBDA suppresses breast cancer metastasis by inhibiting the COX-2 enzyme, down-regulating production of the COX-2 enzyme, and suppressing genes involves in metastasis of cancer cells. As breast cancer metastasis is responsible for 90% of breast cancer deaths, CBDA in a daily raw cannabis juice regimen may be a viable method of breast cancer prevention and treatment, especially in women with a family history of breast cancer. This is especially important as 1 in 8 women will get breast cancer in their lifetime.

CBDA's mechanism as a COX-2 inhibitor and activator of 5-HT1A serotonin receptors may help more than just nausea, pain, and cancer. CBDA is a stronger activator of 5-HT1A serotonin receptors than CBD. CBDA may be an even bigger therapeutic target for mental health treatments than CBD. CBDA treats depression at doses 10-100 times lower than CBD in rodents.[655] In addition, COX-2 inhibitors like CBDA suppress inflammatory pathways involved in mental illness and have shown promise as treatments for schizophrenia and major depressive disorder in clinical trials.

CBD

Cannabidiol (CBD) was isolated in 1940 and its chemical structure was discovered in 1963.[643.656] The "diol" in cannabidiol stands for the presence of two alcoholic groups. There are several rare forms of CBD known including cannabidiol monomethyl ether (CBDM), cannabidiol-C_4 (CBD-C_4), cannabidivarinic acid (CBDVA), cannabidivarin (CBDV), and cannabidiorcol (CBD-C_1).[611] CBDV is of note because it is being investigated as a treatment for epilepsy by GW Pharmaceuticals, but it is such a rare cannabinoid it would have to be synthesized in yeast or other systems to be commercialized.

CBD does not activate the CB1 or CB2 receptor directly, but in the presence of THC, blocks it from binding to the CB1 receptor. This is why CBD can work to reverse THC overdose and help cannabis users titrate their dose. CBD also inhibits the p450 liver enzyme CYP2C9, and thus blocks conversion of THC to 11-OH-THC, which is one of the ways taking CBD with THC can reduce the "high effect."[657] The liver exclusively metabolizes THC, CBD and CBN via the cytochrome p450 family of enzymes, predominately by CYP2C and CYP3A.[658-661]

One misconception is that CBD directly inhibits FAAH, the enzyme that breaks down anandamide, to boosts its levels and increase signaling at the CB1 and CB2 receptors. CBD was shown to inhibit FAAH in rodent studies, however a recent study has shown that CBD does not inhibit FAAH in humans.[638] CBD does boost anandamide levels in humans, and this is by binding to FABPs and preventing anandamide from being transported into the cell and broken down.[638]

CBD is in fact a "dirty" drug because it has so many modes of actions besides the CB1 or CB2 receptor, and it is hard to determine in clinical research which mechanism is causing physiological or behavioral changes in patients. CBD is a more potent antioxidant than Vitamin C or Vitamin E, and the US government holds a patent #6630507 on cannabinoids including CBD as antioxidants and neuroprotectants.[662] CBD inhibits release of inflammatory cytokines and thus inflammation.

CBD directly activates 5HT1-A serotonin receptors, which mediate its anti-anxiety effects. CBD also inhibits breakdown of neurotransmitter adenosine, and increases its activity at receptors, which is the opposite of what caffeine, an antagonist at adenosine receptors, does.[663] This may be why some people find CBD helps them go to sleep. CBD increases the ability for drugs to bind to the glycine receptors, which increases the ability of cannabis to reduce pain.[664] CBD is also a GPR55 antagonist, which may mediate its anti-cancer effects. Likely in the future even more mechanisms of action will be found.

CBD can inhibit breakdown of other drugs taken because it itself inhibits liver enzymes. This can potentially cause increased or decreased levels of drugs, which can be a positive or negative effective depending on the drug. CBD inhibits CYP3A4 and CYP3A5, whereas THC, CBN, and CBD all inhibit CYP3A7 equally.[413] CBD, THC, and CBN inhibit CYP2C9, while CBD also inhibits CYP2C19 and CYP1A1.

CBE

Cannabielsoin (CBE) is very rare and can be formed from CBD and CBDA after exposure to light.[665-666] CBE was discovered in 1973 and its chemical structure was identified in 1974.[667-668] There are four other forms of CBE known, including cannabielsoic acid A (CBEA-A), cannabielsoic acid B (CBEA-B), cannabielsoic acid-C_3 B (CBEA-C_3-B) and cannabielsoin-C_3 (CBE-C_3).[669] CBD can be converted in the body to an intermediate and then through p450 enzymes to CBE.[666]

CBND

Cannabinodiol (CBND or CBDL) is an aromatized version of CBD, discovered in 1977.[670] CBND is formed when CBN is exposed to light. One alternative form of CBND is known, cannabinodivarin (CBVD).[611] CBND is a psychotropic cannabinoid, but little is known about it.

CBCA-DERIVED CANNABINOIDS

CBCA

Cannabichromenic acid (CBCA) is created when CBC-synthase converts CBGA into CBCA.[671-672] CBCA is produced in the immature hemp or cannabis plant one week before THCA is produced.[671] CBCA is a non-psychoactive cannabinoid that is anti-inflammatory, antimicrobial and pain relieving, but little research has been performed on it, likely due to its instability as a cannabinoid. CBCA can be converted to CBC by decarboxylation or to CBLA by aging.

CBC

Cannabichromene (CBC) was discovered in 1966 at the same time by two separate labs.[673-674] There are several rare forms of CBC known including cannabichromevarinic acid (CBCVA), cannabivarichromene, and cannabivarichromevarin (CBCV).[611] Cannabicyclolic acid (CBLA) is not a natural cannabinoid found in cannabis. CBLA forms when CBCA is exposed to light, which occurs when only cannabis is harvested early in the vegetative stage and stored.[671]

CBL

CBC converts to cannabicyclol (CBL) in cannabis when it is exposed to light, or the conversion can occur in raw extract.[675] It was first named THC III in 1964 but then was renamed in 1967 after the structure was identified.[673-677] There are two alternative forms of CBL including cannabicyclolic acid (CBLA) and cannabicyclovarin (CBLV).[611] CBLV was detected in 1972 and isolated in 198.[678] CBLV can be synthetically produced by exposing CBCV to light.

CBGVA-DERIVED CANNABINOIDS

CBGVA

Cannabigerovarinic acid (CBGVA) is similar to CBGA in that other cannabinoids are derived from it. However, CBGVA is not made from CBGA, and instead is formed with geranyl pyrophosphate reacts with divarinolic acid. CBGVA can turn into THCVA with the help of enzyme THCV-synthase, and then decarboxylated into THCV. There are no commercial products with CBGVA, although decarboxylated hemp and cannabis products contain THCV and are on the market.

THCVA

Tetrahydrocannabivarin carboxylic acid (THCVA) is created when THCV-synthase converts CBGVA into THCVA. Not all cannabis strains have high levels of THCV synthase, and in fact strains rich in THCV originated in Asia and Southern Africa before being brought to the United States.

THCV

Tetrahydrocannabivarin (THCV) is created when THCVA is dried or heated (decarboxylated) in cannabis storage or by smoking. Some strains have as high as 50% THCV once decarboxylated, but these strains are hard to grow, and don't grow in commercial indoor sites. Doug's Varin is one of the only strains in the United States reported to have over 20% THCV, but it is hard to find on the commercial market. Durban Poison is a strain that has on average 5% THCV depending on who is producing it.

THCV binds to both CB1 and CB2 receptors but can either an antagonist to the CB1 receptor at low doses or activate the CB1 receptor at higher doses.[679] Its action as a CB1 antagonist may be why strains with THCV reduces appetite. Because CB1 receptor blockade has been associated with psychiatric side effects like depression or suicidal thought with the drug rimonabant, it is recommended that patients with psychiatric conditions avoid strains with high amounts of THCV to avoid negative experiences.

It is also anecdotally reported that cannabis products with THCV are helpful for migraine and other forms of pain relief. THCV anecdotally increases energy and counteracts the sedative effects of terpene myrcene found in most strains. THCV is being studied in clinical trials by GW Pharmaceuticals as a treatment for epilepsy and diabetes.[373,680]

RARE CANNABINOIDS

CBT

In 1976 scientist Hawthorne Watson discovered the chemical structure of cannabitriol (CBT), a rare cannabinoid isolated from marijuana grown in Jamaica , although the chemical was first identified in 1966.[681] CBT has a similar structure to THC, with the addition of two alcohol groups and a phenol group. 8 variations of CBT have been reported in cannabis.

CBT is extremely rare and has only been identified in small amounts. It is unclear whether CBT is psychoactive or what, if any, health benefits it may provide as clinical trials and patient case studies have not been performed. It is also unknown whether CBT is found in strains of cannabis grown outside of Jamaica.

CBF AND OTHER CANNABINOIDS

Cannabifuran (CBF) was discovered in 1972 but incorrectly named cannabinoidiol.[670,678] Another form of CBF is dehydrocannabifuran (DCBF), discovered in 1975. Cannabicitran was first named citrylidene-cannabis in 1971 and then isolated in 1974.[667] Cannabitetrol (CBTT) was discovered in 1984 and cannabioxepane (CBX) was discovered in 2011.[682] Cannabichromanone (CBCN) was discovered in 1975. There are two other forms of CBCN, cannabichromanone-C_3 (CBCN-C_3) and cannabicoumaronone (CBCON). Oxo-tetrahydrocannabinol (OTHC) was discovered in 1975. Cannabiripsol (CBR) was discovered in 1979 from a cannabis strain grown in South Africa.[683]

TERPENES

Besides cannabinoids, cannabis also contains chemicals called terpenes add smell and flavor to cannabis as well as after specific medical benefits. Terpenes are also the active ingredients in essential oils, fragrances, and cleaning products. Some of these terpenes, such as myrcene and beta-caryophyllene, have been reviewed in Chapter 14 on Priming your Endocannabinoid System. There are about 30 terpenes detected in cannabis; many are rare or present in low amounts, and multiple terpenes are found in each strain.

This book will not provide an overview of each terpene and its medical benefits, and they are numerous, and many terpenes have not been researched enough to provide science-based evidence of their effects. Terpenes contribute to the entourage effect seen in cannabis, where ingredients, such as cannabinoids and terpenes, work better together than they do individually.

The numerous terpene and cannabinoid combinations contribute to the broad variety of cannabis strains, uses for cannabis, and individual responses of users to strains. To identify the terpene combination that works best for your condition or symptoms, with or without CBD or THC, is truly personalized medicine and beyond the scope of this book. To work with a professional to determine your unique formulation, contact Infused Health.

WHAT TO DO WHEN CANNABIS DOESN'T WORK FOR YOU

Maybe you've tried cannabis or CBD in the past, and it made you feel weird or it didn't help your pain. Or maybe you have a friend who tried cannabis oil and it didn't cure their cancer. Your prior experience with cannabis or other people's experiences with cannabinoid medicine has nothing to do with your future response to cannabinoid medicine, much like how an antidepressant is highly effective for one depressed patient and causes another patient to commit suicide. There are many factors to how you will respond to cannabinoid therapy, which means treating patients is a true science.

PRODUCT VARIABILITY

The biggest variable is patient response is the cannabis product. A cannabis joint can vary in the strain used, which means the THC, CBD, and other cannabinoid levels will vary depending on what someone rolled up. There can even be toxins like mold or pesticide residue, which accounts for many of the negative effects people can feel from cannabis, including nausea, headache, or anxiety. Even when you try to use the same strain every time you smoke a joint, the same strain can vary in THC level from harvest to harvest due to little changes like weather, plant stress, or a change in grower.

To make things even more confusing, some cannabis strains are mislabeled, meaning that someone could be selling Sour Diesel when it's really Girl Scout Cookies! The consumer certainly can't see or smell the difference between the strains, so they are dependent on the grower or dispensary to do their due diligence on verifying strains. Unfortunately, there are few tools that can cheaply identify the cannabinoid and terpene profile and match it to a standard strain to combat "counterfeit" strains trying to be sold for a higher price or simply mislabeled strains. Because there is no federal government oversight on what is sold to cannabis customers, like there is for alcohol and tobacco (Alcohol and Tobacco Tax and Trade Bureau), there are no consumer protections. Your best protection is to work with a grower or dispensary you trust, and never purchase black market products.

DOSAGE

Always start low and go slow when it comes to edibles. Many states have labeled 10 mg as a starter or single-serving dose for edibles, but even this may be too much for a new user, or one that use doesn't build a tolerance. Breaking a 10 mg piece of chocolate in half or even in quarters could be a great way to adjust and add 2.5 mg or 5 mg each week until you reach your happy or pain-relieving dose.

It may take some time to get used to how THC makes you feel. This is similar to taking any new medication, as anti-depressants or anti-seizure drugs can make patients feel disoriented, sluggish, or overly energetic until your brain chemistry gets used to it. THC is the same way. The first time (or two or three) you use it you might feel dizzy, confused, heart racing, anxious, paranoid, or sleepy to the point you need to take a nap. This may be especially frustrating because other people you know are not seeing the same effects and instead are relaxed, happy, and energetic.

Remember, everyone's brain and body chemistry are different, and you will find what works with your body. After two weeks of regular use, your body will be able to handle small doses of THC, whether oral or smoked. To fine tune the effects you want to have, like pain relief or energy, you can experiment with different strains, products, and CBD ratios.

TERPENE PROFILE

Sometimes it's not the amount of THC or the way you took it (ate an edible versus smoked) that is the issue. Most of the psychoactive effects of cannabis products are actually based on the terpene profile. For example, a cannabis strain or product with myrcene will carry THC through the blood-brain-barrier better, and more THC will be available to bind to your CB1 receptors, making you feel more high and lethargic. Strains with higher THC but less myrcene may make you feel less "high: than the above scenario. Likewise, strains with linalool, beta-caryophyllene or other terpenes that relax and reduce anxiety are less likely to make you feel paranoid, even if you are using a sativa that is prone to induce paranoia.

Taking some time to find the perfect strain or product for you might not be easy, and the same strain may not make you feel the same way each day depending on your mood, stress level, or diet that day. I'm working with an app called StrainConnect that will help you find your perfect strain based on your medical or recreational needs and personality that will help speed this process along so you waste less time and money on cannabis that doesn't work for you.

GENETICS

Another reason why some people have unfavorable responses to cannabis is genetics. No, I'm not talking about the genetics of the cannabis plant, I'm talking about your endocannabinoid genes. Your DNA has mutations that you inherited from your parents, sometimes leading to changes in how your endocannabinoid system functions. These aren't rare mutations, in fact, more than 25% of humans have a mutation in one of the many genes that regulates the endocannabinoid system. If 1 in 4 people have this mutation, now it makes more sense why if four people smoke a joint for the first time in their lives, there's always that odd one out that feels paranoid or anxious instead of relaxed.

The real head scratcher is why twins, who have the same DNA, same weight and even the same disease, don't respond the same to the same cannabis product. There's a secondary layer of complexity to add to the equation: epigenetics. You may have heard of "nature versus nurture", which is the relative contributions of genetics (nature) to our experiences (nurture) in causing individual differences. In this case nurture is epigenetics, the external factors that switch genes on and off.

Epigenetics is why two twins with the same DNA can have individual differences. One twin may have one gene turned off and the other twin has the game gene switched on. Everything from stress, to your mother's stress while she was pregnant with you, to DNA damage, to medications, to diet and exercise, can impact epigenetics. Some of your life's experiences have longer epigenetic changes than others. Some are easily reversible, and some are permanent and even passed on through generations. DNA methylation is one epigenetic mechanism that turns genes off.

Some people are unresponsive to cannabinoid treatment because they have epigenetic changes that prevent their endocannabinoid genes from producing cannabinoid receptors, endocannabinoids, or other critical proteins. There is no way to know your epigenetic history or current state; however certain types of cancers are associated with associated with DNA methylation and gene silencing. It is possible that treatments that demethylate DNA, that is remove methyl groups from DNA, can reactivate silenced genes and kill cancer or promote endocannabinoid function, but that is a relatively new science and a topic for another book.

Understanding how your genetics influence your response to cannabis isn't a simple task, and if you are interested in learning more you should consult an expert in the field, such as our team at Infused Health.

SHOULD YOU CONSIDER THC?

There are several reasons why you might be scared to try THC, and they can be legitimate. If you are in a state or country where medical marijuana or recreational (adult use) marijuana has not yet been legalized, I do not recommend that you grow cannabis at home or purchase cannabis on the black market.

YOU COULD GET DRUG TESTED FOR WORK OR THE COURT SYSTEM

You might be applying for a job or work at a job where you get regularly tested for drugs. Unfortunately, even in states where medical marijuana is legal medically or recreationally, there are no legal protections for an employee firing for you for testing positive for marijuana. When federal and state law conflict, as they do with medical marijuana, federal law takes precedence for employers. Even if marijuana is legalized nationwide, it is still likely some employers, such as hospitals and schools, may still test for marijuana use and fire employees who are positive.

Several high-profile cases of patients being fired over their cannabis use have been reported in the media. One is Cyd Maurer, a television news anchor from Eugene, Oregon. Cyd was involved in an accident involving a work vehicle and was tested for drug use. Unfortunately, because THC can stay in the body weeks and even months in some cases after use, she came up positive for THC and was fired despite not being under the influence or impaired during the accident.

Another example is Brandon Coates, a man from Colorado who used medical marijuana as a quadriplegic at home, not at DIRECTV where he worked. The court ruled in 2013 that because marijuana is illegal under federal law, employees have no protection to use it any time. In fact, the court ruled Colorado's Lawful Off-Duty Activities Statute, which prohibits employers from taking disciplinary action against workers for legal, off-duty activities, does not protect marijuana users in Colorado. New federal and state bills are being proposed to prevent marijuana patients from being fired for being patients.

WHAT DOES A DRUG TEST LOOK FOR?

Urine testing, or urinalysis, is the most common way to screen for drug use, including marijuana use. Drug tests don't test for the active ingredient in the drug, in this case THC. They test for a metabolite of the drug, which shows you took the drug and it was broken down in your body. Urinalysis detects the metabolite 11-nor-9-carboxy-delta-9-tetrahydrocannabinol (THC-COOH), produced when the liver breaks down THC. THC-COOH stays in your body much longer than THC. According to a survey by testing lab Quest Diagnostics, 50% of all drug tests are failed due to marijuana, as opposed to other drugs.

How much THC-COOH do you have to have in urine to fail a drug test? The most common cutoff level is 50 nanograms per milliliter (ng/mL) but can range between 20-100 ng/mL depending on the drug screening company. When a person tests positive for marijuana, a confirmatory Gas Chromatography/Mass Spectrometry (GC/MS) test is performed to verify the positive urine test. The confirmatory GC/MS cutoff is 15 ng/ML and only tests THC-COOH.

Other less common methods of drug testing include hair, blood, and saliva tests. Blood tests are commonly used to detect recent use and impairment but are used less often because of cost and difficulty of getting a sample. Blood tests test THC levels, not THC-COOH, and are often used in investigations of DUIs, accidents and injuries for legal reasons. If you have been abstinent for anywhere between 3-7 days, you will likely pass a blood test for marijuana, but there are no guarantees.

Hair testing for marijuana is controversial because it does not measure current use and tests for non-psychoactive residues that do not appear until 7-10 days after use. What this means is that you can unfairly pass a hair test within a week of smoking, if you smoked or consumed cannabis for the first time. The average hair test goes back 30 days, but some samples can test more than 90 days of past use. Men can get around a hair test by shaving hair and letting new hair grow in. Women are less lucky and have no way of circumventing a hair test, making this test controversial because it is biased for women to fail. 85% of daily cannabis users will fail a hair test, while 52% of occasional smokers will fail it.[657] Users who ate cannabis as opposed to those who smoked it were slightly more likely to pass the hair test.[657]

Saliva testing is a new technology and less reliable than other methods. You can test positive for marijuana use up to 3 days after use. While not widely adopted in the United States by employers, several states, including Michigan and California, have pushed for adoption in roadside DUI testing. This testing becomes controversial as basically makes it illegal for medical marijuana patients to drive, even when patients using other prescription drugs are allowed to drive on them. If you are asked to take a saliva test by a law enforcement officer, call your lawyer and refuse to take it. Roadside saliva tests for marijuana have not been put into law in any state and are only admissible if you voluntarily take it.

HOW LONG DOES THC STAY IN THE BODY?

Daily heavy users of cannabis have tested positive for THC-COOH in urinalysis up to 30 days after last use or even 60 days if they have been using for a decade or more. Thankfully, for frequent users 10 days is the standard for how long you have to abstain for to pass a drug test. For occasional users, it may take only four days to pass a drug test.

There are of course exceptions to these general rules. People who are obese or simply have a high body fat percentage may take months to pass a drug test because THC is fat-soluble and will hide out in your body. You also risk failing a drug test if you have been clean but start burning fat through exercise and diet. Others have claimed liver problems or a history of being on many medications means it takes longer for your body to clear THC from your body.

SHOULD YOU FAKE A DRUG TEST?

If you are concerned you may not pass your urinalysis, you may have searched online for ways to pass your drug tests. These methods include detoxing or drinking lots of water, which are legal but ineffective ways to attempt to pass your drug test. An illegal method of passing your drug testing is buying a fake urine sample to swap out for your own during the test.

All 50 states have laws against possession of a device or substance to interfere with a drug screening test. Many places that drug test know people are trying to fake drug tests and have precautions such as two-way mirrors or personal searches to catch you. If you are caught and you are lucky, you will just not be hired or fired. If you are less lucky because you did this at a state or federal facility, you will face felony charges.

Many employers and agencies are drug testing now that cannabis is legal in so many states. They know people are consuming marijuana and desperate to pass their drug tests. They will catch you. So, the simple answer: don't fake your drug test.

NOT ALL CANNABIS PRODUCTS HAVE THC

The good news is that drug tests do not test for all 138 cannabinoids found in medical marijuana. The standard drug test, urinalysis, only test for THC metabolite THC-COOH. Metabolites of other cannabinoids including CBD, CBG, and CBN show little cross-reactivity and will not cause a false positive if you are using a product that truly does not contain THC. But that's a big if.

CBD only products made from industrial hemp legally have less than 0.3% THC in them. It is possible to test positive if you are taking very high doses of CBD oil, in the range of 1000 mg or more a day. It is also possible to test positive for THC-COOH if your manufacturer of CBD products is not honest. It is actually difficult to meet the legal cutoff for to qualify for industrial hemp instead of marijuana, 0.3% THC. If plants are stressed, they start producing more THC, and can reach up to 1% THC. The hemp grower is supposed to destroy the crop, but some manufacturers still bottle up the product and sell it as 0.3% THC. A secondary GC/MS test should confirm your levels of THC-COOH are under the cutoff, so request this test if you do come up positive on your first, less stringent test.

CBN & CBG isolate products may also still have traces THC in them due to cross-contamination in the manufacturing facilities. Think of it like a wheat-free product that is made at a facility that manufactures wheat products as well; the manufacturer discloses this product was made a facility that also manufacturers wheat products and thus cannot be labeled "gluten-free." In the same way, quality controls in the cannabis industry are not high enough to be 100% certain your CBN, CBD, or CBG isolate products do not a trace of THC in them. Wean yourself off the products if you are expecting an important drug test.

NOT ALL THC PRODUCTS WILL FAIL A DRUG TEST

Some cannabis products will not cause a positive drug test because they are not metabolized through the liver. Topical products are one example. Cannabis creams containing THC applied to the skin are metabolized in the skin, and even if you apply the cream from head to toe daily, you should not test positive for marijuana. Same goes for a cannabis-infused massage, you're in the clear! Just make sure you don't apply cannabis cream and then rub your eyes, mouth, or touch food, you might accidentally eat THC cream, and then accidentally test positive in a drug test. Wash your hands after use!

A more stringent drug test, such as that required for a job with the FBI or DEA, may be more sensitive, so only avoid topicals if you are sure your employer is weeding out people that have even had a happy thought about cannabis in their life.

It is unclear whether novel products, like a spray of THC-containing sexual lubricant Foria, will result in a positive drug test. If you're not sure whether it will affect a drug test, your best bet is to contact the manufacturer or avoid the product completely. Don't just rely on the word of a budtender at a dispensary or a friend. Transdermal products that come in the form of patches or gel pens applied to inside of the wrist close to the veins, do cross the skin barrier to enter your bloodstream. Use of transdermal cannabis products containing THC will absolutely cause a positive drug test for marijuana.

RISKS OF CANNABIS USE

Any prescription drug, herbal supplement, or even food carries a risk for a subset of people. Depending on your genetic makeup, medical conditions you have, or prescription drugs you take, cannabis may not be right for you. Side effects of cannabis are minimal and may include increased appetite ("the munchies"), sleepiness, lethargy, dizziness, nausea, euphoria and laughter, bronchitis from chronic smoking, and paranoia. In the end, the decision to use cannabis or CBD is a personal one that impacts your health and should be a decision that includes your physician.

HEART ISSUES

Cannabis can lower blood pressure in some users, and thus patients who are medications to lower blood pressure or have hypotension should be careful with THC or abstain. Short-term use of cannabis can cause tachycardia, while long-term use can lead to bradycardia and hypotension.[684] Long-term use of cannabis can lead to reduced tachycardia.[685] If you have heart problems, talk to your doctor about whether cannabis is safe your you or abstain completely. Stroke and heart attack survivors may still be able to use cannabis products, particularly CBD instead of THC, because CBD help treat damage from these conditions and prevent new attack.

OVERDOSE

You cannot overdose on cannabis. To die from cannabis, you would have to eat 1,500 pounds of cannabis in 15 minutes, which is impossible. Cannabis is even safer than water, which can kill you. The reason why you cannot overdose or die from cannabis use is that CB1 receptors are virtually undetectable in the brain stem, the brain region that controls involuntary body functions including breathing.

ADDICTION

Can you become addicted to cannabis? It depends. Almost anything you can think of can be addictive, including something as seemingly harmless as playing Candy Crush games on your iPhone. An activity or substance crosses the line into addiction when it meets these three criteria. First, when doing or using it causes harm to yourself, others or your work. Second, when you want to stop but are unable to. Three, when you become tolerant to the substance and suffer withdrawal symptoms.

Addictive drugs of abuse such as cocaine or heroin release large amounts of dopamine in your brain. This makes you feel good and makes you want to consume drugs again. Cannabis also releases dopamine in your brain, but does this automatically mean cannabis is addictive? No. Natural rewards such as food, water, and sex release dopamine so that you do things like eat, live, and reproduce.

About 9% of people who use cannabis can become addicted to the THC in it. Cannabis use disorder (CUD) is the name given to those who struggle with quitting cannabis and have officially sought treatment. The average adult with marijuana use disorder has used cannabis daily for 10 years and attempted to quit over 6 times.[686]

People at risk of becoming addicted to any substance, including cannabis, may have a genetic predisposition to compulsive behavior, an underlying mental health condition, or exposure to a severe amount of stress. Thankfully cannabis does not have the same physical withdrawal syndrome that heroin or methamphetamine withdrawal does and only has mental withdrawal symptoms for those who are seriously dependent including insomnia, anxiety, depression, and changes in appetite.[687-688]

Taking CBD can help reduce symptoms of cannabis withdrawal and is being validated for this purpose in clinical trials. A 1:1 ratio of CBD to THC may be effective at treating short-term withdrawal actually effective at treating withdrawal from THC in cannabis.[689] Finally, cannabis is the exit drug, not the entrance drug. Using cannabis helps users decrease their alcohol, prescription and illegal drug use, not increase it.

CANNABINOID HYPEREMESIS SYNDROME

Cannabinoid hyperemesis syndrome (CHS) develops in a small subset of long-term heavy daily cannabis users as their body, in basic terms, becomes allergic to cannabis. CHS is very rare and is characterized by cyclic episodes of nausea, vomiting, and abdominal pain, which is alleviated only by permanent abstinence from cannabis use. Chronic stimulation of CB1 receptors in the gut by THC may result in toxicity in sensitive patients. CHS may be develop due to a genetic mutation or previous traumatic brain injury, and further research is required to screen for people at risk for the syndrome. There may also be a syndrome being misdiagnosed as CHS that is caused by illegal pesticides on cannabis.

Most patients with CHS do not know their cannabis use is the cause of CHS, because cannabis is normally associated with reduction of nausea and vomiting in people without the syndrome. In fact, these patients will initially use more cannabis to try to control their nausea and vomiting, which makes their symptoms worse as their body rejects the cannabis. One of the symptoms of CHS is constantly taking hot showers because it alleviates the symptoms.

If you think you have CHS, stop cannabis use, see your doctor or go to the hospital if you are severely dehydrated. Once you have CHS, you have it for life. Even after months or years of abstinence, symptoms of CHS will return within weeks of using cannabis regularly. Thankfully, a new study found a lotion containing capsaicin may be a treatment for the disease.[119,690]

BRAIN CHANGES

There are numerous studies suggesting that regular cannabis use changes brain structure. Some of these studies have small sample sizes or flawed methodology. For example, 70% of individuals who use cannabis also use tobacco, and recent studies have shown cannabis plus tobacco use impacts the brain much more than cannabis alone.[691] However, most studies of cannabis and the brain do not separate the confounding effect of cannabis alone or look at users that use it medically instead of recreationally. The only one that did found no correlation between hippocampal size and memory performance in cannabis users.[691] This suggests the old myth that cannabis causes brain damage is just plain wrong.

CONCLUSION

Now that you know the truth about *Vitamin Weed* and may even have experienced the benefits of it yourself, it's time to spread the message. *Vitamin Weed* could save the life of your sister, your dad, your son, your coworker or your best friend. Get active with local and national nonprofits lobbying for cannabis legalization and patients' rights. Participate in clinical research on the medical benefits of cannabis.

SUPPORT CANNABIS RESEARCH

The greatest hurdle to clinical research on the benefits of cannabinoids are political. Most federal funding for cannabis research is earmarked for finding negatives of marijuana including addiction. This is based on cannabis being a Schedule 1 illegal drug considered a substance of abuse instead of a phytocannabinoid that can prevent disease. Another problem is the federal government won't let universities grow their own cannabis to use in clinical research, and researchers must obtain their cannabis from a small farm in Mississippi, the only source legally allowed in the United States.

The U.S. government has no problem approving research for pharmaceutical versions of THC, where one chemical like an ester is added to change the molecular structure for patenting and profiting from it. The government actually owns patents on individual cannabinoids and chemical derivatives of them. The federal government does not fund clinical research on the cannabis plant because it cannot patent or profit from it. While more research is always desirable, we have enough to know cannabinoids and cannabis are not only safe, but prevent and treat disease.

My nonprofit IMPACT Network works with universities, researchers, and patient nonprofits around the world, but is still a grassroots organization lacking the government and traditional donor support that established, mainstream clinical research organizations do. To support clinical research and advocacy programs at IMPACT Network, a 501c3 nonprofit, please donate at www.impactcannabis.org/donate.

REFERENCES

1. Noonan, M.A., et al., *Withdrawal from cocaine self-administration normalizes deficits in proliferation and enhances maturity of adult-generated hippocampal neurons.* J Neurosci, 2008. **28**(10): p. 2516-26.
2. Noonan, M.A., et al., *Reduction of adult hippocampal neurogenesis confers vulnerability in an animal model of cocaine addiction.* J Neurosci, 2010. **30**(1): p. 304-15.
3. Eisch, A.J.a.N., M.A., *Regulation of adult neurogenesis by cannabinoids.* Chimica Oggi, 2006. **24**(5): p. 84-88.
4. De Petrocellis, L., et al., *The endogenous cannabinoid anandamide inhibits human breast cancer cell proliferation.* Proc Natl Acad Sci U S A, 1998. **95**(14): p. 8375-80.
5. Grimaldi, C., et al., *Anandamide inhibits adhesion and migration of breast cancer cells.* Exp Cell Res, 2006. **312**(4): p. 363-73.
6. Xie, C., et al., *Anti-proliferative effects of anandamide in human hepatocellular carcinoma cells.* Oncol Lett, 2012. **4**(3): p. 403-407.
7. Clapper, J.R., et al., *Anandamide suppresses pain initiation through a peripheral endocannabinoid mechanism.* Nat Neurosci, 2010. **13**(10): p. 1265-70.
8. Onaivi, E.S., *Neuropsychobiological evidence for the functional presence and expression of cannabinoid CB2 receptors in the brain.* Neuropsychobiology, 2006. **54**(4): p. 231-46.
9. Iribarne, M., et al., *Cannabinoid receptors in conjunctival epithelium: identification and functional properties.* Invest Ophthalmol Vis Sci, 2008. **49**(10): p. 4535-44.
10. Siegel, A., et al., *Neuropharmacology of brain-stimulation-evoked aggression.* Neurosci Biobehav Rev, 1999. **23**(3): p. 359-89.
11. di Tomaso, E., M. Beltramo, and D. Piomelli, *Brain cannabinoids in chocolate.* Nature, 1996. **382**(6593): p. 677-8.
12. Pacioni, G., et al., *Truffles contain endocannabinoid metabolic enzymes and anandamide.* Phytochemistry, 2015. **110**: p. 104-10.
13. McPartland, J.M., et al., *Evolutionary origins of the endocannabinoid system.* Gene, 2006. **370**: p. 64-74.
14. McPartland, J., et al., *Cannabinoid receptors are absent in insects.* J Comp Neurol, 2001. **436**(4): p. 423-9.
15. McPartland, J.M., et al., *Cannabinoid receptors in invertebrates.* J Evol Biol, 2006. **19**(2): p. 366-73.
16. Matias, I., J.M. McPartland, and V. Di Marzo, *Occurrence and possible biological role of the endocannabinoid system in the sea squirt Ciona intestinalis.* J Neurochem, 2005. **93**(5): p. 1141-56.

17. Min, R., V. Di Marzo, and H.D. Mansvelder, *DAG lipase involvement in depolarization-induced suppression of inhibition: does endocannabinoid biosynthesis always meet the demand?* Neuroscientist, 2010. **16**(6): p. 608-13.
18. Alger, B.E. and J. Kim, *Supply and demand for endocannabinoids.* Trends Neurosci, 2011. **34**(6): p. 304-15.
19. Di Marzo, V., et al., *Formation and inactivation of endogenous cannabinoid anandamide in central neurons.* Nature, 1994. **372**(6507): p. 686-91.
20. Lee, H.C., G.M. Simon, and B.F. Cravatt, *ABHD4 regulates multiple classes of N-acyl phospholipids in the mammalian central nervous system.* Biochemistry, 2015. **54**(15): p. 2539-49.
21. Liu, J., et al., *A biosynthetic pathway for anandamide.* Proc Natl Acad Sci U S A, 2006. **103**(36): p. 13345-50.
22. Bisogno, T., et al., *Cloning of the first sn1-DAG lipases points to the spatial and temporal regulation of endocannabinoid signaling in the brain.* J Cell Biol, 2003. **163**(3): p. 463-8.
23. Nakane, S., et al., *2-Arachidonoyl-sn-glycero-3-phosphate, an arachidonic acid-containing lysophosphatidic acid: occurrence and rapid enzymatic conversion to 2-arachidonoyl-sn-glycerol, a cannabinoid receptor ligand, in rat brain.* Arch Biochem Biophys, 2002. **402**(1): p. 51-8.
24. Higgs, H.N. and J.A. Glomset, *Identification of a phosphatidic acid-preferring phospholipase A1 from bovine brain and testis.* Proc Natl Acad Sci U S A, 1994. **91**(20): p. 9574-8.
25. Gaetani, S., et al., *The endocannabinoid system as a target for novel anxiolytic and antidepressant drugs.* Int Rev Neurobiol, 2009. **85**: p. 57-72.
26. Kim, J. and B.E. Alger, *Reduction in endocannabinoid tone is a homeostatic mechanism for specific inhibitory synapses.* Nat Neurosci, 2010. **13**(5): p. 592-600.
27. Kaczocha, M., S.T. Glaser, and D.G. Deutsch, *Identification of intracellular carriers for the endocannabinoid anandamide.* Proc Natl Acad Sci U S A, 2009. **106**(15): p. 6375-80.
28. Kaczocha, M., et al., *Inhibition of fatty acid binding proteins elevates brain anandamide levels and produces analgesia.* PLoS One, 2014. **9**(4): p. e94200.
29. Kaczocha, M., et al., *Fatty acid-binding proteins transport N-acylethanolamines to nuclear receptors and are targets of endocannabinoid transport inhibitors.* J Biol Chem, 2012. **287**(5): p. 3415-24.
30. Chicca, A., et al., *Evidence for bidirectional endocannabinoid transport across cell membranes.* J Biol Chem, 2012. **287**(41): p. 34660-82.
31. Cravatt, B.F., et al., *Molecular characterization of an enzyme that degrades neuromodulatory fatty-acid amides.* Nature, 1996. **384**(6604): p. 83-7.
32. Cravatt, B.F., et al., *Supersensitivity to anandamide and enhanced endogenous cannabinoid signaling in mice lacking fatty acid amide hydrolase.* Proc Natl Acad Sci U S A, 2001. **98**(16): p. 9371-6.
33. Kaczocha, M., et al., *Lipid droplets are novel sites of N-acylethanolamine inactivation by fatty acid amide hydrolase-2.* J Biol Chem, 2010. **285**(4): p.

2796-806.
34. Blankman, J.L., et al., *ABHD12 controls brain lysophosphatidylserine pathways that are deregulated in a murine model of the neurodegenerative disease PHARC.* Proc Natl Acad Sci U S A, 2013. **110**(4): p. 1500-5.
35. Wei, B.Q., et al., *A second fatty acid amide hydrolase with variable distribution among placental mammals.* J Biol Chem, 2006. **281**(48): p. 36569-78.
36. Nomura, D.K., et al., *Endocannabinoid hydrolysis generates brain prostaglandins that promote neuroinflammation.* Science, 2011. **334**(6057): p. 809-13.
37. Savinainen, J.R., S.M. Saario, and J.T. Laitinen, *The serine hydrolases MAGL, ABHD6 and ABHD12 as guardians of 2-arachidonoylglycerol signalling through cannabinoid receptors.* Acta Physiol (Oxf), 2012. **204**(2): p. 267-76.
38. Blankman, J.L., G.M. Simon, and B.F. Cravatt, *A comprehensive profile of brain enzymes that hydrolyze the endocannabinoid 2-arachidonoylglycerol.* Chem Biol, 2007. **14**(12): p. 1347-56.
39. Marrs, W.R., et al., *The serine hydrolase ABHD6 controls the accumulation and efficacy of 2-AG at cannabinoid receptors.* Nat Neurosci, 2010. **13**(8): p. 951-7.
40. Tchantchou, F. and Y. Zhang, *Selective inhibition of alpha/beta-hydrolase domain 6 attenuates neurodegeneration, alleviates blood brain barrier breakdown, and improves functional recovery in a mouse model of traumatic brain injury.* J Neurotrauma, 2013. **30**(7): p. 565-79.
41. Kozak, K.R., et al., *Metabolism of the endocannabinoids, 2-arachidonylglycerol and anandamide, into prostaglandin, thromboxane, and prostacyclin glycerol esters and ethanolamides.* J Biol Chem, 2002. **277**(47): p. 44877-85.
42. Woodward, D.F., et al., *The pharmacology and therapeutic relevance of endocannabinoid derived cyclo-oxygenase (COX)-2 products.* Pharmacol Ther, 2008. **120**(1): p. 71-80.
43. Alhouayek, M. and G.G. Muccioli, *COX-2-derived endocannabinoid metabolites as novel inflammatory mediators.* Trends Pharmacol Sci, 2014. **35**(6): p. 284-92.
44. Sang, N., et al., *Postsynaptically synthesized prostaglandin E2 (PGE2) modulates hippocampal synaptic transmission via a presynaptic PGE2 EP2 receptor.* J Neurosci, 2005. **25**(43): p. 9858-70.
45. Sang, N., J. Zhang, and C. Chen, *COX-2 oxidative metabolite of endocannabinoid 2-AG enhances excitatory glutamatergic synaptic transmission and induces neurotoxicity.* J Neurochem, 2007. **102**(6): p. 1966-77.
46. Woodward, D.F., J.W. Wang, and N.J. Poloso, *Recent progress in prostaglandin F2alpha ethanolamide (prostamide F2alpha) research and therapeutics.* Pharmacol Rev, 2013. **65**(4): p. 1135-47.
47. Sang, N., J. Zhang, and C. Chen, *PGE2 glycerol ester, a COX-2 oxidative metabolite of 2-arachidonoyl glycerol, modulates inhibitory synaptic*

transmission in mouse hippocampal neurons. J Physiol, 2006. **572**(Pt 3): p. 735-45.

48. Urquhart, P., A. Nicolaou, and D.F. Woodward, *Endocannabinoids and their oxygenation by cyclo-oxygenases, lipoxygenases and other oxygenases.* Biochim Biophys Acta, 2015. **1851**(4): p. 366-76.
49. Devane, W.A., et al., *Isolation and structure of a brain constituent that binds to the cannabinoid receptor.* Science, 1992. **258**(5090): p. 1946-9.
50. Hansen, H.S., *Effect of diet on tissue levels of palmitoylethanolamide.* CNS Neurol Disord Drug Targets, 2013. **12**(1): p. 17-25.
51. Caille, S.A.-J., L.; Polis, I.; Stouffer, D.G.; Parsons, L.H., *Specific Alterations of Extracellular Endocannabinoid Levels in the Nucleus Accumbens by Ethanol, Heroin and Cocaine Self-Administration.* Journal of Neuroscience, 2007. **27**(14): p. 3695-3702.
52. Kearn, C.S., et al., *Relationships between ligand affinities for the cerebellar cannabinoid receptor CB1 and the induction of GDP/GTP exchange.* J Neurochem, 1999. **72**(6): p. 2379-87.
53. Movahed, P., et al., *Vascular effects of anandamide and N-acylvanillylamines in the human forearm and skin microcirculation.* Br J Pharmacol, 2005. **146**(2): p. 171-9.
54. Zygmunt, P.M., et al., *Vanilloid receptors on sensory nerves mediate the vasodilator action of anandamide.* Nature, 1999. **400**(6743): p. 452-7.
55. Sugiura, T., et al., *2-Arachidonoylglycerol: a possible endogenous cannabinoid receptor ligand in brain.* Biochem Biophys Res Commun, 1995. **215**(1): p. 89-97.
56. Patel, S. and C.J. Hillard, *Role of endocannabinoid signaling in anxiety and depression.* Curr Top Behav Neurosci, 2009. **1**: p. 347-71.
57. Du, H., et al., *Inhibition of COX-2 expression by endocannabinoid 2-arachidonoylglycerol is mediated via PPAR-gamma.* Br J Pharmacol, 2011. **163**(7): p. 1533-49.
58. Balvers, M.G., et al., *Measurement of palmitoylethanolamide and other N-acylethanolamines during physiological and pathological conditions.* CNS Neurol Disord Drug Targets, 2013. **12**(1): p. 23-33.
59. Tsuboi, K., N. Takezaki, and N. Ueda, *The N-acylethanolamine-hydrolyzing acid amidase (NAAA).* Chem Biodivers, 2007. **4**(8): p. 1914-25.
60. O'Sullivan, S.E. and D.A. Kendall, *Cannabinoid activation of peroxisome proliferator-activated receptors: potential for modulation of inflammatory disease.* Immunobiology, 2010. **215**(8): p. 611-6.
61. Jonsson, K.O., et al., *Effects of homologues and analogues of palmitoylethanolamide upon the inactivation of the endocannabinoid anandamide.* Br J Pharmacol, 2001. **133**(8): p. 1263-75.
62. Ho, W.S., D.A. Barrett, and M.D. Randall, *'Entourage' effects of N-palmitoylethanolamide and N-oleoylethanolamide on vasorelaxation to anandamide occur through TRPV1 receptors.* Br J Pharmacol, 2008. **155**(6): p. 837-46.
63. De Petrocellis, L., J.B. Davis, and V. Di Marzo, *Palmitoylethanolamide enhances anandamide stimulation of human vanilloid VR1 receptors.* FEBS

Lett, 2001. **506**(3): p. 253-6.
64. De Petrocellis, L., et al., *Effect on cancer cell proliferation of palmitoylethanolamide, a fatty acid amide interacting with both the cannabinoid and vanilloid signalling systems.* Fundam Clin Pharmacol, 2002. **16**(4): p. 297-302.
65. Di Marzo, V., et al., *Palmitoylethanolamide inhibits the expression of fatty acid amide hydrolase and enhances the anti-proliferative effect of anandamide in human breast cancer cells.* Biochem J, 2001. **358**(Pt 1): p. 249-55.
66. Ghafouri, N., et al., *Palmitoylethanolamide and stearoylethanolamide levels in the interstitium of the trapezius muscle of women with chronic widespread pain and chronic neck-shoulder pain correlate with pain intensity and sensitivity.* Pain, 2013. **154**(9): p. 1649-58.
67. Marini, I., et al., *Palmitoylethanolamide versus a nonsteroidal anti-inflammatory drug in the treatment of temporomandibular joint inflammatory pain.* J Orofac Pain, 2012. **26**(2): p. 99-104.
68. Giugliano, E., et al., *The adjuvant use of N-palmitoylethanolamine and transpolydatin in the treatment of endometriotic pain.* Eur J Obstet Gynecol Reprod Biol, 2013. **168**(2): p. 209-13.
69. Lambert, D.M., et al., *Anticonvulsant activity of N-palmitoylethanolamide, a putative endocannabinoid, in mice.* Epilepsia, 2001. **42**(3): p. 321-7.
70. Sheerin, A.H., et al., *Selective antiepileptic effects of N-palmitoylethanolamide, a putative endocannabinoid.* Epilepsia, 2004. **45**(10): p. 1184-8.
71. Hansen, H.S., *Role of anorectic N-acylethanolamines in intestinal physiology and satiety control with respect to dietary fat.* Pharmacol Res, 2014. **86**: p. 18-25.
72. Magotti, P., et al., *Structure of human N-acylphosphatidylethanolamine-hydrolyzing phospholipase D: regulation of fatty acid ethanolamide biosynthesis by bile acids.* Structure, 2015. **23**(3): p. 598-604.
73. Fu, J., et al., *Oleylethanolamide regulates feeding and body weight through activation of the nuclear receptor PPAR-alpha.* Nature, 2003. **425**(6953): p. 90-3.
74. Hansen, H.S. and T.A. Diep, *N-acylethanolamines, anandamide and food intake.* Biochem Pharmacol, 2009. **78**(6): p. 553-60.
75. Overton, H.A., et al., *Deorphanization of a G protein-coupled receptor for oleoylethanolamide and its use in the discovery of small-molecule hypophagic agents.* Cell Metab, 2006. **3**(3): p. 167-75.
76. Artmann, A., et al., *Influence of dietary fatty acids on endocannabinoid and N-acylethanolamine levels in rat brain, liver and small intestine.* Biochim Biophys Acta, 2008. **1781**(4): p. 200-12.
77. Hansen, H.S., *Palmitoylethanolamide and other anandamide congeners. Proposed role in the diseased brain.* Exp Neurol, 2010. **224**(1): p. 48-55.
78. Dalle Carbonare, M., et. al., *A saturated N-acylethanolamine other than N-palmitoyl ethanolamine with anti-inflammatory properties: a neglected story...* J Neuroendocrinol, 2008. **20**(Suppl 1): p. 26-34.

79. Bisogno, T., et al., *Brain regional distribution of endocannabinoids: implications for their biosynthesis and biological function.* Biochem Biophys Res Commun, 1999. **256**(2): p. 377-80.
80. Bisogno, T., et al., *Biosynthesis and inactivation of N-arachidonoylethanolamine (anandamide) and N-docosahexaenoylethanolamine in bovine retina.* Arch Biochem Biophys, 1999. **370**(2): p. 300-7.
81. Sheskin, T., et al., *Structural requirements for binding of anandamide-type compounds to the brain cannabinoid receptor.* J Med Chem, 1997. **40**(5): p. 659-67.
82. Poling, J.S., et al., *Docosahexaenoic acid block of neuronal voltage-gated K+ channels: subunit selective antagonism by zinc.* Neuropharmacology, 1996. **35**(7): p. 969-82.
83. Walter, L., et al., *Astrocytes in culture produce anandamide and other acylethanolamides.* J Biol Chem, 2002. **277**(23): p. 20869-76.
84. Berger, A., et al., *Anandamide and diet: inclusion of dietary arachidonate and docosahexaenoate leads to increased brain levels of the corresponding N-acylethanolamines in piglets.* Proc Natl Acad Sci U S A, 2001. **98**(11): p. 6402-6.
85. Kim, H.S., et al., *Marijuana Tourism and Emergency Department Visits in Colorado.* N Engl J Med, 2016. **374**(8): p. 797-8.
86. Yang, R., et al., *Decoding functional metabolomics with docosahexaenoyl ethanolamide (DHEA) identifies novel bioactive signals.* J Biol Chem, 2011. **286**(36): p. 31532-41.
87. Park, S.W., et al., *5-lipoxygenase mediates docosahexaenoyl ethanolamide and N-arachidonoyl-L-alanine-induced reactive oxygen species production and inhibition of proliferation of head and neck squamous cell carcinoma cells.* BMC Cancer, 2016. **16**: p. 458.
88. Di Marzo, V., et al., *Cannabimimetic fatty acid derivatives in cancer and inflammation.* Prostaglandins Other Lipid Mediat, 2000. **61**(1-2): p. 43-61.
89. Howes, J., et al., *Long-term pharmacokinetics of an extract of isoflavones from red clover (Trifolium pratense).* J Altern Complement Med, 2002. **8**(2): p. 135-42.
90. Grabiec, U. and F. Dehghani, *N-Arachidonoyl Dopamine: A Novel Endocannabinoid and Endovanilloid with Widespread Physiological and Pharmacological Activities.* Cannabis Cannabinoid Res, 2017. **2**(1): p. 183-196.
91. Huang, S.M., et al., *An endogenous capsaicin-like substance with high potency at recombinant and native vanilloid VR1 receptors.* Proc Natl Acad Sci U S A, 2002. **99**(12): p. 8400-5.
92. Price, T.J., et al., *Modulation of trigeminal sensory neuron activity by the dual cannabinoid-vanilloid agonists anandamide, N-arachidonoyl-dopamine and arachidonyl-2-chloroethylamide.* Br J Pharmacol, 2004. **141**(7): p. 1118-30.
93. Marinelli, S., et al., *N-arachidonoyl-dopamine tunes synaptic transmission onto dopaminergic neurons by activating both cannabinoid and vanilloid*

receptors. Neuropsychopharmacology, 2007. **32**(2): p. 298-308.
94. Sagar, D.R., et al., *TRPV1 and CB(1) receptor-mediated effects of the endovanilloid/endocannabinoid N-arachidonoyl-dopamine on primary afferent fibre and spinal cord neuronal responses in the rat.* Eur J Neurosci, 2004. **20**(1): p. 175-84.
95. Sancho, R., et al., *Mechanisms of HIV-1 inhibition by the lipid mediator N-arachidonoyldopamine.* J Immunol, 2005. **175**(6): p. 3990-9.
96. Porter, A.C., et al., *Characterization of a novel endocannabinoid, virodhamine, with antagonist activity at the CB1 receptor.* J Pharmacol Exp Ther, 2002. **301**(3): p. 1020-4.
97. Kozlowska, H., et al., *Virodhamine relaxes the human pulmonary artery through the endothelial cannabinoid receptor and indirectly through a COX product.* Br J Pharmacol, 2008. **155**(7): p. 1034-42.
98. Sharir, H., et al., *The endocannabinoids anandamide and virodhamine modulate the activity of the candidate cannabinoid receptor GPR55.* J Neuroimmune Pharmacol, 2012. **7**(4): p. 856-65.
99. Hanus, L., et al., *2-arachidonyl glyceryl ether, an endogenous agonist of the cannabinoid CB1 receptor.* Proc Natl Acad Sci U S A, 2001. **98**(7): p. 3662-5.
100. Fezza, F., et al., *Noladin ether, a putative novel endocannabinoid: inactivation mechanisms and a sensitive method for its quantification in rat tissues.* FEBS Lett, 2002. **513**(2-3): p. 294-8.
101. Appendino, G., et al., *Homologues and isomers of noladin ether, a putative novel endocannabinoid: interaction with rat cannabinoid CB(1) receptors.* Bioorg Med Chem Lett, 2003. **13**(1): p. 43-6.
102. Shoemaker, J.L., et al., *The endocannabinoid noladin ether acts as a full agonist at human CB2 cannabinoid receptors.* J Pharmacol Exp Ther, 2005. **314**(2): p. 868-75.
103. Duncan, M., et al., *Noladin ether, a putative endocannabinoid, attenuates sensory neurotransmission in the rat isolated mesenteric arterial bed via a non-CB1/CB2 G(i/o) linked receptor.* Br J Pharmacol, 2004. **142**(3): p. 509-18.
104. Jones, E.K. and T.C. Kirkham, *Noladin ether, a putative endocannabinoid, enhances motivation to eat after acute systemic administration in rats.* Br J Pharmacol, 2012. **166**(6): p. 1815-21.
105. Freund, T.F. and N. Hajos, *Excitement reduces inhibition via endocannabinoids.* Neuron, 2003. **38**(3): p. 362-5.
106. Bennetzen, M.F., et al., *Reduced cannabinoid receptor 1 protein in subcutaneous adipose tissue of obese.* Eur J Clin Invest, 2010. **40**(2): p. 121-6.
107. Bab, I., A. Zimmer, and E. Melamed, *Cannabinoids and the skeleton: from marijuana to reversal of bone loss.* Ann Med, 2009. **41**(8): p. 560-7.
108. Howlett, A.C., et al., *International Union of Pharmacology. XXVII. Classification of cannabinoid receptors.* Pharmacol Rev, 2002. **54**(2): p. 161-202.
109. Malan, T.P., Jr., et al., *CB2 cannabinoid receptor agonists: pain relief without psychoactive effects?* Curr Opin Pharmacol, 2003. **3**(1): p. 62-7.

110. Kim, J. and Y. Li, *Chronic activation of CB2 cannabinoid receptors in the hippocampus increases excitatory synaptic transmission.* J Physiol, 2015. **593**(4): p. 871-86.
111. Onaivi, E.S., et al., *Discovery of the presence and functional expression of cannabinoid CB2 receptors in brain.* Ann N Y Acad Sci, 2006. **1074**: p. 514-36.
112. Whiteside, G.T., G.P. Lee, and K.J. Valenzano, *The role of the cannabinoid CB2 receptor in pain transmission and therapeutic potential of small molecule CB2 receptor agonists.* Curr Med Chem, 2007. **14**(8): p. 917-36.
113. Ibrahim, M.M., et al., *CB2 cannabinoid receptor mediation of antinociception.* Pain, 2006. **122**(1-2): p. 36-42.
114. Quartilho, A., et al., *Inhibition of inflammatory hyperalgesia by activation of peripheral CB2 cannabinoid receptors.* Anesthesiology, 2003. **99**(4): p. 955-60.
115. Onaivi, E.S., et al., *Behavioral effects of CB2 cannabinoid receptor activation and its influence on food and alcohol consumption.* Ann N Y Acad Sci, 2008. **1139**: p. 426-33.
116. Starowicz, K.M., et al., *Endocannabinoid dysregulation in the pancreas and adipose tissue of mice fed with a high-fat diet.* Obesity (Silver Spring), 2008. **16**(3): p. 553-65.
117. Everaerts, W., et al., *The capsaicin receptor TRPV1 is a crucial mediator of the noxious effects of mustard oil.* Curr Biol, 2011. **21**(4): p. 316-21.
118. Eberhardt, M.J., et al., *Reactive metabolites of acetaminophen activate and sensitize the capsaicin receptor TRPV1.* Sci Rep, 2017. **7**(1): p. 12775.
119. Dezieck, L., et al., *Resolution of cannabis hyperemesis syndrome with topical capsaicin in the emergency department: a case series.* Clin Toxicol (Phila), 2017. **55**(8): p. 908-913.
120. Gunthorpe, M.J. and A. Szallasi, *Peripheral TRPV1 receptors as targets for drug development: new molecules and mechanisms.* Curr Pharm Des, 2008. **14**(1): p. 32-41.
121. McHugh, D., et al., *N-arachidonoyl glycine, an abundant endogenous lipid, potently drives directed cellular migration through GPR18, the putative abnormal cannabidiol receptor.* BMC Neurosci, 2010. **11**: p. 44.
122. McHugh, D., et al., *Delta(9) -Tetrahydrocannabinol and N-arachidonyl glycine are full agonists at GPR18 receptors and induce migration in human endometrial HEC-1B cells.* Br J Pharmacol, 2012. **165**(8): p. 2414-24.
123. Calder, P.C., *Marine omega-3 fatty acids and inflammatory processes: Effects, mechanisms and clinical relevance.* Biochim Biophys Acta, 2015. **1851**(4): p. 469-84.
124. Flegel, C., et al., *Characterization of non-olfactory GPCRs in human sperm with a focus on GPR18.* Sci Rep, 2016. **6**: p. 32255.
125. Ashton, J.C., *The atypical cannabinoid O-1602: targets, actions, and the central nervous system.* Cent Nerv Syst Agents Med Chem, 2012. **12**(3): p. 233-9.
126. Morgan, D.J., et al., *Delta9-Tetrahydrocannabinol (Delta9-THC) attenuates mouse sperm motility and male fecundity.* Br J Pharmacol, 2012. **165**(8): p.

2575-83.
127. Wise, L.A., et al., *Marijuana use and fecundability in a North American preconception cohort study.* J Epidemiol Community Health, 2018. **72**(3): p. 208-215.
128. Bradshaw, H.B., S.H. Lee, and D. McHugh, *Orphan endogenous lipids and orphan GPCRs: a good match.* Prostaglandins Other Lipid Mediat, 2009. **89**(3-4): p. 131-4.
129. Aneetha, H., et al., *Alcohol dehydrogenase-catalyzed in vitro oxidation of anandamide to N-arachidonoyl glycine, a lipid mediator: synthesis of N-acyl glycinals.* Bioorg Med Chem Lett, 2009. **19**(1): p. 237-41.
130. Huang, S.M., et al., *Identification of a new class of molecules, the arachidonyl amino acids, and characterization of one member that inhibits pain.* J Biol Chem, 2001. **276**(46): p. 42639-44.
131. Miller, S., et al., *Evidence for a GPR18 Role in Diurnal Regulation of Intraocular Pressure.* Invest Ophthalmol Vis Sci, 2016. **57**(14): p. 6419-6426.
132. O'Dowd, B.F., et al., *Discovery of three novel G-protein-coupled receptor genes.* Genomics, 1998. **47**(2): p. 310-3.
133. Wang, J., et al., *Kynurenic acid as a ligand for orphan G protein-coupled receptor GPR35.* J Biol Chem, 2006. **281**(31): p. 22021-8.
134. Yu, T., et al., *Beneficial effects of cannabinoid receptor type 2 (CB2R) in injured skeletal muscle post-contusion.* Histol Histopathol, 2015. **30**(6): p. 737-49.
135. Shore, D.M. and P.H. Reggio, *The therapeutic potential of orphan GPCRs, GPR35 and GPR55.* Front Pharmacol, 2015. **6**: p. 69.
136. Imielinski, M., et al., *Common variants at five new loci associated with early-onset inflammatory bowel disease.* Nat Genet, 2009. **41**(12): p. 1335-40.
137. Yang, Y., et al., *G-protein-coupled receptor 35 is a target of the asthma drugs cromolyn disodium and nedocromil sodium.* Pharmacology, 2010. **86**(1): p. 1-5.
138. Sawzdargo, M., et al., *Identification and cloning of three novel human G protein-coupled receptor genes GPR52, PsiGPR53 and GPR55: GPR55 is extensively expressed in human brain.* Brain Res Mol Brain Res, 1999. **64**(2): p. 193-8.
139. Ryberg, E., et al., *The orphan receptor GPR55 is a novel cannabinoid receptor.* Br J Pharmacol, 2007. **152**(7): p. 1092-101.
140. Whyte, L.S., et al., *The putative cannabinoid receptor GPR55 affects osteoclast function in vitro and bone mass in vivo.* Proc Natl Acad Sci U S A, 2009. **106**(38): p. 16511-6.
141. Arifin, S.A. and M. Falasca, *Lysophosphatidylinositol Signalling and Metabolic Diseases.* Metabolites, 2016. **6**(1).
142. Pertwee, R.G., *Pharmacological actions of cannabinoids.* Handb Exp Pharmacol, 2005(168): p. 1-51.
143. Kapur, A., et al., *Atypical responsiveness of the orphan receptor GPR55 to cannabinoid ligands.* J Biol Chem, 2009. **284**(43): p. 29817-27.
144. Overton, H.A., M.C. Fyfe, and C. Reynet, *GPR119, a novel G protein-coupled receptor target for the treatment of type 2 diabetes and obesity.* Br J

Pharmacol, 2008. **153 Suppl 1**: p. S76-81.
145. Brown, A.J., *Novel cannabinoid receptors.* Br J Pharmacol, 2007. **152**(5): p. 567-75.
146. Lan, H., et al., *GPR119 is required for physiological regulation of glucagon-like peptide-1 secretion but not for metabolic homeostasis.* J Endocrinol, 2009. **201**(2): p. 219-30.
147. Swaminath, G., *Fatty acid binding receptors and their physiological role in type 2 diabetes.* Arch Pharm (Weinheim), 2008. **341**(12): p. 753-61.
148. Hillig, K.W. and P.G. Mahlberg, *A chemotaxonomic analysis of cannabinoid variation in Cannabis (Cannabaceae).* Am J Bot, 2004. **91**(6): p. 966-75.
149. Cabral, G.A., T.J. Rogers, and A.H. Lichtman, *Turning Over a New Leaf: Cannabinoid and Endocannabinoid Modulation of Immune Function.* J Neuroimmune Pharmacol, 2015. **10**(2): p. 193-203.
150. Pertwee, R.G., *Emerging strategies for exploiting cannabinoid receptor agonists as medicines.* Br J Pharmacol, 2009. **156**(3): p. 397-411.
151. Syed, Y.Y., K. McKeage, and L.J. Scott, *Delta-9-tetrahydrocannabinol/cannabidiol (Sativex(R)): a review of its use in patients with moderate to severe spasticity due to multiple sclerosis.* Drugs, 2014. **74**(5): p. 563-78.
152. Gofshteyn, J.S., et al., *Cannabidiol as a Potential Treatment for Febrile Infection-Related Epilepsy Syndrome (FIRES) in the Acute and Chronic Phases.* J Child Neurol, 2017. **32**(1): p. 35-40.
153. Hess, E.J., et al., *Cannabidiol as a new treatment for drug-resistant epilepsy in tuberous sclerosis complex.* Epilepsia, 2016. **57**(10): p. 1617-1624.
154. Devinsky, O., et al., *Cannabidiol in patients with treatment-resistant epilepsy: an open-label interventional trial.* Lancet Neurol, 2016. **15**(3): p. 270-8.
155. Schinasi, L. and M.E. Leon, *Non-Hodgkin lymphoma and occupational exposure to agricultural pesticide chemical groups and active ingredients: a systematic review and meta-analysis.* Int J Environ Res Public Health, 2014. **11**(4): p. 4449-527.
156. Tam, J., et al., *Peripheral CB1 cannabinoid receptor blockade improves cardiometabolic risk in mouse models of obesity.* J Clin Invest, 2010. **120**(8): p. 2953-66.
157. Schlosburg, J.E., et al., *Chronic monoacylglycerol lipase blockade causes functional antagonism of the endocannabinoid system.* Nat Neurosci, 2010. **13**(9): p. 1113-9.
158. Long, J.Z., et al., *Selective blockade of 2-arachidonoylglycerol hydrolysis produces cannabinoid behavioral effects.* Nat Chem Biol, 2009. **5**(1): p. 37-44.
159. Ramesh, D., et al., *Dual inhibition of endocannabinoid catabolic enzymes produces enhanced antiwithdrawal effects in morphine-dependent mice.* Neuropsychopharmacology, 2013. **38**(6): p. 1039-49.
160. Piomelli, D., et al., *Pharmacological profile of the selective FAAH inhibitor KDS-4103 (URB597).* CNS Drug Rev, 2006. **12**(1): p. 21-38.
161. Gunduz-Cinar, O., et al., *Amygdala FAAH and anandamide: mediating protection and recovery from stress.* Trends Pharmacol Sci, 2013. **34**(11): p.

637-44.
162. Schlosburg, J.E., et al., *Inhibitors of endocannabinoid-metabolizing enzymes reduce precipitated withdrawal responses in THC-dependent mice.* AAPS J, 2009. **11**(2): p. 342-52.
163. Panlilio, L.V., Z. Justinova, and S.R. Goldberg, *Inhibition of FAAH and activation of PPAR: new approaches to the treatment of cognitive dysfunction and drug addiction.* Pharmacol Ther, 2013. **138**(1): p. 84-102.
164. Solinas, M., et al., *The endogenous cannabinoid anandamide produces delta-9-tetrahydrocannabinol-like discriminative and neurochemical effects that are enhanced by inhibition of fatty acid amide hydrolase but not by inhibition of anandamide transport.* J Pharmacol Exp Ther, 2007. **321**(1): p. 370-80.
165. Fegley, D., et al., *Anandamide transport is independent of fatty-acid amide hydrolase activity and is blocked by the hydrolysis-resistant inhibitor AM1172.* Proc Natl Acad Sci U S A, 2004. **101**(23): p. 8756-61.
166. Deplanque, X., A. Wullens, and L. Norberciak, *Prevalence and risk factors of vitamin D deficiency in healthy adults aged 18-65 years in northern France.* Rev Med Interne, 2017.
167. Holick, M.F. and T.C. Chen, *Vitamin D deficiency: a worldwide problem with health consequences.* Am J Clin Nutr, 2008. **87**(4): p. 1080S-6S.
168. Garland, C.F., et al., *Vitamin D and prevention of breast cancer: pooled analysis.* J Steroid Biochem Mol Biol, 2007. **103**(3-5): p. 708-11.
169. Prakash, S., et al., *The prevalence of headache may be related with the latitude: a possible role of Vitamin D insufficiency?* J Headache Pain, 2010. **11**(4): p. 301-7.
170. Vinkhuyzen, A.A., et al., *Gestational vitamin D deficiency and autism-related traits: the Generation R Study.* Mol Psychiatry, 2016.
171. McGrath, J.J., et al., *Developmental vitamin D deficiency and risk of schizophrenia: a 10-year update.* Schizophr Bull, 2010. **36**(6): p. 1073-8.
172. Basatemur, E., et al., *Trends in the Diagnosis of Vitamin D Deficiency.* Pediatrics, 2017.
173. Russo, E.B., *Clinical endocannabinoid deficiency (CECD): can this concept explain therapeutic benefits of cannabis in migraine, fibromyalgia, irritable bowel syndrome and other treatment-resistant conditions?* Neuro Endocrinol Lett, 2004. **25**(1-2): p. 31-9.
174. Baron, E.P., *Comprehensive Review of Medicinal Marijuana, Cannabinoids, and Therapeutic Implications in Medicine and Headache: What a Long Strange Trip It's Been.* Headache, 2015. **55**(6): p. 885-916.
175. Volfe, Z., A. Dvilansky, and I. Nathan, *Cannabinoids block release of serotonin from platelets induced by plasma from migraine patients.* Int J Clin Pharmacol Res, 1985. **5**(4): p. 243-6.
176. Fride, E., et al., *Critical role of the endogenous cannabinoid system in mouse pup suckling and growth.* Eur J Pharmacol, 2001. **419**(2-3): p. 207-14.
177. Di Marzo, V., et al., *Trick or treat from food endocannabinoids?* Nature, 1998. **396**(6712): p. 636-7.

178. Wu, J., et al., *Oxylipins, endocannabinoids, and related compounds in human milk: Levels and effects of storage conditions.* Prostaglandins Other Lipid Mediat, 2016. **122**: p. 28-36.
179. Diaz-Alonso, J., M. Guzman, and I. Galve-Roperh, *Endocannabinoids via CB(1) receptors act as neurogenic niche cues during cortical development.* Philos Trans R Soc Lond B Biol Sci, 2012. **367**(1607): p. 3229-41.
180. Hibbeln, J.R., et al., *Maternal seafood consumption in pregnancy and neurodevelopmental outcomes in childhood (ALSPAC study): an observational cohort study.* Lancet, 2007. **369**(9561): p. 578-85.
181. Doenni, V.M., et al., *Deficient adolescent social behavior following early-life inflammation is ameliorated by augmentation of anandamide signaling.* Brain Behav Immun, 2016. **58**: p. 237-247.
182. El-Talatini, M.R., A.H. Taylor, and J.C. Konje, *The relationship between plasma levels of the endocannabinoid, anandamide, sex steroids, and gonadotrophins during the menstrual cycle.* Fertil Steril, 2010. **93**(6): p. 1989-96.
183. El-Talatini, M.R., et al., *Localisation and function of the endocannabinoid system in the human ovary.* PLoS One, 2009. **4**(2): p. e4579.
184. El-Talatini, M.R., A.H. Taylor, and J.C. Konje, *Fluctuation in anandamide levels from ovulation to early pregnancy in in-vitro fertilization-embryo transfer women, and its hormonal regulation.* Hum Reprod, 2009. **24**(8): p. 1989-98.
185. Maccarrone, M., et al., *Endogenous cannabinoids in neuronal and immune cells: toxic effects, levels and degradation.* Funct Neurol, 2001. **16**(4 Suppl): p. 53-60.
186. Ribeiro, M.L., et al., *17beta-oestradiol and progesterone regulate anandamide synthesis in the rat uterus.* Reprod Biomed Online, 2009. **18**(2): p. 209-18.
187. Nallendran, V., et al., *The plasma levels of the endocannabinoid, anandamide, increase with the induction of labour.* BJOG, 2010. **117**(7): p. 863-9.
188. Fattore, L. and W. Fratta, *How important are sex differences in cannabinoid action?* Br J Pharmacol, 2010. **160**(3): p. 544-8.
189. Rubino, T. and D. Parolaro, *Sexually dimorphic effects of cannabinoid compounds on emotion and cognition.* Front Behav Neurosci, 2011. **5**: p. 64.
190. Pascual, A.C., et al., *Cannabinoid receptor-dependent metabolism of 2-arachidonoylglycerol during aging.* Exp Gerontol, 2014. **55**: p. 134-42.
191. Pascual, A.C., et al., *Aging modifies the enzymatic activities involved in 2-arachidonoylglycerol metabolism.* Biofactors, 2013. **39**(2): p. 209-20.
192. Bilkei-Gorzo, A., *The endocannabinoid system in normal and pathological brain ageing.* Philos Trans R Soc Lond B Biol Sci, 2012. **367**(1607): p. 3326-41.
193. Katayama, K., et al., *Distribution of anandamide amidohydrolase in rat tissues with special reference to small intestine.* Biochim Biophys Acta, 1997. **1347**(2-3): p. 212-8.
194. Alvheim, A.R., et al., *Dietary linoleic acid elevates the endocannabinoids 2-*

AG and anandamide and promotes weight gain in mice fed a low fat diet. Lipids, 2014. **49**(1): p. 59-69.

195. Calder, P.C., *Immunomodulation by omega-3 fatty acids.* Prostaglandins Leukot Essent Fatty Acids, 2007. **77**(5-6): p. 327-35.
196. Annuzzi, G., et al., *Differential alterations of the concentrations of endocannabinoids and related lipids in the subcutaneous adipose tissue of obese diabetic patients.* Lipids Health Dis, 2010. **9**: p. 43.
197. Pu, S., et al., *Interactions between dietary oil treatments and genetic variants modulate fatty acid ethanolamides in plasma and body weight composition.* Br J Nutr, 2016. **115**(6): p. 1012-23.
198. Abdulnour, J., et al., *Circulating endocannabinoids in insulin sensitive vs. insulin resistant obese postmenopausal women. A MONET group study.* Obesity (Silver Spring), 2014. **22**(1): p. 211-6.
199. Cote, M., et al., *Circulating endocannabinoid levels, abdominal adiposity and related cardiometabolic risk factors in obese men.* Int J Obes (Lond), 2007. **31**(4): p. 692-9.
200. Nicholson, J., et al., *Leptin levels are negatively correlated with 2-arachidonoylglycerol in the cerebrospinal fluid of patients with osteoarthritis.* PLoS One, 2015. **10**(4): p. e0123132.
201. Matias, I., et al., *Endocannabinoids measurement in human saliva as potential biomarker of obesity.* PLoS One, 2012. **7**(7): p. e42399.
202. Engeli, S., et al., *Activation of the peripheral endocannabinoid system in human obesity.* Diabetes, 2005. **54**(10): p. 2838-43.
203. Di Marzo, V., et al., *Role of insulin as a negative regulator of plasma endocannabinoid levels in obese and nonobese subjects.* Eur J Endocrinol, 2009. **161**(5): p. 715-22.
204. Mallipedhi, A., et al., *Changes in plasma levels of N-arachidonoyl ethanolamine and N-palmitoylethanolamine following bariatric surgery in morbidly obese females with impaired glucose homeostasis.* J Diabetes Res, 2015. **2015**: p. 680867.
205. Heyman, E., et al., *Intense exercise increases circulating endocannabinoid and BDNF levels in humans--possible implications for reward and depression.* Psychoneuroendocrinology, 2012. **37**(6): p. 844-51.
206. Gasperi, V., et al., *The fatty acid amide hydrolase in lymphocytes from sedentary and active subjects.* Med Sci Sports Exerc, 2014. **46**(1): p. 24-32.
207. Galdino, G., et al., *Acute resistance exercise induces antinociception by activation of the endocannabinoid system in rats.* Anesth Analg, 2014. **119**(3): p. 702-15.
208. Ferreira-Vieira, T.H., et al., *A role for the endocannabinoid system in exercise-induced spatial memory enhancement in mice.* Hippocampus, 2014. **24**(1): p. 79-88.
209. Berdyshev, E.V., et al., *Stress-induced generation of N-acylethanolamines in mouse epidermal JB6 P+ cells.* Biochem J, 2000. **346 Pt 2**: p. 369-74.
210. Magina, S., et al., *Inhibition of basal and ultraviolet B-induced melanogenesis by cannabinoid CB(1) receptors: a keratinocyte-dependent effect.* Arch Dermatol Res, 2011. **303**(3): p. 201-10.

211. Wang, X., et al., *Circulating Endocannabinoids and Insulin Resistance in Patients with Obstructive Sleep Apnea.* Biomed Res Int, 2016. **2016**: p. 9782031.
212. Hanlon, E.C., et al., *Sleep Restriction Enhances the Daily Rhythm of Circulating Levels of Endocannabinoid 2-Arachidonoylglycerol.* Sleep, 2016. **39**(3): p. 653-64.
213. Maple, K.E., et al., *Dose-dependent cannabis use, depressive symptoms, and FAAH genotype predict sleep quality in emerging adults: a pilot study.* Am J Drug Alcohol Abuse, 2016. **42**(4): p. 431-40.
214. Prospero-Garcia, O., et al., *Endocannabinoids and sleep.* Neurosci Biobehav Rev, 2016. **71**: p. 671-679.
215. Pava, M.J., A. Makriyannis, and D.M. Lovinger, *Endocannabinoid Signaling Regulates Sleep Stability.* PLoS One, 2016. **11**(3): p. e0152473.
216. Murillo-Rodriguez, E., et al., *The anandamide membrane transporter inhibitor, VDM-11, modulates sleep and c-Fos expression in the rat brain.* Neuroscience, 2008. **157**(1): p. 1-11.
217. de Kloet, A.D. and S.C. Woods, *Minireview: Endocannabinoids and their receptors as targets for obesity therapy.* Endocrinology, 2009. **150**(6): p. 2531-6.
218. Maccarrone, M. and T. Wenger, *Effects of cannabinoids on hypothalamic and reproductive function.* Handb Exp Pharmacol, 2005(168): p. 555-71.
219. Solinas, M., S.R. Goldberg, and D. Piomelli, *The endocannabinoid system in brain reward processes.* Br J Pharmacol, 2008. **154**(2): p. 369-83.
220. Aviello, G., et al., *Inhibitory effect of the anorexic compound oleoylethanolamide on gastric emptying in control and overweight mice.* J Mol Med (Berl), 2008. **86**(4): p. 413-22.
221. Valenti, M., et al., *Differential diurnal variations of anandamide and 2-arachidonoyl-glycerol levels in rat brain.* Cell Mol Life Sci, 2004. **61**(7-8): p. 945-50.
222. Murillo-Rodriguez, E., et al., *Cannabidiol, a constituent of Cannabis sativa, modulates sleep in rats.* FEBS Lett, 2006. **580**(18): p. 4337-45.
223. Martinez-Vargas, M., et al., *Sleep modulates cannabinoid receptor 1 expression in the pons of rats.* Neuroscience, 2003. **117**(1): p. 197-201.
224. Rueda-Orozco, P.E., et al., *Impairment of endocannabinoids activity in the dorsolateral striatum delays extinction of behavior in a procedural memory task in rats.* Neuropharmacology, 2008. **55**(1): p. 55-62.
225. Karatsoreos, I.N., *Links between Circadian Rhythms and Psychiatric Disease.* Front Behav Neurosci, 2014. **8**: p. 162.
226. Acuna-Goycolea, C., K. Obrietan, and A.N. van den Pol, *Cannabinoids excite circadian clock neurons.* J Neurosci, 2010. **30**(30): p. 10061-6.
227. Dasgupta, P., et al., *Nicotine inhibits apoptosis induced by chemotherapeutic drugs by up-regulating XIAP and survivin.* Proc Natl Acad Sci U S A, 2006. **103**(16): p. 6332-7.
228. Ravi, J., et al., *FAAH inhibition enhances anandamide mediated anti-tumorigenic effects in non-small cell lung cancer by downregulating the EGF/EGFR pathway.* Oncotarget, 2014. **5**(9): p. 2475-86.

229. Ferrer, B., et al., *Regulation of brain anandamide by acute administration of ethanol.* Biochem J, 2007. **404**(1): p. 97-104.
230. Rubio, M., et al., *Short-term exposure to alcohol in rats affects brain levels of anandamide, other N-acylethanolamines and 2-arachidonoyl-glycerol.* Neurosci Lett, 2007. **421**(3): p. 270-4.
231. Robinson, S.L., et al., *Acute and chronic ethanol exposure differentially regulate CB1 receptor function at glutamatergic synapses in the rat basolateral amygdala.* Neuropharmacology, 2016. **108**: p. 474-84.
232. Varodayan, F.P., et al., *Chronic ethanol exposure decreases CB1 receptor function at GABAergic synapses in the rat central amygdala.* Addict Biol, 2016. **21**(4): p. 788-801.
233. Henderson-Redmond, A.N., J. Guindon, and D.J. Morgan, *Roles for the endocannabinoid system in ethanol-motivated behavior.* Prog Neuropsychopharmacol Biol Psychiatry, 2016. **65**: p. 330-9.
234. Palomino, A., et al., *Effects of acute versus repeated cocaine exposure on the expression of endocannabinoid signaling-related proteins in the mouse cerebellum.* Front Integr Neurosci, 2014. **8**: p. 22.
235. Chouker, A., et al., *Motion sickness, stress and the endocannabinoid system.* PLoS One, 2010. **5**(5): p. e10752.
236. Hill, M.N., et al., *Circulating endocannabinoids and N-acyl ethanolamines are differentially regulated in major depression and following exposure to social stress.* Psychoneuroendocrinology, 2009. **34**(8): p. 1257-62.
237. Demers, C.H., et al., *Interactions Between Anandamide and Corticotropin-Releasing Factor Signaling Modulate Human Amygdala Function and Risk for Anxiety Disorders: An Imaging Genetics Strategy for Modeling Molecular Interactions.* Biol Psychiatry, 2016. **80**(5): p. 356-62.
238. Qin, Z., et al., *Chronic stress induces anxiety via an amygdalar intracellular cascade that impairs endocannabinoid signaling.* Neuron, 2015. **85**(6): p. 1319-31.
239. Gray, J.M., et al., *Corticotropin-releasing hormone drives anandamide hydrolysis in the amygdala to promote anxiety.* J Neurosci, 2015. **35**(9): p. 3879-92.
240. Hill, M.N., et al., *Disruption of fatty acid amide hydrolase activity prevents the effects of chronic stress on anxiety and amygdalar microstructure.* Mol Psychiatry, 2013. **18**(10): p. 1125-35.
241. Lomazzo, E., et al., *Chronic stress leads to epigenetic dysregulation in the neuropeptide-Y and cannabinoid CB1 receptor genes in the mouse cingulate cortex.* Neuropharmacology, 2017. **113**(Pt A): p. 301-313.
242. Neumeister, A., et al., *Translational evidence for a role of endocannabinoids in the etiology and treatment of posttraumatic stress disorder.* Psychoneuroendocrinology, 2015. **51**: p. 577-84.
243. Pietrzak, R.H., et al., *Cannabinoid type 1 receptor availability in the amygdala mediates threat processing in trauma survivors.* Neuropsychopharmacology, 2014. **39**(11): p. 2519-28.
244. Lazary, J., et al., *Genetically reduced FAAH activity may be a risk for the development of anxiety and depression in persons with repetitive childhood*

trauma. Eur Neuropsychopharmacol, 2016. **26**(6): p. 1020-8.
245. Zhong, W., et al., *Age and sex patterns of drug prescribing in a defined American population.* Mayo Clin Proc, 2013. **88**(7): p. 697-707.
246. Daniels, K. and W.D. Mosher, *Contraceptive methods women have ever used: United States, 1982-2010.* Natl Health Stat Report, 2013(62): p. 1-15.
247. Guindon, J., et al., *Alterations in endocannabinoid tone following chemotherapy-induced peripheral neuropathy: effects of endocannabinoid deactivation inhibitors targeting fatty-acid amide hydrolase and monoacylglycerol lipase in comparison to reference analgesics following cisplatin treatment.* Pharmacol Res, 2013. **67**(1): p. 94-109.
248. Pridgen, W.L., et al., *A famciclovir + celecoxib combination treatment is safe and efficacious in the treatment of fibromyalgia.* J Pain Res, 2017. **10**: p. 451-460.
249. Giuffrida, A., et al., *Cerebrospinal anandamide levels are elevated in acute schizophrenia and are inversely correlated with psychotic symptoms.* Neuropsychopharmacology, 2004. **29**(11): p. 2108-14.
250. Buczynski, M.W. and L.H. Parsons, *Quantification of brain endocannabinoid levels: methods, interpretations and pitfalls.* Br J Pharmacol, 2010. **160**(3): p. 423-42.
251. Vaughn, L.K., et al., *Endocannabinoid signalling: has it got rhythm?* Br J Pharmacol, 2010. **160**(3): p. 530-43.
252. Adler, J.N. and J.A. Colbert, *Clinical decisions. Medicinal use of marijuana--polling results.* N Engl J Med, 2013. **368**(22): p. e30.
253. Chan, M.H., et al., *Colorado Medical Students' Attitudes and Beliefs About Marijuana.* J Gen Intern Med, 2017.
254. Kondrad, E. and A. Reid, *Colorado family physicians' attitudes toward medical marijuana.* J Am Board Fam Med, 2013. **26**(1): p. 52-60.
255. Ananth, P.J., M. Clement, and J. Wolfe, *Pediatric oncology providers and use of medical marijuana in children with cancer.* 2016.
256. Ware, M.A. and D. Ziemianski, *Medical education on cannabis and cannabinoids: Perspectives, challenges, and opportunities.* Clin Pharmacol Ther, 2015. **97**(6): p. 548-50.
257. HelloMD. *Medical Marijuana Patient Survey Results.* 2016; Available from: https://s3-us-west-2.amazonaws.com/hellomd-news/HelloMD_Medical_Marijuana_Patient_Survey.pdf.
258. Burggren, A. *Cannabis Effects on Brain Morphology in Aging (CAN).* 2017 [cited 2018; Available from: clinicaltrials.gov/ct2/show/NCT01874886.
259. Westlake, T.M., et al., *Cannabinoid receptor binding and messenger RNA expression in human brain: an in vitro receptor autoradiography and in situ hybridization histochemistry study of normal aged and Alzheimer's brains.* Neuroscience, 1994. **63**(3): p. 637-52.
260. Ramirez, B.G., et al., *Prevention of Alzheimer's disease pathology by cannabinoids: neuroprotection mediated by blockade of microglial activation.* J Neurosci, 2005. **25**(8): p. 1904-13.
261. Solas, M., et al., *CB2 receptor and amyloid pathology in frontal cortex of Alzheimer's disease patients.* Neurobiol Aging, 2013. **34**(3): p. 805-8.

262. Palazuelos, J., et al., *CB2 cannabinoid receptors promote neural progenitor cell proliferation via mTORC1 signaling.* J Biol Chem, 2012. **287**(2): p. 1198-209.
263. Bravo-Ferrer, I., et al., *Cannabinoid Type-2 Receptor Drives Neurogenesis and Improves Functional Outcome After Stroke.* Stroke, 2017. **48**(1): p. 204-212.
264. Koppel, J., et al., *CB2 receptor deficiency increases amyloid pathology and alters tau processing in a transgenic mouse model of Alzheimer's disease.* Mol Med, 2014. **20**: p. 29-36.
265. Watt, G. and T. Karl, *In vivo Evidence for Therapeutic Properties of Cannabidiol (CBD) for Alzheimer's Disease.* Front Pharmacol, 2017. **8**: p. 20.
266. Janefjord, E., et al., *Cannabinoid effects on beta amyloid fibril and aggregate formation, neuronal and microglial-activated neurotoxicity in vitro.* Cell Mol Neurobiol, 2014. **34**(1): p. 31-42.
267. Harvey, B.S., et al., *Contrasting protective effects of cannabinoids against oxidative stress and amyloid-beta evoked neurotoxicity in vitro.* Neurotoxicology, 2012. **33**(1): p. 138-46.
268. Zhang, J., et al., *Monoacylglycerol Lipase: A Novel Potential Therapeutic Target and Prognostic Indicator for Hepatocellular Carcinoma.* Sci Rep, 2016. **6**: p. 35784.
269. Zhang, J., et al., *Synaptic and cognitive improvements by inhibition of 2-AG metabolism are through upregulation of microRNA-188-3p in a mouse model of Alzheimer's disease.* J Neurosci, 2014. **34**(45): p. 14919-33.
270. Chen, R., et al., *Monoacylglycerol lipase is a therapeutic target for Alzheimer's disease.* Cell Rep, 2012. **2**(5): p. 1329-39.
271. Piro, J.R., et al., *A dysregulated endocannabinoid-eicosanoid network supports pathogenesis in a mouse model of Alzheimer's disease.* Cell Rep, 2012. **1**(6): p. 617-23.
272. Rosenberg, P.a.F., B. *Trial of Dronabinol Adjunctive Treatment of Agitation in Alzheimer's Disease (AD) (THC-AD) (THC-AD).* 2017 [cited 2018; Available from: https://clinicaltrials.gov/ct2/show/NCT02792257.
273. Volicer, L., et al., *Effects of dronabinol on anorexia and disturbed behavior in patients with Alzheimer's disease.* Int J Geriatr Psychiatry, 1997. **12**(9): p. 913-9.
274. Zajac, D.M., S.R. Sikkema, and R. Chandrasena, *Nabilone for the Treatment of Dementia-Associated Sexual Disinhibition.* Prim Care Companion CNS Disord, 2015. **17**(1).
275. Lanctot, K.L., and Herrman, N. *Safety and Efficacy of Nabilone in Alzheimer's Disease.* 2017 [cited 2018; Available from: https://clinicaltrials.gov/ct2/show/NCT02351882.
276. in t' Veld, B.A., et al., *Nonsteroidal antiinflammatory drugs and the risk of Alzheimer's disease.* N Engl J Med, 2001. **345**(21): p. 1515-21.
277. Moreira, F.A. and B. Lutz, *The endocannabinoid system: emotion, learning and addiction.* Addict Biol, 2008. **13**(2): p. 196-212.
278. Fernandez-Ruiz, J. and S. Gonzales, *Cannabinoid control of motor function*

at the basal ganglia. Handb Exp Pharmacol, 2005(168): p. 479-507.

279. Martin, A.B., et al., *Expression and function of CB1 receptor in the rat striatum: localization and effects on D1 and D2 dopamine receptor-mediated motor behaviors.* Neuropsychopharmacology, 2008. **33**(7): p. 1667-79.
280. Finseth, T.A., et al., *Self-reported efficacy of cannabis and other complementary medicine modalities by Parkinson's disease patients in colorado.* Evid Based Complement Alternat Med, 2015. **2015**: p. 874849.
281. Venderova, K., et al., *Survey on cannabis use in Parkinson's disease: subjective improvement of motor symptoms.* Mov Disord, 2004. **19**(9): p. 1102-6.
282. Lotan, I., et al., *Cannabis (medical marijuana) treatment for motor and non-motor symptoms of Parkinson disease: an open-label observational study.* Clin Neuropharmacol, 2014. **37**(2): p. 41-4.
283. Garcia, C., et al., *Symptom-relieving and neuroprotective effects of the phytocannabinoid Delta(9)-THCV in animal models of Parkinson's disease.* Br J Pharmacol, 2011. **163**(7): p. 1495-506.
284. Leehey, M.A. *A Study of Tolerability and Efficacy of Cannabidiol on Tremor in Parkinson's Disease.* 2017 [cited 2018; Available from: http://www.clinicaltrials.gov/ct2/show/NCT02818777.
285. Chagas, M.H., et al., *Effects of cannabidiol in the treatment of patients with Parkinson's disease: an exploratory double-blind trial.* J Psychopharmacol, 2014. **28**(11): p. 1088-98.
286. Chagas, M.H., et al., *Cannabidiol can improve complex sleep-related behaviours associated with rapid eye movement sleep behaviour disorder in Parkinson's disease patients: a case series.* J Clin Pharm Ther, 2014. **39**(5): p. 564-6.
287. Zuardi, A.W., et al., *Cannabidiol for the treatment of psychosis in Parkinson's disease.* J Psychopharmacol, 2009. **23**(8): p. 979-83.
288. Bassi, M.S., Sancesario, A., Morace, R., Centonze, D., and Iezzi, E., *Cannabinoids in Parkinson's Disease.* Cannabis and Cannabinoid Research, 2017. **2**(1): p. 21-29.
289. Kim, Y. and Y.Y. He, *Ultraviolet radiation-induced non-melanoma skin cancer: Regulation of DNA damage repair and inflammation.* Genes Dis, 2014. **1**(2): p. 188-198.
290. Hybertson, B.M., et al., *Oxidative stress in health and disease: the therapeutic potential of Nrf2 activation.* Mol Aspects Med, 2011. **32**(4-6): p. 234-46.
291. Gao, B., A. Doan, and B.M. Hybertson, *The clinical potential of influencing Nrf2 signaling in degenerative and immunological disorders.* Clin Pharmacol, 2014. **6**: p. 19-34.
292. Sailler, S., et al., *Regulation of circulating endocannabinoids associated with cancer and metastases in mice and humans.* Oncoscience, 2014. **1**(4): p. 272-82.
293. Contassot, E., et al., *Arachidonyl ethanolamide induces apoptosis of uterine cervix cancer cells via aberrantly expressed vanilloid receptor-1.* Gynecol Oncol, 2004. **93**(1): p. 182-8.

294. Juknat, A., et al., *Differential transcriptional profiles mediated by exposure to the cannabinoids cannabidiol and Delta9-tetrahydrocannabinol in BV-2 microglial cells.* Br J Pharmacol, 2012. **165**(8): p. 2512-28.
295. Hasenoehrl, C., et al., *G protein-coupled receptor GPR55 promotes colorectal cancer and has opposing effects to cannabinoid receptor 1.* Int J Cancer, 2018. **142**(1): p. 121-132.
296. Massa, F., et al., *The endogenous cannabinoid system protects against colonic inflammation.* J Clin Invest, 2004. **113**(8): p. 1202-9.
297. Takeda, S., et al., *Cannabidiolic acid, a major cannabinoid in fiber-type cannabis, is an inhibitor of MDA-MB-231 breast cancer cell migration.* Toxicol Lett, 2012. **214**(3): p. 314-9.
298. National Toxicology, P., *NTP Toxicology and Carcinogenesis Studies of 1-Trans-Delta(9)-Tetrahydrocannabinol (CAS No. 1972-08-3) in F344 Rats and B6C3F1 Mice (Gavage Studies).* Natl Toxicol Program Tech Rep Ser, 1996. **446**: p. 1-317.
299. Bifulco, M., et al., *Cannabinoids and cancer: pros and cons of an antitumour strategy.* Br J Pharmacol, 2006. **148**(2): p. 123-35.
300. Starowicz, K., et al., *Full inhibition of spinal FAAH leads to TRPV1-mediated analgesic effects in neuropathic rats and possible lipoxygenase-mediated remodeling of anandamide metabolism.* PLoS One, 2013. **8**(4): p. e60040.
301. Pergam, S.A., et al., *Cannabis use among patients at a comprehensive cancer center in a state with legalized medicinal and recreational use.* Cancer, 2017. **123**(22): p. 4488-4497.
302. Kampa-Schittenhelm, K.M., et al., *Dronabinol has preferential antileukemic activity in acute lymphoblastic and myeloid leukemia with lymphoid differentiation patterns.* BMC Cancer, 2016. **16**: p. 25.
303. McAllister, S.D., et al., *Pathways mediating the effects of cannabidiol on the reduction of breast cancer cell proliferation, invasion, and metastasis.* Breast Cancer Res Treat, 2011. **129**(1): p. 37-47.
304. Hanlon, K.E., et al., *Modulation of breast cancer cell viability by a cannabinoid receptor 2 agonist, JWH-015, is calcium dependent.* Breast Cancer (Dove Med Press), 2016. **8**: p. 59-71.
305. Morales, P., et al., *Selective, nontoxic CB(2) cannabinoid o-quinone with in vivo activity against triple-negative breast cancer.* J Med Chem, 2015. **58**(5): p. 2256-64.
306. Siegel, R.L., K.D. Miller, and A. Jemal, *Cancer statistics, 2016.* CA Cancer J Clin, 2016. **66**(1): p. 7-30.
307. Torres, S., et al., *A combined preclinical therapy of cannabinoids and temozolomide against glioma.* Mol Cancer Ther, 2011. **10**(1): p. 90-103.
308. Martinez, D. *Investigation of Cannabis for Pain and Inflammation in Lung Cancer.* 2016 [cited 2018; Available from: https://clinicaltrials.gov/ct2/show/NCT02675842.
309. Portenoy, R.K., et al., *Nabiximols for opioid-treated cancer patients with poorly-controlled chronic pain: a randomized, placebo-controlled, graded-dose trial.* J Pain, 2012. **13**(5): p. 438-49.
310. Feigenbaum, J.J., et al., *Nonpsychotropic cannabinoid acts as a functional*

N-methyl-D-aspartate receptor blocker. Proc Natl Acad Sci U S A, 1989. **86**(23): p. 9584-7.
311. PLC, E.T. *A Study of Dexanabinol in Combination With Chemotherapy in Patients With Advanced Tumours.* 2016 [cited 2018; Available from: https://clinicaltrials.gov/ct2/show/NCT02423239.
312. Kesari, S. *Dexanabinol in Patients With Brain Cancer.* 2017 [cited 2018; Available from: https://clinicaltrials.gov/ct2/show/NCT01654497.
313. Bar-Sela, G., et al., *Is the clinical use of cannabis by oncology patients advisable?* Curr Med Chem, 2014. **21**(17): p. 1923-30.
314. Bar-Lev Schleider, L., et al., *Prospective analysis of safety and efficacy of medical cannabis in large unselected population of patients with cancer.* Eur J Intern Med, 2018. **49**: p. 37-43.
315. Whiting, P.F., et al., *Cannabinoids for Medical Use: A Systematic Review and Meta-analysis.* JAMA, 2015. **313**(24): p. 2456-73.
316. Bar-Sela, G. *Evaluation Prospectively the Level of Reduction in Cognitive Functions of Cancer Patients Who Are on Active Oncology Treatments and Use Cannabis. The Second Goal is to Identify High-risk Groups for Cognitive Impairment Due to Cannabis Use.* 2017 [cited 2018; Available from: https://clinicaltrials.gov/ct2/show/NCT01983267.
317. Pergolizzi, J.V. *Evaluation of the Efficacy of Cesamet™ for the Treatment of Pain in Patients With Chemotherapy-Induced Neuropathy.* 2008 [cited 2018; Available from: https://clinicaltrials.gov/ct2/show/NCT00380965.
318. Singh, Y. and C. Bali, *Cannabis extract treatment for terminal acute lymphoblastic leukemia with a Philadelphia chromosome mutation.* Case Rep Oncol, 2013. **6**(3): p. 585-92.
319. Tan, H., et al., *The role of cannabinoid transmission in emotional memory formation: implications for addiction and schizophrenia.* Front Psychiatry, 2014. **5**: p. 73.
320. Sirrs, S., et al., *Defects in fatty acid amide hydrolase 2 in a male with neurologic and psychiatric symptoms.* Orphanet J Rare Dis, 2015. **10**: p. 38.
321. Zuardi, A.W., F.S. Guimaraes, and A.C. Moreira, *Effect of cannabidiol on plasma prolactin, growth hormone and cortisol in human volunteers.* Braz J Med Biol Res, 1993. **26**(2): p. 213-7.
322. Bergamaschi, M.M., et al., *Cannabidiol reduces the anxiety induced by simulated public speaking in treatment-naive social phobia patients.* Neuropsychopharmacology, 2011. **36**(6): p. 1219-26.
323. Crippa, J.A., et al., *Neural basis of anxiolytic effects of cannabidiol (CBD) in generalized social anxiety disorder: a preliminary report.* J Psychopharmacol, 2011. **25**(1): p. 121-30.
324. Gruber, S. *Sublingual Cannabidiol for Anxiety.* 2017 [cited 2018; Available from: https://clinicaltrials.gov/ct2/show/NCT02548559.
325. Nazario, L.R., et al., *Caffeine protects against memory loss induced by high and non-anxiolytic dose of cannabidiol in adult zebrafish (Danio rerio).* Pharmacol Biochem Behav, 2015. **135**: p. 210-6.
326. Martin-Santos, R., et al., *Acute effects of a single, oral dose of d9-tetrahydrocannabinol (THC) and cannabidiol (CBD) administration in healthy*

volunteers. Curr Pharm Des, 2012. **18**(32): p. 4966-79.
327. Fitzgibbon, M., D.P. Finn, and M. Roche, *High Times for Painful Blues: The Endocannabinoid System in Pain-Depression Comorbidity.* Int J Neuropsychopharmacol, 2015. **19**(3): p. pyv095.
328. Cornelius, J.R., et al., *Double-blind fluoxetine trial in comorbid MDD-CUD youth and young adults.* Drug Alcohol Depend, 2010. **112**(1-2): p. 39-45.
329. Levin, F.R., et al., *A randomized double-blind, placebo-controlled trial of venlafaxine-extended release for co-occurring cannabis dependence and depressive disorders.* Addiction, 2013. **108**(6): p. 1084-94.
330. Nishiguchi, K.M., et al., *Exome sequencing extends the phenotypic spectrum for ABHD12 mutations: from syndromic to nonsyndromic retinal degeneration.* Ophthalmology, 2014. **121**(8): p. 1620-7.
331. Monteleone, P., et al., *Investigation of CNR1 and FAAH endocannabinoid gene polymorphisms in bipolar disorder and major depression.* Pharmacol Res, 2010. **61**(5): p. 400-4.
332. Mitjans, M., et al., *Genetic variability in the endocannabinoid system and 12-week clinical response to citalopram treatment: the role of the CNR1, CNR2 and FAAH genes.* J Psychopharmacol, 2012. **26**(10): p. 1391-8.
333. Onaivi, E.S., et al., *Functional expression of brain neuronal CB2 cannabinoid receptors are involved in the effects of drugs of abuse and in depression.* Ann N Y Acad Sci, 2008. **1139**: p. 434-49.
334. Schmidt, M., et al., *Consensus: soy isoflavones as a first-line approach to the treatment of menopausal vasomotor complaints.* Gynecol Endocrinol, 2016. **32**(6): p. 427-30.
335. Morgan, C.J., et al., *Impact of cannabidiol on the acute memory and psychotomimetic effects of smoked cannabis: naturalistic study: naturalistic study [corrected].* Br J Psychiatry, 2010. **197**(4): p. 285-90.
336. Lawn, W., et al., *Acute and chronic effects of cannabinoids on effort-related decision-making and reward learning: an evaluation of the cannabis 'amotivational' hypotheses.* Psychopharmacology (Berl), 2016. **233**(19-20): p. 3537-52.
337. Al Mansouri, S., et al., *The cannabinoid receptor 2 agonist, beta-caryophyllene, reduced voluntary alcohol intake and attenuated ethanol-induced place preference and sensitivity in mice.* Pharmacol Biochem Behav, 2014. **124**: p. 260-8.
338. Hill, M.N., et al., *Reductions in circulating endocannabinoid levels in individuals with post-traumatic stress disorder following exposure to the World Trade Center attacks.* Psychoneuroendocrinology, 2013. **38**(12): p. 2952-61.
339. Neumeister, A., et al., *Elevated brain cannabinoid CB1 receptor availability in post-traumatic stress disorder: a positron emission tomography study.* Mol Psychiatry, 2013. **18**(9): p. 1034-40.
340. Felmingham, K.L., et al., *The brain-derived neurotrophic factor Val66Met polymorphism predicts response to exposure therapy in posttraumatic stress disorder.* Biol Psychiatry, 2013. **73**(11): p. 1059-63.
341. Mota, N., et al., *The rs1049353 polymorphism in the CNR1 gene interacts*

with childhood abuse to predict posttraumatic threat symptoms. J Clin Psychiatry, 2015. **76**(12): p. e1622-3.
342. Jetly, R., et al., *The efficacy of nabilone, a synthetic cannabinoid, in the treatment of PTSD-associated nightmares: A preliminary randomized, double-blind, placebo-controlled cross-over design study.* Psychoneuroendocrinology, 2015. **51**: p. 585-8.
343. Cameron, C., D. Watson, and J. Robinson, *Use of a synthetic cannabinoid in a correctional population for posttraumatic stress disorder-related insomnia and nightmares, chronic pain, harm reduction, and other indications: a retrospective evaluation.* J Clin Psychopharmacol, 2014. **34**(5): p. 559-64.
344. Roitman, P., et al., *Preliminary, open-label, pilot study of add-on oral Delta9-tetrahydrocannabinol in chronic post-traumatic stress disorder.* Clin Drug Investig, 2014. **34**(8): p. 587-91.
345. Shannon, S. and J. Opila-Lehman, *Effectiveness of Cannabidiol Oil for Pediatric Anxiety and Insomnia as Part of Posttraumatic Stress Disorder: A Case Report.* Perm J, 2016. **20**(4): p. 108-111.
346. Ware, M.A. and E. St Arnaud-Trempe, *The abuse potential of the synthetic cannabinoid nabilone.* Addiction, 2010. **105**(3): p. 494-503.
347. Veitenhansl, M., et al., *40(th) EASD Annual Meeting of the European Association for the Study of Diabetes : Munich, Germany, 5-9 September 2004.* Diabetologia, 2004. **47**(Suppl 1): p. A1-A464.
348. Rudd, R.A., et al., *Increases in Drug and Opioid Overdose Deaths--United States, 2000-2014.* MMWR Morb Mortal Wkly Rep, 2016. **64**(50-51): p. 1378-82.
349. Cicero, T.J. and B.M. Kuehn, *Driven by prescription drug abuse, heroin use increases among suburban and rural whites.* JAMA, 2014. **312**(2): p. 118-9.
350. Lipton, R.B., et al., *Prevalence and burden of migraine in the United States: data from the American Migraine Study II.* Headache, 2001. **41**(7): p. 646-57.
351. Hazard, E., et al., *The burden of migraine in the United States: current and emerging perspectives on disease management and economic analysis.* Value Health, 2009. **12**(1): p. 55-64.
352. Goldberg, L.D., *The cost of migraine and its treatment.* Am J Manag Care, 2005. **11**(2 Suppl): p. S62-7.
353. Russo, E.B., *Clinical endocannabinoid deficiency (CECD): can this concept explain therapeutic benefits of cannabis in migraine, fibromyalgia, irritable bowel syndrome and other treatment-resistant conditions?* Neuro Endocrinol Lett, 2008. **29**(2): p. 192-200.
354. Cupini, L.M., et al., *Degradation of endocannabinoids in chronic migraine and medication overuse headache.* Neurobiol Dis, 2008. **30**(2): p. 186-9.
355. Durham, P. and S. Papapetropoulos, *Biomarkers associated with migraine and their potential role in migraine management.* Headache, 2013. **53**(8): p. 1262-77.
356. Hamel, E., *Serotonin and migraine: biology and clinical implications.* Cephalalgia, 2007. **27**(11): p. 1293-300.
357. Lee, S.T., J.H. Park, and M. Kim, *Efficacy of the 5-HT1A agonist, buspirone*

hydrochloride, in migraineurs with anxiety: a randomized, prospective, parallel group, double-blind, placebo-controlled study. Headache, 2005. **45**(8): p. 1004-11.

358. Pascual, J. and J. Berciano, *An open trial of buspirone in migraine prophylaxis. Preliminary report.* Clin Neuropharmacol, 1991. **14**(3): p. 245-50.
359. Leone, M., et al., *5-HT1A receptor hypersensitivity in migraine is suggested by the m-chlorophenylpiperazine test.* Neuroreport, 1998. **9**(11): p. 2605-8.
360. Cassidy, E.M., et al., *Central 5-HT receptor hypersensitivity in migraine without aura.* Cephalalgia, 2003. **23**(1): p. 29-34.
361. Cassidy, E.M., et al., *Differing central amine receptor sensitivity in different migraine subtypes? A neuroendocrine study using buspirone.* Pain, 2003. **101**(3): p. 283-90.
362. Buse, D.C., et al., *Chronic migraine prevalence, disability, and sociodemographic factors: results from the American Migraine Prevalence and Prevention Study.* Headache, 2012. **52**(10): p. 1456-70.
363. Juhasz, G., et al., *Variations in the cannabinoid receptor 1 gene predispose to migraine.* Neurosci Lett, 2009. **461**(2): p. 116-20.
364. Akerman, S., et al., *Endocannabinoids in the brainstem modulate dural trigeminovascular nociceptive traffic via CB1 and "triptan" receptors: implications in migraine.* J Neurosci, 2013. **33**(37): p. 14869-77.
365. Greco, R., et al., *Effects of anandamide in migraine: data from an animal model.* J Headache Pain, 2011. **12**(2): p. 177-83.
366. Greco, R., et al., *Activation of CB2 receptors as a potential therapeutic target for migraine: evaluation in an animal model.* J Headache Pain, 2014. **15**: p. 14.
367. Lochte, B.C., et al., *The Use of Cannabis for Headache Disorders.* Cannabis Cannabinoid Res, 2017. **2**(1): p. 61-71.
368. Mikuriya, T.H. *Chronic migraine headache: five cases successfully treated with Marinol and/or illicit cannabis.* Available from: http://druglibrary.org/schaffer/hemp/migrn1.htm.
369. Rhyne, D.N., et al., *Effects of Medical Marijuana on Migraine Headache Frequency in an Adult Population.* Pharmacotherapy, 2016. **36**(5): p. 505-10.
370. Tudge, L., et al., *Neural effects of cannabinoid CB1 neutral antagonist tetrahydrocannabivarin on food reward and aversion in healthy volunteers.* Int J Neuropsychopharmacol, 2014. **18**(6).
371. Rzepa, E., L. Tudge, and C. McCabe, *The CB1 Neutral Antagonist Tetrahydrocannabivarin Reduces Default Mode Network and Increases Executive Control Network Resting State Functional Connectivity in Healthy Volunteers.* Int J Neuropsychopharmacol, 2015. **19**(2).
372. Englund, A., et al., *The effect of five day dosing with THCV on THC-induced cognitive, psychological and physiological effects in healthy male human volunteers: A placebo-controlled, double-blind, crossover pilot trial.* J Psychopharmacol, 2016. **30**(2): p. 140-51.
373. Wargent, E.T., et al., *The cannabinoid Delta(9)-tetrahydrocannabivarin (THCV) ameliorates insulin sensitivity in two mouse models of obesity.* Nutr

Diabetes, 2013. **3**: p. e68.

374. Bolognini, D., et al., *The plant cannabinoid Delta9-tetrahydrocannabivarin can decrease signs of inflammation and inflammatory pain in mice.* Br J Pharmacol, 2010. **160**(3): p. 677-87.

375. Cascio, M.G., et al., *The phytocannabinoid, Delta(9)-tetrahydrocannabivarin, can act through 5-HT(1)A receptors to produce antipsychotic effects.* Br J Pharmacol, 2015. **172**(5): p. 1305-18.

376. Antonaci, F., et al., *Migraine and psychiatric comorbidity: a review of clinical findings.* J Headache Pain, 2011. **12**(2): p. 115-25.

377. Rock, E.M., et al., *Evaluation of the potential of the phytocannabinoids, cannabidivarin (CBDV) and Delta(9) -tetrahydrocannabivarin (THCV), to produce CB1 receptor inverse agonism symptoms of nausea in rats.* Br J Pharmacol, 2013. **170**(3): p. 671-8.

378. Xiong, W., et al., *Cannabinoids suppress inflammatory and neuropathic pain by targeting alpha3 glycine receptors.* J Exp Med, 2012. **209**(6): p. 1121-34.

379. Fine, P.G. and M.J. Rosenfeld, *Cannabinoids for neuropathic pain.* Curr Pain Headache Rep, 2014. **18**(10): p. 451.

380. Grace, P.M., et al., *Morphine paradoxically prolongs neuropathic pain in rats by amplifying spinal NLRP3 inflammasome activation.* Proc Natl Acad Sci U S A, 2016. **113**(24): p. E3441-50.

381. Cajanus, K., et al., *Effect of endocannabinoid degradation on pain: role of FAAH polymorphisms in experimental and postoperative pain in women treated for breast cancer.* Pain, 2016. **157**(2): p. 361-9.

382. Lucas, P. and Z. Walsh, *Medical cannabis access, use, and substitution for prescription opioids and other substances: A survey of authorized medical cannabis patients.* Int J Drug Policy, 2017. **42**: p. 30-35.

383. Reiman, A., M. Welty, and P. Solomon, *Cannabis as a Substitute for Opioid-Based Pain Medication: Patient Self-Report.* Cannabis Cannabinoid Res, 2017. **2**(1): p. 160-166.

384. Hill, K.P., *Medical Marijuana for Treatment of Chronic Pain and Other Medical and Psychiatric Problems: A Clinical Review.* JAMA, 2015. **313**(24): p. 2474-83.

385. Piper, B.J., et al., *Chronic pain patients' perspectives of medical cannabis.* Pain, 2017. **158**(7): p. 1373-1379.

386. Russo, R., et al., *Synergistic antinociception by the cannabinoid receptor agonist anandamide and the PPAR-alpha receptor agonist GW7647.* Eur J Pharmacol, 2007. **566**(1-3): p. 117-9.

387. Abrams, D.I., et al., *Cannabinoid-opioid interaction in chronic pain.* Clin Pharmacol Ther, 2011. **90**(6): p. 844-51.

388. Chambers, J., et al., *An Online Survey of Patients' Experiences Since the Rescheduling of Hydrocodone: The First 100 Days.* Pain Med, 2016. **17**(9): p. 1686-93.

389. Ste-Marie, P.A., et al., *Association of herbal cannabis use with negative psychosocial parameters in patients with fibromyalgia.* Arthritis Care Res (Hoboken), 2012. **64**(8): p. 1202-8.

390. Schley, M., et al., *Delta-9-THC based monotherapy in fibromyalgia patients*

on experimentally induced pain, axon reflex flare, and pain relief. Curr Med Res Opin, 2006. **22**(7): p. 1269-76.
391. Skrabek, R.Q., et al., *Nabilone for the treatment of pain in fibromyalgia.* J Pain, 2008. **9**(2): p. 164-73.
392. Fiz, J., et al., *Cannabis use in patients with fibromyalgia: effect on symptoms relief and health-related quality of life.* PLoS One, 2011. **6**(4): p. e18440.
393. Habib, G. and S. Artul, *Medical Cannabis for the Treatment of Fibromyalgia.* J Clin Rheumatol, 2018.
394. Grandi, G., et al., *Prevalence of menstrual pain in young women: what is dysmenorrhea?* J Pain Res, 2012. **5**: p. 169-74.
395. Mathias, S.D., et al., *Chronic pelvic pain: prevalence, health-related quality of life, and economic correlates.* Obstet Gynecol, 1996. **87**(3): p. 321-7.
396. Cravatt, B.F., et al., *Functional disassociation of the central and peripheral fatty acid amide signaling systems.* Proc Natl Acad Sci U S A, 2004. **101**(29): p. 10821-6.
397. Benedetti, F., et al., *Nonopioid placebo analgesia is mediated by CB1 cannabinoid receptors.* Nat Med, 2011. **17**(10): p. 1228-30.
398. Pecina, M., et al., *FAAH selectively influences placebo effects.* Mol Psychiatry, 2014. **19**(3): p. 385-91.
399. Yildiz, M., et al., *Lack of association of DRD3 and CNR1 polymorphisms with premenstrual dysphoric disorders.* Iran J Reprod Med, 2015. **13**(4): p. 221-6.
400. Tripp, D.A., et al., *A survey of cannabis (marijuana) use and self-reported benefit in men with chronic prostatitis/chronic pelvic pain syndrome.* Can Urol Assoc J, 2014. **8**(11-12): p. E901-5.
401. Sadhasivam, S., et al., *Novel associations between FAAH genetic variants and postoperative central opioid-related adverse effects.* Pharmacogenomics J, 2015. **15**(5): p. 436-42.
402. Parazzini, F., et al., *Epidemiology of endometriosis and its comorbidities.* Eur J Obstet Gynecol Reprod Biol, 2017. **209**: p. 3-7.
403. Sanchez, A.M., et al., *Elevated Systemic Levels of Endocannabinoids and Related Mediators Across the Menstrual Cycle in Women With Endometriosis.* Reprod Sci, 2016. **23**(8): p. 1071-9.
404. Resuehr, D., et al., *Progesterone-dependent regulation of endometrial cannabinoid receptor type 1 (CB1-R) expression is disrupted in women with endometriosis and in isolated stromal cells exposed to 2,3,7,8-tetrachlorodibenzo-p-dioxin (TCDD).* Fertil Steril, 2012. **98**(4): p. 948-56 e1.
405. Dmitrieva, N., et al., *Endocannabinoid involvement in endometriosis.* Pain, 2010. **151**(3): p. 703-10.
406. Leconte, M., et al., *Antiproliferative effects of cannabinoid agonists on deep infiltrating endometriosis.* Am J Pathol, 2010. **177**(6): p. 2963-70.
407. Sharma, C., et al., *Polypharmacological Properties and Therapeutic Potential of beta-Caryophyllene: A Dietary Phytocannabinoid of Pharmaceutical Promise.* Curr Pharm Des, 2016. **22**(21): p. 3237-64.
408. Abbas, M.A., et al., *beta-Caryophyllene causes regression of endometrial implants in a rat model of endometriosis without affecting fertility.* Eur J Pharmacol, 2013. **702**(1-3): p. 12-9.

409. Martinez-Zamora, M.A., et al., *Increased levels of dioxin-like substances in adipose tissue in patients with deep infiltrating endometriosis.* Hum Reprod, 2015. **30**(5): p. 1059-68.
410. Cobellis, L., et al., *Effectiveness of the association micronized N-Palmitoylethanolamine (PEA)-transpolydatin in the treatment of chronic pelvic pain related to endometriosis after laparoscopic assessment: a pilot study.* Eur J Obstet Gynecol Reprod Biol, 2011. **158**(1): p. 82-6.
411. Lo Monte, G., I. Soave, and R. Marci, *[Administration of micronized palmitoylethanolamide (PEA)-transpolydatin in the treatment of chronic pelvic pain in women affected by endometriosis: preliminary results].* Minerva Ginecol, 2013. **65**(4): p. 453-63.
412. Tartaglia, E., et al., *Effectiveness of the Association N-Palmitoylethanolamine and Transpolydatin in the Treatment of Primary Dysmenorrhea.* J Pediatr Adolesc Gynecol, 2015. **28**(6): p. 447-50.
413. Yamaori, S., et al., *Potent inhibition of human cytochrome P450 3A isoforms by cannabidiol: role of phenolic hydroxyl groups in the resorcinol moiety.* Life Sci, 2011. **88**(15-16): p. 730-6.
414. Lee, C.R., *Drug interactions and hormonal contraception.* Trends in Urology Gynaecology & Sexual Health, 2009: p. 23-26.
415. Grayson, L., et al., *An interaction between warfarin and cannabidiol, a case report.* Epilepsy Behav Case Rep, 2018. **9**: p. 10-11.
416. Maccarrone, M., et al., *Progesterone activates fatty acid amide hydrolase (FAAH) promoter in human T lymphocytes through the transcription factor Ikaros. Evidence for a synergistic effect of leptin.* J Biol Chem, 2003. **278**(35): p. 32726-32.
417. Grimaldi, P., et al., *The faah gene is the first direct target of estrogen in the testis: role of histone demethylase LSD1.* Cell Mol Life Sci, 2012. **69**(24): p. 4177-90.
418. Hojnik, M., et al., *A synergistic interaction of 17-beta-estradiol with specific cannabinoid receptor type 2 antagonist/inverse agonist on proliferation activity in primary human osteoblasts.* Biomed Rep, 2015. **3**(4): p. 554-558.
419. Galanopoulou, A.S., *Stirring the pot with estrogens.* Epilepsy Curr, 2013. **13**(3): p. 129-31.
420. Woo, J.H., et al., *Cannabinoid receptor gene polymorphisms and bone mineral density in Korean postmenopausal women.* Menopause, 2015. **22**(5): p. 512-9.
421. Heiss, G., et al., *Health risks and benefits 3 years after stopping randomized treatment with estrogen and progestin.* JAMA, 2008. **299**(9): p. 1036-45.
422. Shan, J., L. Chen, and K. Lu, *Protective effects of trans-caryophyllene on maintaining osteoblast function.* IUBMB Life, 2017. **69**(1): p. 22-29.
423. Grimaldi, P., et al., *Modulation of the endocannabinoid-degrading enzyme fatty acid amide hydrolase by follicle-stimulating hormone.* Vitam Horm, 2009. **81**: p. 231-61.
424. Hegde, V.L., M. Nagarkatti, and P.S. Nagarkatti, *Cannabinoid receptor activation leads to massive mobilization of myeloid-derived suppressor cells with potent immunosuppressive properties.* Eur J Immunol, 2010. **40**(12): p.

3358-71.

425. Mounessa, J.S., et al., *The role of cannabinoids in dermatology.* J Am Acad Dermatol, 2017. **77**(1): p. 188-190.

426. Zheng, D., et al., *The cannabinoid receptors are required for ultraviolet-induced inflammation and skin cancer development.* Cancer Res, 2008. **68**(10): p. 3992-8.

427. Dobrosi, N., et al., *Endocannabinoids enhance lipid synthesis and apoptosis of human sebocytes via cannabinoid receptor-2-mediated signaling.* FASEB J, 2008. **22**(10): p. 3685-95.

428. Olah, A., et al., *Cannabidiol exerts sebostatic and antiinflammatory effects on human sebocytes.* J Clin Invest, 2014. **124**(9): p. 3713-24.

429. Yun, J.W., et al., *Antipruritic effects of TRPV1 antagonist in murine atopic dermatitis and itching models.* J Invest Dermatol, 2011. **131**(7): p. 1576-9.

430. Caterina, M.J., *TRP channel cannabinoid receptors in skin sensation, homeostasis, and inflammation.* ACS Chem Neurosci, 2014. **5**(11): p. 1107-16.

431. Szepietowski, J.C., T. Szepietowski, and A. Reich, *Efficacy and tolerance of the cream containing structured physiological lipids with endocannabinoids in the treatment of uremic pruritus: a preliminary study.* Acta Dermatovenerol Croat, 2005. **13**(2): p. 97-103.

432. Rukwied, R., et al., *Cannabinoid agonists attenuate capsaicin-induced responses in human skin.* Pain, 2003. **102**(3): p. 283-8.

433. Yuan, C., et al., *N-palmitoylethanolamine and N-acetylethanolamine are effective in asteatotic eczema: results of a randomized, double-blind, controlled study in 60 patients.* Clin Interv Aging, 2014. **9**: p. 1163-9.

434. Wilkinson, J.D. and E.M. Williamson, *Cannabinoids inhibit human keratinocyte proliferation through a non-CB1/CB2 mechanism and have a potential therapeutic value in the treatment of psoriasis.* J Dermatol Sci, 2007. **45**(2): p. 87-92.

435. Telek, A., et al., *Inhibition of human hair follicle growth by endo- and exocannabinoids.* FASEB J, 2007. **21**(13): p. 3534-41.

436. Garza, L.A., et al., *Prostaglandin D2 inhibits hair growth and is elevated in bald scalp of men with androgenetic alopecia.* Sci Transl Med, 2012. **4**(126): p. 126ra34.

437. Morgan, C.J., et al., *Hyper-priming in cannabis users: a naturalistic study of the effects of cannabis on semantic memory function.* Psychiatry Res, 2010. **176**(2-3): p. 213-8.

438. Flaherty, A.W., *Frontotemporal and dopaminergic control of idea generation and creative drive.* J Comp Neurol, 2005. **493**(1): p. 147-53.

439. Mathew, R.J., et al., *Regional cerebral blood flow after marijuana smoking.* J Cereb Blood Flow Metab, 1992. **12**(5): p. 750-8.

440. Mathew, R.J., et al., *Marijuana intoxication and brain activation in marijuana smokers.* Life Sci, 1997. **60**(23): p. 2075-89.

441. Mathew, R.J., et al., *Time course of tetrahydrocannabinol-induced changes in regional cerebral blood flow measured with positron emission tomography.* Psychiatry Res, 2002. **116**(3): p. 173-85.

442. Lundqvist, T., S. Jonsson, and S. Warkentin, *Frontal lobe dysfunction in long-term cannabis users.* Neurotoxicol Teratol, 2001. **23**(5): p. 437-43.
443. Kowal, M.A., et al., *Cannabis and creativity: highly potent cannabis impairs divergent thinking in regular cannabis users.* Psychopharmacology (Berl), 2015. **232**(6): p. 1123-34.
444. Holton, K.F., et al., *The effect of dietary glutamate on fibromyalgia and irritable bowel symptoms.* Clin Exp Rheumatol, 2012. **30**(6 Suppl 74): p. 10-7.
445. Ashok, I. and R. Sheeladevi, *Biochemical responses and mitochondrial mediated activation of apoptosis on long-term effect of aspartame in rat brain.* Redox Biol, 2014. **2**: p. 820-31.
446. Janaky, R., et al., *Mechanisms of L-cysteine neurotoxicity.* Neurochem Res, 2000. **25**(9-10): p. 1397-405.
447. Ravindranath, V., *Neurolathyrism: mitochondrial dysfunction in excitotoxicity mediated by L-beta-oxalyl aminoalanine.* Neurochem Int, 2002. **40**(6): p. 505-9.
448. Abou-Donia, M.B., et al., *Imidacloprid induces neurobehavioral deficits and increases expression of glial fibrillary acidic protein in the motor cortex and hippocampus in offspring rats following in utero exposure.* J Toxicol Environ Health A, 2008. **71**(2): p. 119-30.
449. Sylvetsky, A.C., J.E. Blau, and K.I. Rother, *Understanding the metabolic and health effects of low-calorie sweeteners: methodological considerations and implications for future research.* Rev Endocr Metab Disord, 2016. **17**(2): p. 187-94.
450. Attina, T.M., et al., *Exposure to endocrine-disrupting chemicals in the USA: a population-based disease burden and cost analysis.* Lancet Diabetes Endocrinol, 2016. **4**(12): p. 996-1003.
451. Wilcox, C.M., B. Cryer, and G. Triadafilopoulos, *Patterns of use and public perception of over-the-counter pain relievers: focus on nonsteroidal antiinflammatory drugs.* J Rheumatol, 2005. **32**(11): p. 2218-24.
452. Dimova, S., et al., *Acetaminophen decreases intracellular glutathione levels and modulates cytokine production in human alveolar macrophages and type II pneumocytes in vitro.* Int J Biochem Cell Biol, 2005. **37**(8): p. 1727-37.
453. Shaw, W., *Evidence that Increased Acetaminophen use in Genetically Vulnerable Children Appears to be a Major Cause of the Epidemics of Autism, Attention Deficit with Hyperactivity, and Asthma.* Journal of Restorative Medicine, 2013. **2**: p. 14.
454. Oshnouei, S., et al., *Effects of Acetaminophen consumption in asthmatic children.* Iran Red Crescent Med J, 2012. **14**(10): p. 641-6.
455. Bauer, A.Z. and D. Kriebel, *Prenatal and perinatal analgesic exposure and autism: an ecological link.* Environ Health, 2013. **12**: p. 41.
456. Headley, J. and K. Northstone, *Medication administered to children from 0 to 7.5 years in the Avon Longitudinal Study of Parents and Children (ALSPAC).* Eur J Clin Pharmacol, 2007. **63**(2): p. 189-95.
457. Kharb, S., et al., *Glutathione levels in health and sickness.* Indian J Med Sci,

2000. **54**(2): p. 52-4.
458. Masubuchi, Y., C. Suda, and T. Horie, *Involvement of mitochondrial permeability transition in acetaminophen-induced liver injury in mice.* J Hepatol, 2005. **42**(1): p. 110-6.
459. Sekhar, R.V., et al., *Deficient synthesis of glutathione underlies oxidative stress in aging and can be corrected by dietary cysteine and glycine supplementation.* Am J Clin Nutr, 2011. **94**(3): p. 847-53.
460. Dewall, C.N., et al., *Acetaminophen reduces social pain: behavioral and neural evidence.* Psychol Sci, 2010. **21**(7): p. 931-7.
461. Pickering, G., et al., *The brain signature of paracetamol in healthy volunteers: a double-blind randomized trial.* Drug Des Devel Ther, 2015. **9**: p. 3853-62.
462. Pallone, S.R. and G.R. Bergus, *Fertility awareness-based methods: another option for family planning.* J Am Board Fam Med, 2009. **22**(2): p. 147-57.
463. Sarafian, T.A., et al., *Oxidative stress produced by marijuana smoke. An adverse effect enhanced by cannabinoids.* Am J Respir Cell Mol Biol, 1999. **20**(6): p. 1286-93.
464. Owumi, S.E., et al., *Co-administration of N-Acetylcysteine and Acetaminophen Efficiently Blocks Acetaminophen Toxicity.* Drug Dev Res, 2015. **76**(5): p. 251-8.
465. Swiderska-Kolacz, G., J. Klusek, and A. Kolataj, *The effect of melatonin on glutathione and glutathione transferase and glutathione peroxidase activities in the mouse liver and kidney in vivo.* Neuro Endocrinol Lett, 2006. **27**(3): p. 365-8.
466. Baker, R.D., et al., *Selenium regulation of glutathione peroxidase in human hepatoma cell line Hep3B.* Arch Biochem Biophys, 1993. **304**(1): p. 53-7.
467. Das, S.K. and D.M. Vasudevan, *Protective effects of silymarin, a milk thistle (Silybium marianum) derivative on ethanol-induced oxidative stress in liver.* Indian J Biochem Biophys, 2006. **43**(5): p. 306-11.
468. Turner, C.E. and M.A. Elsohly, *Biological activity of cannabichromene, its homologs and isomers.* J Clin Pharmacol, 1981. **21**(8-9 Suppl): p. 283S-291S.
469. Gertsch, J., et al., *Beta-caryophyllene is a dietary cannabinoid.* Proc Natl Acad Sci U S A, 2008. **105**(26): p. 9099-104.
470. Bento, A.F., et al., *beta-Caryophyllene inhibits dextran sulfate sodium-induced colitis in mice through CB2 receptor activation and PPARgamma pathway.* Am J Pathol, 2011. **178**(3): p. 1153-66.
471. Paula-Freire, L.I., et al., *The oral administration of trans-caryophyllene attenuates acute and chronic pain in mice.* Phytomedicine, 2014. **21**(3): p. 356-62.
472. Katsuyama, S., et al., *Involvement of peripheral cannabinoid and opioid receptors in beta-caryophyllene-induced antinociception.* Eur J Pain, 2013. **17**(5): p. 664-75.
473. Galdino, P.M., et al., *The anxiolytic-like effect of an essential oil derived from Spiranthera odoratissima A. St. Hil. leaves and its major component, beta-caryophyllene, in male mice.* Prog Neuropsychopharmacol Biol Psychiatry,

2012. **38**(2): p. 276-84.
474. Vinholes, J., et al., *Assessment of the antioxidant and antiproliferative effects of sesquiterpenic compounds in in vitro Caco-2 cell models.* Food Chem, 2014. **156**: p. 204-11.
475. Legault, J. and A. Pichette, *Potentiating effect of beta-caryophyllene on anticancer activity of alpha-humulene, isocaryophyllene and paclitaxel.* J Pharm Pharmacol, 2007. **59**(12): p. 1643-7.
476. Klauke, A.L., et al., *The cannabinoid CB(2) receptor-selective phytocannabinoid beta-caryophyllene exerts analgesic effects in mouse models of inflammatory and neuropathic pain.* Eur Neuropsychopharmacol, 2014. **24**(4): p. 608-20.
477. Fiorenzani, P., et al., *In vitro and in vivo characterization of the new analgesic combination Beta-caryophyllene and docosahexaenoic Acid.* Evid Based Complement Alternat Med, 2014. **2014**: p. 596312.
478. Aracil-Fernandez, A., et al., *Decreased cocaine motor sensitization and self-administration in mice overexpressing cannabinoid CB(2) receptors.* Neuropsychopharmacology, 2012. **37**(7): p. 1749-63.
479. Viveros-Paredes, J.M., et al., *Neuroprotective Effects of beta-Caryophyllene against Dopaminergic Neuron Injury in a Murine Model of Parkinson's Disease Induced by MPTP.* Pharmaceuticals (Basel), 2017. **10**(3).
480. Pant, A., et al., *Beta-caryophyllene modulates expression of stress response genes and mediates longevity in Caenorhabditis elegans.* Exp Gerontol, 2014. **57**: p. 81-95.
481. Oz, M., et al., *Additive effects of endogenous cannabinoid anandamide and ethanol on alpha7-nicotinic acetylcholine receptor-mediated responses in Xenopus Oocytes.* J Pharmacol Exp Ther, 2005. **313**(3): p. 1272-80.
482. Guida, F., et al., *Palmitoylethanolamide induces microglia changes associated with increased migration and phagocytic activity: involvement of the CB2 receptor.* Sci Rep, 2017. **7**(1): p. 375.
483. Deciga-Campos, M. and R. Ortiz-Andrade, *Enhancement of Antihyperalgesia by the Coadministration of N-palmitoylethanolamide and Acetaminophen in Diabetic Rats.* Drug Dev Res, 2015. **76**(5): p. 228-34.
484. Deciga-Campos, M., P.M. Ramirez-Marin, and F.J. Lopez-Munoz, *Synergistic antinociceptive interaction between palmitoylethanolamide and tramadol in the mouse formalin test.* Eur J Pharmacol, 2015. **765**: p. 68-74.
485. Grillo, S.L., et al., *N-Palmitoylethanolamine depot injection increased its tissue levels and those of other acylethanolamide lipids.* Drug Des Devel Ther, 2013. **7**: p. 747-52.
486. Schifilliti, C., et al., *Micronized palmitoylethanolamide reduces the symptoms of neuropathic pain in diabetic patients.* Pain Res Treat, 2014. **2014**: p. 849623.
487. Hesselink, J.M., *Chronic idiopathic axonal neuropathy and pain, treated with the endogenous lipid mediator palmitoylethanolamide: a case collection.* Int Med Case Rep J, 2013. **6**: p. 49-53.
488. Hesselink, J.M., *Evolution in pharmacologic thinking around the natural analgesic palmitoylethanolamide: from nonspecific resistance to PPAR-*

alpha agonist and effective nutraceutical. J Pain Res, 2013. **6**: p. 625-34.
489. D'Agostino, G., et al., *Central administration of palmitoylethanolamide reduces hyperalgesia in mice via inhibition of NF-kappaB nuclear signalling in dorsal root ganglia.* Eur J Pharmacol, 2009. **613**(1-3): p. 54-9.
490. Banni, S. and V. Di Marzo, *Effect of dietary fat on endocannabinoids and related mediators: consequences on energy homeostasis, inflammation and mood.* Mol Nutr Food Res, 2010. **54**(1): p. 82-92.
491. Dawid, C., et al., *Bioactive C(1)(7)-Polyacetylenes in Carrots (Daucus carota L.): Current Knowledge and Future Perspectives.* J Agric Food Chem, 2015. **63**(42): p. 9211-22.
492. Kobaek-Larsen, M., et al., *Inhibitory effects of feeding with carrots or (-)-falcarinol on development of azoxymethane-induced preneoplastic lesions in the rat colon.* J Agric Food Chem, 2005. **53**(5): p. 1823-7.
493. Kobaek-Larsen, M., et al., *Dietary polyacetylenes, falcarinol and falcarindiol, isolated from carrots prevents the formation of neoplastic lesions in the colon of azoxymethane-induced rats.* Food Funct, 2017. **8**(3): p. 964-974.
494. Tan, K.W., et al., *Dietary polyacetylenes of the falcarinol type are inhibitors of breast cancer resistance protein (BCRP/ABCG2).* Eur J Pharmacol, 2014. **723**: p. 346-52.
495. Machado, S., E. Silva, and A. Massa, *Occupational allergic contact dermatitis from falcarinol.* Contact Dermatitis, 2002. **47**(2): p. 113-4.
496. Leonti, M., et al., *Falcarinol is a covalent cannabinoid CB1 receptor antagonist and induces pro-allergic effects in skin.* Biochem Pharmacol, 2010. **79**(12): p. 1815-26.
497. Gertsch, J., S. Raduner, and K.H. Altmann, *New natural noncannabinoid ligands for cannabinoid type-2 (CB2) receptors.* J Recept Signal Transduct Res, 2006. **26**(5-6): p. 709-30.
498. Raduner, S., et al., *Alkylamides from Echinacea are a new class of cannabinomimetics. Cannabinoid type 2 receptor-dependent and -independent immunomodulatory effects.* J Biol Chem, 2006. **281**(20): p. 14192-206.
499. Spelman, K., et al., *Role for PPARgamma in IL-2 inhibition in T cells by Echinacea-derived undeca-2E-ene-8,10-diynoic acid isobutylamide.* Int Immunopharmacol, 2009. **9**(11): p. 1260-4.
500. Woelkart, K., O.M. Salo-Ahen, and R. Bauer, *CB receptor ligands from plants.* Curr Top Med Chem, 2008. **8**(3): p. 173-86.
501. Shah, S.A., et al., *Evaluation of echinacea for the prevention and treatment of the common cold: a meta-analysis.* Lancet Infect Dis, 2007. **7**(7): p. 473-80.
502. Yin, H., et al., *Lipid G protein-coupled receptor ligand identification using beta-arrestin PathHunter assay.* J Biol Chem, 2009. **284**(18): p. 12328-38.
503. Vivar, O.I., et al., *3,3'-Diindolylmethane induces a G(1) arrest in human prostate cancer cells irrespective of androgen receptor and p53 status.* Biochem Pharmacol, 2009. **78**(5): p. 469-76.
504. G, W.W., et al., *Phytochemicals from cruciferous vegetables, epigenetics, and prostate cancer prevention.* AAPS J, 2013. **15**(4): p. 951-61.

505. Mahmud, Z.A., et al., *Three classes of ligands each bind to distinct sites on the orphan G protein-coupled receptor GPR84.* Sci Rep, 2017. **7**(1): p. 17953.
506. Reed, G.A., et al., *Single-dose and multiple-dose administration of indole-3-carbinol to women: pharmacokinetics based on 3,3'-diindolylmethane.* Cancer Epidemiol Biomarkers Prev, 2006. **15**(12): p. 2477-81.
507. Minker, E., et al., *Antispasmogenic effect of rutamarin and arborinine on isolated smooth muscle organs.* Planta Med, 1979. **37**(2): p. 156-60.
508. Zhang, Y., et al., *(+)-Rutamarin as a dual inducer of both GLUT4 translocation and expression efficiently ameliorates glucose homeostasis in insulin-resistant mice.* PLoS One, 2012. **7**(2): p. e31811.
509. Yang, Q.Y., X.Y. Tian, and W.S. Fang, *Bioactive coumarins from Boenninghausenia sessilicarpa.* J Asian Nat Prod Res, 2007. **9**(1): p. 59-65.
510. Xu, B., et al., *Antiviral activity of (+)-rutamarin against Kaposi's sarcoma-associated herpesvirus by inhibition of the catalytic activity of human topoisomerase II.* Antimicrob Agents Chemother, 2014. **58**(1): p. 563-73.
511. Kogan, N.M., et al., *HU-331, a novel cannabinoid-based anticancer topoisomerase II inhibitor.* Mol Cancer Ther, 2007. **6**(1): p. 173-83.
512. Pucci, M., et al., *Endocannabinoids stimulate human melanogenesis via type-1 cannabinoid receptor.* J Biol Chem, 2012. **287**(19): p. 15466-78.
513. Djuric, Z., et al., *Effect of soy isoflavone supplementation on markers of oxidative stress in men and women.* Cancer Lett, 2001. **172**(1): p. 1-6.
514. Sehdev, V., J.C. Lai, and A. Bhushan, *Biochanin A Modulates Cell Viability, Invasion, and Growth Promoting Signaling Pathways in HER-2-Positive Breast Cancer Cells.* J Oncol, 2009. **2009**: p. 121458.
515. Thors, L., et al., *Biochanin A, a naturally occurring inhibitor of fatty acid amide hydrolase.* Br J Pharmacol, 2010. **160**(3): p. 549-60.
516. Chundi, V., et al., *Biochanin-A attenuates neuropathic pain in diabetic rats.* J Ayurveda Integr Med, 2016. **7**(4): p. 231-237.
517. Wang, J., et al., *Biochanin A protects dopaminergic neurons against lipopolysaccharide-induced damage and oxidative stress in a rat model of Parkinson's disease.* Pharmacol Biochem Behav, 2015. **138**: p. 96-103.
518. Pang, T., et al., *Identification and determination of glycosides in tobacco leaves by liquid chromatography with atmospheric pressure chemical ionization tandem mass spectrometry.* J Sep Sci, 2007. **30**(3): p. 289-96.
519. Chen, A.Y. and Y.C. Chen, *A review of the dietary flavonoid, kaempferol on human health and cancer chemoprevention.* Food Chem, 2013. **138**(4): p. 2099-107.
520. Arai, Y., et al., *Dietary intakes of flavonols, flavones and isoflavones by Japanese women and the inverse correlation between quercetin intake and plasma LDL cholesterol concentration.* J Nutr, 2000. **130**(9): p. 2243-50.
521. DuPont, M.S., et al., *Absorption of kaempferol from endive, a source of kaempferol-3-glucuronide, in humans.* Eur J Clin Nutr, 2004. **58**(6): p. 947-54.
522. de Vries, J.H., et al., *Plasma concentrations and urinary excretion of the antioxidant flavonols quercetin and kaempferol as biomarkers for dietary*

intake. Am J Clin Nutr, 1998. **68**(1): p. 60-5.
523. Thors, L., M. Belghiti, and C.J. Fowler, *Inhibition of fatty acid amide hydrolase by kaempferol and related naturally occurring flavonoids.* Br J Pharmacol, 2008. **155**(2): p. 244-52.
524. Gertsch, J., R.G. Pertwee, and V. Di Marzo, *Phytocannabinoids beyond the Cannabis plant - do they exist?* Br J Pharmacol, 2010. **160**(3): p. 523-9.
525. Calderon-Montano, J.M., et al., *A review on the dietary flavonoid kaempferol.* Mini Rev Med Chem, 2011. **11**(4): p. 298-344.
526. Wang, C., et al., *Lignans and flavonoids inhibit aromatase enzyme in human preadipocytes.* J Steroid Biochem Mol Biol, 1994. **50**(3-4): p. 205-12.
527. Aiyer, H.S., et al., *Influence of berry polyphenols on receptor signaling and cell-death pathways: implications for breast cancer prevention.* J Agric Food Chem, 2012. **60**(23): p. 5693-708.
528. Nothlings, U., et al., *Flavonols and pancreatic cancer risk: the multiethnic cohort study.* Am J Epidemiol, 2007. **166**(8): p. 924-31.
529. Jaganathan, S.K. and M. Mandal, *Antiproliferative effects of honey and of its polyphenols: a review.* J Biomed Biotechnol, 2009. **2009**: p. 830616.
530. Kim, S.H. and K.C. Choi, *Anti-cancer Effect and Underlying Mechanism(s) of Kaempferol, a Phytoestrogen, on the Regulation of Apoptosis in Diverse Cancer Cell Models.* Toxicol Res, 2013. **29**(4): p. 229-34.
531. Toker, G., et al., *Flavonoids with antinociceptive and anti-inflammatory activities from the leaves of Tilia argentea (silver linden).* J Ethnopharmacol, 2004. **95**(2-3): p. 393-7.
532. Liggins, J., et al., *Daidzein and genistein content of cereals.* Eur J Clin Nutr, 2002. **56**(10): p. 961-6.
533. Thors, L., J. Eriksson, and C.J. Fowler, *Inhibition of the cellular uptake of anandamide by genistein and its analogue daidzein in cells with different levels of fatty acid amide hydrolase-driven uptake.* Br J Pharmacol, 2007. **152**(5): p. 744-50.
534. Jin, S., et al., *Daidzein induces MCF-7 breast cancer cell apoptosis via the mitochondrial pathway.* Ann Oncol, 2010. **21**(2): p. 263-8.
535. Constantinou, A.I., et al., *The soy isoflavone daidzein improves the capacity of tamoxifen to prevent mammary tumours.* Eur J Cancer, 2005. **41**(4): p. 647-54.
536. McCarty, M.F., *Isoflavones made simple - genistein's agonist activity for the beta-type estrogen receptor mediates their health benefits.* Med Hypotheses, 2006. **66**(6): p. 1093-114.
537. Matthies, A., et al., *Daidzein and genistein are converted to equol and 5-hydroxy-equol by human intestinal Slackia isoflavoniconvertens in gnotobiotic rats.* J Nutr, 2012. **142**(1): p. 40-6.
538. Alves, R.C., et al., *Isoflavones in coffee: influence of species, roast degree, and brewing method.* J Agric Food Chem, 2010. **58**(5): p. 3002-7.
539. GolKhoo, S., et al., *Determination of daidzein and genistein in soy milk in Iran by using HPLC analysis method.* Pak J Biol Sci, 2008. **11**(18): p. 2254-8.
540. Li, J., et al., *Puerarin attenuates amyloid-beta-induced cognitive impairment*

through suppression of apoptosis in rat hippocampus in vivo. Eur J Pharmacol, 2010. **649**(1-3): p. 195-201.
541. Morton, M.S., et al., *Phytoestrogen concentrations in serum from Japanese men and women over forty years of age.* J Nutr, 2002. **132**(10): p. 3168-71.
542. Piotrowska, E., et al., *Genistin-rich soy isoflavone extract in substrate reduction therapy for Sanfilippo syndrome: An open-label, pilot study in 10 pediatric patients.* Curr Ther Res Clin Exp, 2008. **69**(2): p. 166-79.
543. Moskot, M., et al., *The phytoestrogen genistein modulates lysosomal metabolism and transcription factor EB (TFEB) activation.* J Biol Chem, 2014. **289**(24): p. 17054-69.
544. Anderson, J.W., B.M. Johnstone, and M.E. Cook-Newell, *Meta-analysis of the effects of soy protein intake on serum lipids.* N Engl J Med, 1995. **333**(5): p. 276-82.
545. Colacurci, N., et al., *Effects of soy isoflavones on endothelial function in healthy postmenopausal women.* Menopause, 2005. **12**(3): p. 299-307.
546. Drews, K., et al., *[The safety and tolerance of isoflavones (Soyfem) administration in postmenopausal women].* Ginekol Pol, 2007. **78**(5): p. 361-5.
547. Nahas, E.A., et al., *Efficacy and safety of a soy isoflavone extract in postmenopausal women: a randomized, double-blind, and placebo-controlled study.* Maturitas, 2007. **58**(3): p. 249-58.
548. Spagnuolo, P., *Interactions Between Nutraceutical Supplements and Standard Acute Myeloid Leukemia Chemotherapeutics.* J Pharm Pharm Sci, 2015. **18**(4): p. 339-43.
549. Tsai, T.H., *Concurrent measurement of unbound genistein in the blood, brain and bile of anesthetized rats using microdialysis and its pharmacokinetic application.* J Chromatogr A, 2005. **1073**(1-2): p. 317-22.
550. Malinova, V., G. Wegrzyn, and M. Narajczyk, *The use of elevated doses of genistein-rich soy extract in the gene expression-targeted isoflavone therapy for Sanfilippo disease patients.* JIMD Rep, 2012. **5**: p. 21-5.
551. Piotrowska, E., et al., *Two-year follow-up of Sanfilippo Disease patients treated with a genistein-rich isoflavone extract: assessment of effects on cognitive functions and general status of patients.* Med Sci Monit, 2011. **17**(4): p. CR196-202.
552. Adlercreutz, H., et al., *Dietary phyto-oestrogens and the menopause in Japan.* Lancet, 1992. **339**(8803): p. 1233.
553. de Kleijn, M.J., et al., *Hormone replacement therapy and endothelial function. Results of a randomized controlled trial in healthy postmenopausal women.* Atherosclerosis, 2001. **159**(2): p. 357-65.
554. Cornwell, T., W. Cohick, and I. Raskin, *Dietary phytoestrogens and health.* Phytochemistry, 2004. **65**(8): p. 995-1016.
555. Welty, F.K., et al., *The association between soy nut consumption and decreased menopausal symptoms.* J Womens Health (Larchmt), 2007. **16**(3): p. 361-9.
556. Brink, E., et al., *Long-term consumption of isoflavone-enriched foods does not affect bone mineral density, bone metabolism, or hormonal status in*

early postmenopausal women: a randomized, double-blind, placebo controlled study. Am J Clin Nutr, 2008. **87**(3): p. 761-70.
557. Bawa, S., *The significance of soy protein and soy bioactive compounds in the prophylaxis and treatment of osteoporosis.* J Osteoporos, 2010. **2010**: p. 891058.
558. Cao, Y., et al., *Isoflavones in urine, saliva, and blood of infants: data from a pilot study on the estrogenic activity of soy formula.* J Expo Sci Environ Epidemiol, 2009. **19**(2): p. 223-34.
559. Setchell, K.D., et al., *Exposure of infants to phyto-oestrogens from soy-based infant formula.* Lancet, 1997. **350**(9070): p. 23-7.
560. Westmark, C.J., P.R. Westmark, and J.S. Malter, *Soy-based diet exacerbates seizures in mouse models of neurological disease.* J Alzheimers Dis, 2013. **33**(3): p. 797-805.
561. Westmark, C.J., *Soy infant formula and seizures in children with autism: a retrospective study.* PLoS One, 2014. **9**(3): p. e80488.
562. Wu, J., et al., *Formononetin, an active compound of Astragalus membranaceus (Fisch) Bunge, inhibits hypoxia-induced retinal neovascularization via the HIF-1alpha/VEGF signaling pathway.* Drug Des Devel Ther, 2016. **10**: p. 3071-3081.
563. Kaczmarczyk-Sedlak, I., et al., *Effect of formononetin on mechanical properties and chemical composition of bones in rats with ovariectomy-induced osteoporosis.* Evid Based Complement Alternat Med, 2013. **2013**: p. 457052.
564. Singh, K.B., et al., *Formononetin, a methoxy isoflavone, enhances bone regeneration in a mouse model of cortical bone defect.* Br J Nutr, 2017. **117**(11): p. 1511-1522.
565. das Neves, M.V., et al., *Isoflavone formononetin from red propolis acts as a fungicide against Candida sp.* Braz J Microbiol, 2016. **47**(1): p. 159-66.
566. Bertolacci, L., et al., *A binding site for nonsteroidal anti-inflammatory drugs in fatty acid amide hydrolase.* J Am Chem Soc, 2013. **135**(1): p. 22-5.
567. Ungprasert, P., et al., *Non-steroidal anti-inflammatory drugs and risk of venous thromboembolism: a systematic review and meta-analysis.* Rheumatology (Oxford), 2015. **54**(4): p. 736-42.
568. Bancos, S., et al., *Ibuprofen and other widely used non-steroidal anti-inflammatory drugs inhibit antibody production in human cells.* Cell Immunol, 2009. **258**(1): p. 18-28.
569. Nicolussi, S., et al., *Guineensine is a novel inhibitor of endocannabinoid uptake showing cannabimimetic behavioral effects in BALB/c mice.* Pharmacol Res, 2014. **80**: p. 52-65.
570. Sharma, C., et al., *Small Molecules from Nature Targeting G-Protein Coupled Cannabinoid Receptors: Potential Leads for Drug Discovery and Development.* Evid Based Complement Alternat Med, 2015. **2015**: p. 238482.
571. Tou, W.I., et al., *Drug design for neuropathic pain regulation from traditional s.* Sci Rep, 2013. **3**: p. 844.
572. Lee, S.A., et al., *Methylpiperate derivatives from Piper longum and their*

inhibition of monoamine oxidase. Arch Pharm Res, 2008. **31**(6): p. 679-83.
573. Lee, S.W., et al., *Guineensine, an Acyl-CoA: cholesterol acyltransferase inhibitor, from the fruits of Piper longum.* Planta Med, 2004. **70**(7): p. 678-9.
574. Reynoso-Moreno, I., et al., *An Endocannabinoid Uptake Inhibitor from Black Pepper Exerts Pronounced Anti-Inflammatory Effects in Mice.* J Agric Food Chem, 2017. **65**(43): p. 9435-9442.
575. Rao, V.S., A.M. Menezes, and G.S. Viana, *Effect of myrcene on nociception in mice.* J Pharm Pharmacol, 1990. **42**(12): p. 877-8.
576. Sengupta, B., et al., *Differential roles of 3-Hydroxyflavone and 7-Hydroxyflavone against nicotine-induced oxidative stress in rat renal proximal tubule cells.* PLoS One, 2017. **12**(6): p. e0179777.
577. Smaga, I., et al., *Antidepressants and changes in concentration of endocannabinoids and N-acylethanolamines in rat brain structures.* Neurotox Res, 2014. **26**(2): p. 190-206.
578. Holmes, T.H. and R.H. Rahe, *The Social Readjustment Rating Scale.* J Psychosom Res, 1967. **11**(2): p. 213-8.
579. Murphy, L.R., *Stress management in work settings: a critical review of the health effects.* Am J Health Promot, 1996. **11**(2): p. 112-35.
580. Gorelick, D.A., et al., *Around-the-clock oral THC effects on sleep in male chronic daily cannabis smokers.* Am J Addict, 2013. **22**(5): p. 510-4.
581. Cousens, K. and A. DiMascio, *(-) Delta 9 THC as an hypnotic. An experimental study of three dose levels.* Psychopharmacologia, 1973. **33**(4): p. 355-64.
582. Carley, D.W., et al., *Pharmacotherapy of Apnea by Cannabimimetic Enhancement, the PACE Clinical Trial: Effects of Dronabinol in Obstructive Sleep Apnea.* Sleep, 2018. **41**(1).
583. Fuss, J., et al., *Masturbation to Orgasm Stimulates the Release of the Endocannabinoid 2-Arachidonoylglycerol in Humans.* J Sex Med, 2017. **14**(11): p. 1372-1379.
584. Brody, S., *Blood pressure reactivity to stress is better for people who recently had penile-vaginal intercourse than for people who had other or no sexual activity.* Biol Psychol, 2006. **71**(2): p. 214-22.
585. Leuner, B., E.R. Glasper, and E. Gould, *Sexual experience promotes adult neurogenesis in the hippocampus despite an initial elevation in stress hormones.* PLoS One, 2010. **5**(7): p. e11597.
586. Sun, A.J. and M.L. Eisenberg, *Association Between Marijuana Use and Sexual Frequency in the United States: A Population-Based Study.* J Sex Med, 2017. **14**(11): p. 1342-1347.
587. Wise, L.A., et al., *Marijuana use and fecundability in a North American preconception cohort study.* J Epidemiol Community Health, 2017.
588. Chellew, K., et al., *The effect of progressive muscle relaxation on daily cortisol secretion.* Stress, 2015. **18**(5): p. 538-44.
589. Ratanasiripong, P., et al., *Biofeedback Intervention for Stress, Anxiety, and Depression among Graduate Students in Public Health Nursing.* Nurs Res Pract, 2015. **2015**: p. 160746.
590. McPartland, J.M., et al., *Cannabimimetic effects of osteopathic manipulative*

treatment. J Am Osteopath Assoc, 2005. **105**(6): p. 283-91.
591. Field, T., et al., *Cortisol decreases and serotonin and dopamine increase following massage therapy.* Int J Neurosci, 2005. **115**(10): p. 1397-413.
592. Sherman, K.J., et al., *Effectiveness of therapeutic massage for generalized anxiety disorder: a randomized controlled trial.* Depress Anxiety, 2010. **27**(5): p. 441-50.
593. Kim, I.H., T.Y. Kim, and Y.W. Ko, *The effect of a scalp massage on stress hormone, blood pressure, and heart rate of healthy female.* J Phys Ther Sci, 2016. **28**(10): p. 2703-2707.
594. Cheatham, S.W., et al., *The Effects of Self-Myofascial Release Using a Foam Roll or Roller Massager on Joint Range of Motion, Muscle Recovery, and Performance: A Systematic Review.* Int J Sports Phys Ther, 2015. **10**(6): p. 827-38.
595. Dong, B., et al., *The Efficacy of Acupuncture for Treating Depression-Related Insomnia Compared with a Control Group: A Systematic Review and Meta-Analysis.* Biomed Res Int, 2017. **2017**: p. 9614810.
596. Sniezek, D.P. and I.J. Siddiqui, *Acupuncture for Treating Anxiety and Depression in Women: A Clinical Systematic Review.* Med Acupunct, 2013. **25**(3): p. 164-172.
597. Thirthalli, J., et al., *Cortisol and antidepressant effects of yoga.* Indian J Psychiatry, 2013. **55**(Suppl 3): p. S405-8.
598. Hill, E.E., et al., *Exercise and circulating cortisol levels: the intensity threshold effect.* J Endocrinol Invest, 2008. **31**(7): p. 587-91.
599. Fuss, J., et al., *A runner's high depends on cannabinoid receptors in mice.* Proc Natl Acad Sci U S A, 2015. **112**(42): p. 13105-8.
600. Beulaygue, I.C. and M.T. French, *Got Munchies? Estimating the Relationship between Marijuana Use and Body Mass Index.* J Ment Health Policy Econ, 2016. **19**(3): p. 123-40.
601. Lisano, J.K., et al., *Performance and Health Related Characteristics of Male Athletes Using Marijuana.* J Strength Cond Res, 2017.
602. Thoma, M.V., et al., *The effect of music on the human stress response.* PLoS One, 2013. **8**(8): p. e70156.
603. Brinol, P., et al., *Treating thoughts as material objects can increase or decrease their impact on evaluation.* Psychol Sci, 2013. **24**(1): p. 41-7.
604. Holt-Lunstad, J., T.B. Smith, and J.B. Layton, *Social relationships and mortality risk: a meta-analytic review.* PLoS Med, 2010. **7**(7): p. e1000316.
605. Cohen, S., et al., *Does hugging provide stress-buffering social support? A study of susceptibility to upper respiratory infection and illness.* Psychol Sci, 2015. **26**(2): p. 135-47.
606. Bains, G.S., et al., *The effect of humor on short-term memory in older adults: a new component for whole-person wellness.* Adv Mind Body Med, 2014. **28**(2): p. 16-24.
607. Sneider, J.T., et al., *Altered regional blood volume in chronic cannabis smokers.* Exp Clin Psychopharmacol, 2006. **14**(4): p. 422-8.
608. Frech, A. and K. Williams, *Depression and the psychological benefits of entering marriage.* J Health Soc Behav, 2007. **48**(2): p. 149-63.

609. Smith, P.H., et al., *Couples' marijuana use is inversely related to their intimate partner violence over the first 9 years of marriage.* Psychol Addict Behav, 2014. **28**(3): p. 734-42.
610. Hasin, D.S., et al., *Prevalence of Marijuana Use Disorders in the United States Between 2001-2002 and 2012-2013.* JAMA Psychiatry, 2015. **72**(12): p. 1235-42.
611. Elsohly, M.A. and D. Slade, *Chemical constituents of marijuana: the complex mixture of natural cannabinoids.* Life Sci, 2005. **78**(5): p. 539-48.
612. Cascio, M.G., et al., *Evidence that the plant cannabinoid cannabigerol is a highly potent alpha2-adrenoceptor agonist and moderately potent 5HT1A receptor antagonist.* Br J Pharmacol, 2010. **159**(1): p. 129-41.
613. Elsohly, H.N. and C.E. Turner, *Constituents of Cannabis sativa L. XXII: isolation of spiro-indan and dihydrostilbene compounds from a Panamanian variant grown in Mississippi, United States of America.* Bull Narc, 1982. **34**(2): p. 51-6.
614. Borrelli, F., et al., *Colon carcinogenesis is inhibited by the TRPM8 antagonist cannabigerol, a Cannabis-derived non-psychotropic cannabinoid.* Carcinogenesis, 2014. **35**(12): p. 2787-97.
615. Borrelli, F., et al., *Beneficial effect of the non-psychotropic plant cannabinoid cannabigerol on experimental inflammatory bowel disease.* Biochem Pharmacol, 2013. **85**(9): p. 1306-16.
616. Baek, S.H., et al., *Boron trifluoride etherate on silica-A modified Lewis acid reagent (VII). Antitumor activity of cannabigerol against human oral epitheloid carcinoma cells.* Arch Pharm Res, 1998. **21**(3): p. 353-6.
617. Colasanti, B.K., C.R. Craig, and R.D. Allara, *Intraocular pressure, ocular toxicity and neurotoxicity after administration of cannabinol or cannabigerol.* Exp Eye Res, 1984. **39**(3): p. 251-9.
618. Colasanti, B.K., *A comparison of the ocular and central effects of delta 9-tetrahydrocannabinol and cannabigerol.* J Ocul Pharmacol, 1990. **6**(4): p. 259-69.
619. Valdeolivas, S., et al., *Neuroprotective properties of cannabigerol in Huntington's disease: studies in R6/2 mice and 3-nitropropionate-lesioned mice.* Neurotherapeutics, 2015. **12**(1): p. 185-99.
620. Granja, A.G., et al., *A cannabigerol quinone alleviates neuroinflammation in a chronic model of multiple sclerosis.* J Neuroimmune Pharmacol, 2012. **7**(4): p. 1002-16.
621. Korte, F., M. Haag, and U. Claussen, *Tetrahydrocannabinolcarboxylic acid, a component of hashish. 1.* Angew Chem Int Ed Engl, 1965. **4**(10): p. 872.
622. Moreno-Sanz, G., *Can You Pass the Acid Test? Critical Review and Novel Therapeutic Perspectives of Delta(9)-Tetrahydrocannabinolic Acid A.* Cannabis Cannabinoid Res, 2016. **1**(1): p. 124-130.
623. McPartland, J.M., et al., *Affinity and Efficacy Studies of Tetrahydrocannabinolic Acid A at Cannabinoid Receptor Types One and Two.* Cannabis Cannabinoid Res, 2017. **2**(1): p. 87-95.
624. Alozie, S.O., et al., *3H-delta 9-Tetrahydrocannabinol, 3H-cannabinol and 3H-cannabidiol: penetration and regional distribution in rat brain.* Pharmacol

Biochem Behav, 1980. **12**(2): p. 217-21.
625. Deiana, S., et al., *Plasma and brain pharmacokinetic profile of cannabidiol (CBD), cannabidivarine (CBDV), Delta(9)-tetrahydrocannabivarin (THCV) and cannabigerol (CBG) in rats and mice following oral and intraperitoneal administration and CBD action on obsessive-compulsive behaviour.* Psychopharmacology (Berl), 2012. **219**(3): p. 859-73.
626. Rock, E.M., et al., *Tetrahydrocannabinolic acid reduces nausea-induced conditioned gaping in rats and vomiting in Suncus murinus.* Br J Pharmacol, 2013. **170**(3): p. 641-8.
627. Parker, L.A., E.M. Rock, and C.L. Limebeer, *Regulation of nausea and vomiting by cannabinoids.* Br J Pharmacol, 2011. **163**(7): p. 1411-22.
628. Ruhaak, L.R., et al., *Evaluation of the cyclooxygenase inhibiting effects of six major cannabinoids isolated from Cannabis sativa.* Biol Pharm Bull, 2011. **34**(5): p. 774-8.
629. De Petrocellis, L., et al., *Effects of cannabinoids and cannabinoid-enriched Cannabis extracts on TRP channels and endocannabinoid metabolic enzymes.* Br J Pharmacol, 2011. **163**(7): p. 1479-94.
630. Ligresti, A., et al., *Antitumor activity of plant cannabinoids with emphasis on the effect of cannabidiol on human breast carcinoma.* J Pharmacol Exp Ther, 2006. **318**(3): p. 1375-87.
631. Moldzio, R., et al., *Effects of cannabinoids Delta(9)-tetrahydrocannabinol, Delta(9)-tetrahydrocannabinolic acid and cannabidiol in MPP+ affected murine mesencephalic cultures.* Phytomedicine, 2012. **19**(8-9): p. 819-24.
632. Russo, E.B., *Beyond Cannabis: Plants and the Endocannabinoid System.* Trends Pharmacol Sci, 2016. **37**(7): p. 594-605.
633. Sulak, D., R. Saneto, and B. Goldstein, *The current status of artisanal cannabis for the treatment of epilepsy in the United States.* Epilepsy Behav, 2017. **70**(Pt B): p. 328-333.
634. Hazekamp, A., et al., *Cannabis tea revisited: a systematic evaluation of the cannabinoid composition of cannabis tea.* J Ethnopharmacol, 2007. **113**(1): p. 85-90.
635. Citti, C., et al., *Medicinal cannabis: Principal cannabinoids concentration and their stability evaluated by a high performance liquid chromatography coupled to diode array and quadrupole time of flight mass spectrometry method.* J Pharm Biomed Anal, 2016. **128**: p. 201-209.
636. Peschel, W., *Quality Control of Traditional Cannabis Tinctures: Pattern, Markers, and Stability.* Sci Pharm, 2016. **84**(3): p. 567-584.
637. Mechoulam, R. and Y. Gaoni, *Hashish. IV. The isolation and structure of cannabinolic cannabidiolic and cannabigerolic acids.* Tetrahedron, 1965. **21**(5): p. 1223-9.
638. Elmes, M.W., et al., *Fatty acid-binding proteins (FABPs) are intracellular carriers for Delta9-tetrahydrocannabinol (THC) and cannabidiol (CBD).* J Biol Chem, 2015. **290**(14): p. 8711-21.
639. Huestis, M.A., et al., *Characterization of the absorption phase of marijuana smoking.* Clin Pharmacol Ther, 1992. **52**(1): p. 31-41.
640. Wall, M.E. and M. Perez-Reyes, *The metabolism of delta 9-*

tetrahydrocannabinol and related cannabinoids in man. J Clin Pharmacol, 1981. **21**(8-9 Suppl): p. 178S-189S.

641. Grotenhermen, F., *Pharmacokinetics and pharmacodynamics of cannabinoids.* Clin Pharmacokinet, 2003. **42**(4): p. 327-60.

642. Wood T, S.W., and Easterfield T, *The Resin of Indian Hemp.* Journal of the American Chemical Society, 1896. **69**: p. 539.

643. Adams, R., M. Hunt, and J.H. Clark, *Structure of Cannabidiol, a Product Isolated from the Marihuana Extract of Minnesota Wild Hemp. I.* Journal of the American Chemical Society, 1940. **62**(1): p. 196-200.

644. Cecinato, A., C. Balducci, and M. Perilli, *Illicit psychotropic substances in the air: The state-of-art.* Sci Total Environ, 2016. **539**: p. 1-6.

645. Mahadevan, A., et al., *Novel cannabinol probes for CB1 and CB2 cannabinoid receptors.* J Med Chem, 2000. **43**(20): p. 3778-85.

646. Petitet, F., et al., *Complex pharmacology of natural cannabinoids: evidence for partial agonist activity of delta9-tetrahydrocannabinol and antagonist activity of cannabidiol on rat brain cannabinoid receptors.* Life Sci, 1998. **63**(1): p. PL1-6.

647. Sofia, R.D., et al., *Comparative anti-phlogistic activity of delta 9-tetrahydrocannabinol, hydrocortisone and aspirin in various rat paw edema models.* Life Sci, 1974. **15**(2): p. 251-60.

648. Tian, Z., et al., *Study on the interaction between cannabinol and DNA using acridine orange as a fluorescence probe.* J Mol Recognit, 2018. **31**(2).

649. Karniol, I.G., et al., *Effects of delta9-tetrahydrocannabinol and cannabinol in man.* Pharmacology, 1975. **13**(6): p. 502-12.

650. Vergara, D., et al., *Compromised External Validity: Federally Produced Cannabis Does Not Reflect Legal Markets.* Sci Rep, 2017. **7**: p. 46528.

651. Abrahamov, A., A. Abrahamov, and R. Mechoulam, *An efficient new cannabinoid antiemetic in pediatric oncology.* Life Sci, 1995. **56**(23-24): p. 2097-102.

652. Avraham, Y., et al., *Very low doses of delta 8-THC increase food consumption and alter neurotransmitter levels following weight loss.* Pharmacol Biochem Behav, 2004. **77**(4): p. 675-84.

653. Munson, A.E., W.C. Rose, and S.G. Bradley, *Synergistic lethal action of alkylating agents and sodium pentobarbital in the mouse.* Pharmacology, 1974. **11**(4): p. 231-40.

654. Bolognini, D., et al., *Cannabidiolic acid prevents vomiting in Suncus murinus and nausea-induced behaviour in rats by enhancing 5-HT1A receptor activation.* Br J Pharmacol, 2013. **168**(6): p. 1456-70.

655. Shbiro, L., et al., *Anti-depressant-like effects of cannabidiol and cannabidiolic acid in genetic rat models of depression.* European Neuropsychopharmacology., 2017. **27**: p. S783-S784.

656. Michoulam, R. and Y. Shvo, *Hashish. I. The structure of cannabidiol.* Tetrahedron, 1963. **19**(12): p. 2073-8.

657. Huestis, M.A., et al., *Cannabinoid concentrations in hair from documented cannabis users.* Forensic Sci Int, 2007. **169**(2-3): p. 129-36.

658. Bornheim, L.M. and M.A. Correia, *Purification and characterization of the*

major hepatic cannabinoid hydroxylase in the mouse: a possible member of the cytochrome P-450IIC subfamily. Mol Pharmacol, 1991. **40**(2): p. 228-34.

659. Swanson, B.A., et al., *Topological analysis of the active sites of cytochromes P450IIB4 (rabbit), P450IIB10 (mouse), and P450IIB11 (dog) by in situ rearrangement of phenyl-iron complexes.* Arch Biochem Biophys, 1992. **292**(1): p. 42-6.
660. Watanabe, K., et al., *Involvement of CYP2C in the metabolism of cannabinoids by human hepatic microsomes from an old woman.* Biol Pharm Bull, 1995. **18**(8): p. 1138-41.
661. Watanabe, K., et al., *Cytochrome P450 enzymes involved in the metabolism of tetrahydrocannabinols and cannabinol by human hepatic microsomes.* Life Sci, 2007. **80**(15): p. 1415-9.
662. Hampson, A.J., et al., *Cannabidiol and (-)Delta9-tetrahydrocannabinol are neuroprotective antioxidants.* Proc Natl Acad Sci U S A, 1998. **95**(14): p. 8268-73.
663. El Yacoubi, M., et al., *The anxiogenic-like effect of caffeine in two experimental procedures measuring anxiety in the mouse is not shared by selective A(2A) adenosine receptor antagonists.* Psychopharmacology (Berl), 2000. **148**(2): p. 153-63.
664. Wang, Q., et al., *Activation of epsilon protein kinase C-mediated anti-apoptosis is involved in rapid tolerance induced by electroacupuncture pretreatment through cannabinoid receptor type 1.* Stroke, 2011. **42**(2): p. 389-96.
665. Shani, A., *Cannabielsoic acids : Isolation and synthesis by a novel oxidative cyclization.* Tetrahedron, 1974. **30**(15): p. 2437-2446.
666. Yamamoto, I., et al., *Cannabielsoin as a new metabolite of cannabidiol in mammals.* Pharmacol Biochem Behav, 1991. **40**(3): p. 541-6.
667. Bercht, C.A., et al., *Cannabis. VII. Identification of cannabinol methyl ether from hashish.* J Chromatogr, 1973. **81**(1): p. 163-6.
668. Uliss, D.B., R.K. Razdan, and H.C. Dalzell, *Letter: Stereospecific intramolecular epoxide cleavage by phenolate anion. Synthesis of novel and biologically active cannabinsids.* J Am Chem Soc, 1974. **96**(23): p. 7372-4.
669. Ross, S.A. and M.A. ElSohly, *The volatile oil composition of fresh and air-dried buds of Cannabis sativa.* J Nat Prod, 1996. **59**(1): p. 49-51.
670. Spronck, H.J. and R.J. Lousberg, *Pyrolysis of cannabidiol. Structure elucidation of a major pyrolytic conversion product.* Experientia, 1977. **33**(6): p. 705-6.
671. Shoyama, Y., et al., *Cannabichromenic acid, a genuine substance of cannabichromene.* Chem Pharm Bull (Tokyo), 1968. **16**(6): p. 1157-8.
672. Morimoto, S., et al., *Purification and characterization of cannabichromenic acid synthase from Cannabis sativa.* Phytochemistry, 1998. **49**(6): p. 1525-9.
673. Claussen, U., F. von Spulak, and F. Korte, *[Hashish. XIV. Information on the substance of hashish].* Tetrahedron, 1968. **24**(2): p. 1021-3.
674. Mechoulam, R., B. Yagnitinsky, and Y. Gaoni, *Stereoelectronic factor in the chloranil dehydrogenation of cannabinoids. Total synthesis of dl-cannabichromene.* J Am Chem Soc, 1968. **90**(9): p. 2418-20.

675. Crombie, L., et al., *Hashish components. Photochemical production of cannabicyclol from cannabichromene.* Tetrahedron Lett, 1968(55): p. 5771-2.
676. Korte, F. and H. Sieper, *[on the Chemical Classification of Plants. Xxiv. Investigation of Hashish Constituents by Thin-Layer Chromatography].* J Chromatogr, 1964. **13**: p. 90-8.
677. Mechoulam, R., P. Braun, and Y. Gaoni, *A stereospecific synthesis of (-)-delta 1- and (-)-delta 1(6)-tetrahydrocannabinols.* J Am Chem Soc, 1967. **89**(17): p. 4552-4.
678. Vree, T.B., et al., *Gas chromatography of cannabis constituents and their synthetic derivatives.* J Chromatogr, 1972. **74**(2): p. 209-24.
679. Pertwee, R.G., *The diverse CB1 and CB2 receptor pharmacology of three plant cannabinoids: delta9-tetrahydrocannabinol, cannabidiol and delta9-tetrahydrocannabivarin.* Br J Pharmacol, 2008. **153**(2): p. 199-215.
680. Hill, A.J., et al., *Delta(9)-Tetrahydrocannabivarin suppresses in vitro epileptiform and in vivo seizure activity in adult rats.* Epilepsia, 2010. **51**(8): p. 1522-32.
681. Chan, W.R., K.E. Magnus, and H.A. Watson, *The structure of cannabitriol.* Experientia, 1976. **32**(3): p. 283-4.
682. ElSohly, H.N., et al., *Constituents of Cannabis sativa, XXV. Isolation of two new dihydrostilbenes from a Panamanian variant.* J Nat Prod, 1984. **47**(3): p. 445-52.
683. Boeren, E.G., M.A. Elsohly, and C.E. Turner, *Cannabiripsol: a novel Cannabis constituent.* Experientia, 1979. **35**(10): p. 1278-9.
684. Pacher, P., S. Batkai, and G. Kunos, *The endocannabinoid system as an emerging target of pharmacotherapy.* Pharmacol Rev, 2006. **58**(3): p. 389-462.
685. Wolff, V. and E. Jouanjus, *Strokes are possible complications of cannabinoids use.* Epilepsy Behav, 2017. **70**(Pt B): p. 355-363.
686. Budney, A.J., et al., *Marijuana dependence and its treatment.* Addict Sci Clin Pract, 2007. **4**(1): p. 4-16.
687. Haney, M., et al., *Abstinence symptoms following smoked marijuana in humans.* Psychopharmacology (Berl), 1999. **141**(4): p. 395-404.
688. Budney, A.J., et al., *The time course and significance of cannabis withdrawal.* J Abnorm Psychol, 2003. **112**(3): p. 393-402.
689. Allsop, D.J., et al., *Nabiximols as an agonist replacement therapy during cannabis withdrawal: a randomized clinical trial.* JAMA Psychiatry, 2014. **71**(3): p. 281-91.
690. Graham, J., M. Barberio, and G.S. Wang, *Capsaicin Cream for Treatment of Cannabinoid Hyperemesis Syndrome in Adolescents: A Case Series.* Pediatrics, 2017. **140**(6).
691. Filbey, F.M., et al., *Combined effects of marijuana and nicotine on memory performance and hippocampal volume.* Behav Brain Res, 2015. **293**: p. 46-53.

INDEX

ABOUT THE AUTHOR

For more information about the author including speaking engagement and media requests, please visit www.drmicheleross.com. To request a cannabis consultation, please visit www.infused.health.

Dr. Michele Ross is Founder and Executive Director of the Denver-based cannabis research & education 501c3 nonprofit IMPACT Network. As a neuroscientist, she was frustrated by the lack of education on the endocannabinoid system both doctors and scientists received, despite medical cannabis being used by millions of patients nationwide. In 2013, she founded the "Endocannabinoid Deficiency Foundation," now known as IMPACT Network, with the mission to drive clinical research on cannabis for women's health. To donate or learn more about IMPACT Network, visit www.impactcannabis.org.

Dr. Ross is both a cannabinoid medicine researcher and a cannabis patient. After being diagnosed with fibromyalgia, neuropathy, and chronic pelvic pain, cannabis was the only thing that reduced her symptoms and allowed her to return to work. After hearing thousands of extraordinary patient stories just like hers, Dr. Ross was compelled to ensure cannabis becomes part of the American healthcare system.

Dr. Ross is a proud advocate of botanical and psychedelic medicine and has formulated and marketed nutraceuticals for companies around the globe. She has also been a leader in digital health and education, crafting continuing medical education for health professionals as well as creating online communities for patients. She is also author of two books, “Train Your Brain to Get Thin” and “Vitamin Weed: A 4-Step Plan to Prevent and Reverse Endocannabinoid Deficiency.”

Dr. Ross holds a Doctorate in Neuroscience from the University of Texas Southwestern Medical Center and has researched addiction, mental health, and psychopharmacology for over a decade. Fun fact: she was the first scientist to star on a reality television show, starring on Big Brother 11 on CBS in 2009.

Made in the USA
Middletown, DE
12 April 2018